SPINAL CORD COMPRESSION: Diagnosis And Principles Of Management

CONTEMPORARY NEUROLOGY SERIES AVAILABLE:

Fred Plum, M.D., *Editor-in-Chief*
Series Editors: Sid Gilman, M.D.
Joseph B. Martin, M.D., Ph.D.
Robert B. Daroff, M.D.
Stephen G. Waxman, M.D., Ph.D.
M-Marsel Mesulam, M.D.

SPINAL CORD COMPRESSION: Diagnosis And Principles Of Management

THOMAS N. BYRNE, M.D.
Associate Clinical Professor of Neurology
Yale University School of Medicine
Assistant Chief, Department of Neurology,
Yale-New Haven Hospital
Co-Director, Neuro-Oncology Unit,
Yale Comprehensive Cancer Center
New Haven, Connecticut

STEPHEN G. WAXMAN, M.D., PH.D.
Professor and Chairman,
Department of Neurology
Yale University School of Medicine
Neurologist-in-Chief,
Yale-New Haven Hospital
Director, PVA/EPVA Neuroscience Research Center,
VA Medical Center
West Haven, Connecticut

 F.A. Davis Company • Philadelphia

Printed in the United States of America

Last digit indicates print number: 10 9 8 7 6 5 4 3 2 1

NOTE: As new scientific information becomes available through basic and clinical research, recommended treatments and drug therapies undergo changes. The author(s) and publisher have done everything possible to make this book accurate, up-to-date, and in accord with accepted standards at the time of publication. However, the reader is advised always to check product information (package inserts) for changes and new information regarding dose and contraindications before administering any drug. Caution is especially urged when using new or infrequently ordered drugs.

Library of Congress Cataloging-in-Publication Data

Byrne, Thomas N.
    Spinal cord compression: Diagnosis and principles of management
    Thomas N. Byrne, Stephen G. Waxman,
        p. cm.—(Contemporary neurology series: 33)
    Includes bibliographical references.
    ISBN 0-8036-1465-9
    1. Spinal cord compression.   I. Waxman, Stephen G.   II. Title.
    III. Series.
    [DNLM: 1. Spinal Cord Compression—diagnosis. 2. Spinal Cord
    Compression—etiology. 3. Spinal Cord Neoplasms—complications.
    W1 CO769N v. 33/WL 400 B995s]
    RC406.C66B97   1990
    617.4'82—dc20
    DNLM/DLC
    for Library of Congress

PREFACE

This book had its origin when, on rounds, one of us was presented with an all-too-common scenario: A 50-year-old man with known prostatic cancer presented to the emergency room paraplegic. Tragically, the patient had been seen in another clinic 2 weeks before, complaining of back pain and leg weakness. The outcome in this case may have been preventable.

Spinal cord compression from neoplastic or nonneoplastic disease is a common clinical problem. As in the case cited above, if undiagnosed and untreated it frequently progresses to permanent paraparesis and sphincter disturbances. Alternatively, spinal cord compression constitutes a treatable cause of paraparesis and quadriparesis. This book is an attempt to communicate to house officers and to practicing clinicians an approach to the diagnosis of spinal cord compression.

Until recently, myelography was the only definitive imaging technique to evaluate the spinal cord. In the past few years, however, computerized tomography (CT) and magnetic resonance imaging (MRI) have emerged as the imaging studies of choice in many diseases of the spine. In fact, the full potential of MRI is rapidly evolving at the time of this writing, and it is expected to replace myelography in most clinical situations. These rapid technologic advances are welcome but we believe that they cannot replace clinical judgment. For example, since most individuals over 50 years of age demonstrate radiographic evidence of spondylosis, the clinician must often decide whether such a finding is incidental or responsible for the patient's neurologic symptoms and signs. In those cases where the findings are not recognized as only incidental, the patient may undergo unnecessary surgery for these "abnormalities" when the actual cause of the clinical syndrome remains undiagnosed and untreated. We believe that an understanding of the pathophysiology of various spinal cord disorders is an essential prerequisite to clinical judgment.

In writing this volume, we have first reviewed the relevant anatomy of the spine and the clinical pathophysiology of spinal cord compression. Since pain is the most common presenting complaint of spinal cord compression, we have devoted a chapter to pain and its evaluation. Subsequent chapters examine nonneoplastic and neoplastic forms of spinal cord compression. The final chapter reviews noncompressive forms of myelopathy. Since at our Medical Center traumatic spinal cord injuries usually fall into the province of neurosurgery, we have not dealt with this area. Similarly, we have not attempted to discuss congenital or developmental forms of spinal cord compression. Finally, we have chosen to emphasize the diagnostic aspects of spinal cord disease and review only the principles of therapeutic management, since we recognize that a comprehensive discussion of the treatment of spinal disease requires the expertise of physicians from several disciplines.

The two authors bring different backgrounds to this book. Following a fellowship in neuro-oncology at Memorial Sloan-Kettering Cancer Center, one of us has been engaged in clinical aspects of neurology and neuro-oncology at Yale; the other has spent the past decade at Stanford and Yale combining a university-based practice with research focusing on molecular aspects of neurologic disease. In bringing together perspectives gained from each of our professional experiences, we have attempted to present a single, coherent approach to the diagnosis of spinal cord compression.

Many colleagues have helped in the writing of this volume and we are indebted to them. Dr. Jerome B. Posner, an inspiring teacher and physician, deserves special thanks. Several other individuals who gave time and thought in reviewing draft versions of a number of chapters include Drs. Susan Hockfield, Joseph Piepmeier, Gordon Sze, John Booss, John Ryan, Frank Bia, and Charles DiSabatino. In addition, Drs. Helmuth Gehbauer, Lysia Forno and Jung Kim contributed previously unpublished material. We acknowledge the help of Dr. Sylvia Fields and Ms. Bernice Wissler of the F.A. Davis Company and Ms. Virginia Simon of the Yale Medical Illustration Department for the careful attention they gave to the preparation of the manuscript and illustrations. We are grateful to Mr. David Chang, Ms. Valerie Degley, and Ms. Louise Leader for their help in the preparation of this volume. We owe particular thanks to the administrations of Yale University School of Medicine and Yale-New Haven Hospital for their encouragement and support during the writing of this book. We are especially grateful to our many colleagues in the basic and clinical neurosciences who have helped to build at Yale an atmosphere conducive to the writing of this book.

Finally we thank Susan Hockfield, Merle Waxman, Matthew Waxman, and David Waxman. They know why we thank them.

Thomas N. Byrne, M.D.
Stephen G. Waxman, M.D., Ph.D.

CONTENTS

Chapter 1

ANATOMY OF THE SPINE

The spine is a segmented structure consisting of a precisely aligned column of vertebrae and their intervertebral articulations. Its primary functions are to: 1) provide support for the trunk and head; 2) provide a protective covering for the spinal cord; and yet, 3) permit enough flexibility to allow movement. These functions are achieved through an architecture based, in humans, on a column of articulated vertebrae that afford both structural support and mobility.

The spinal cord is, similarly, a segmented structure both functionally and anatomically. Sherrington recognized the hierarchical organization of the nervous system and suggested that the spinal cord was the first level of organization, where the most primitive motor reflexes are mediated through the principle of the common path (spinal roots).[67] Disease processes affecting the spine and spinal cord often are manifested by disturbed function of these spinal roots, of the ascending and descending pathways within the spinal cord, or both. For example, spinal mass lesions frequently present with radicular pain at the level of the injured nerve root, with radicular motor, sensory, and reflex disturbances occurring as well. As spinal cord compression ensues, ascending and descending tracts are injured, resulting in neurological disturbances caudal to the level of the lesion. Although the localization and differentiation of these diseases is frequently a vexing problem, requiring radiologic and other laboratory studies for confirmation, the physician is guided by the patient's clinical history and physical examination of symptoms and signs.

VERTEBRAL COLUMN

The vertebral column (Fig. 1–1), normally consists of 7 cervical, 12 thoracic, and 5 lumbar individual vertebrae; the sacrum, which is usually formed by fusion of 5 vertebrae; and the coccyx. Variations in the number and distribution of the presacral vertebrae have been found in approximately 10 percent of skeletons.[41] These variations are, in many cases, radiographically confusing but clinically insignificant. Congenital bony abnormalities have been described in the region of the foramen magnum; some of the abnormalities are associated with clinical symptoms and others are entirely asymptomatic.[51] Other congenital abnormalities that may have major clinical manifestations include Klippel-Feil syndrome, spina bifida, scoliosis, kyphosis, and other dysraphic states. These congenital anomalies of the spine represent a major area of pediatric and orthopedic practice and the reader is referred elsewhere for a more complete discussion of their anatomical and clinical features.[37]

Anterior Segment and Intervertebral Disc

The functional anterior segment consists of two vertebral bodies separated by an intervertebral disc (Fig. 1–2). The intervertebral disc, which unites the adjacent vertebral bodies to complete the functional anterior segment, is attached to the apposing vertebral end-plates. Each intervertebral disc is given the same number as the vertebra immediately above it; for ex-

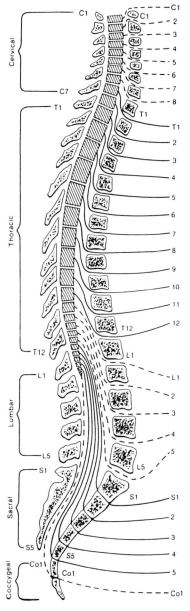

Figure 1—1. The anatomical relationships between the spinal cord segments, vertebral bodies, and intervertebral foraminae. Note the disparity between spinal segmental level and localization of corresponding vertebrae. (From DeJong, RN, [20] p 61, with permission.)

ample, the disc between the L4 and L5 vertebrae is identified as the L4 disc.

The combined height of the intervertebral discs normally contributes approximately 25 percent of the length of the spine

above the sacrum. There is a difference in the vertical shape of the intervertebral discs in the cervical region compared with that in the lumbar region. In the lumbar region the vertical height of the intervertebral discs is slightly greater anteriorly than posteriorly, which helps to contribute to the lumbar lordosis. In the cervical spine this difference is even greater, with the vertical height of the intervertebral disc anteriorly measuring approximately two times that in the posterior region.[13] This greater height in the anterior region contributes to the curve of the cervical spine.

The intervertebral disc is composed of a central nucleus pulposus encircled by the annulus fibrosus (see Fig. 1—4). Fibers of the annulus fibrosus of the intervertebral disc insert into the cartilaginous end-plates of the vertebral bodies and into the bony rim of the vertebral body. The hyaline cartilaginous end-plates form the cephalad and caudal borders of the nucleus pulposus, and the encircling annulus fibrosus forms the lateral border. The annulus consists of a series of concentric rings of fibroelastic fibers that course obliquely between the vertebral bodies. The obliquity of each successive ring is different from that of the adjacent rings, providing for a strong and elastic annulus that unites the vertebral bodies and confines the nucleus pulposus.

In addition to weight-bearing, the anterior segment provides for shock absorption. This is accomplished through the nucleus pulposus, which is placed slightly posterior to the center of the intervertebral disc space in the lumbar spine. The nucleus pulposus, a mucopolysaccharide gel, is composed of 70 to 88 percent water in the young healthy adult[41] and is a deformable but not compressible structure. The incompressible nucleus pulposus surrounded by the elastic annulus permits the intervertebral disc to change its shape and thereby permit movement between the vertebral bodies. For example, when the spine is flexed, the fluid of the nucleus moves from anterior to posterior. The direction of movement is not limited by the intervertebral discs.

The mechanical stresses experienced by the lumbar intervertebral discs have great practical importance. Using a needle con-

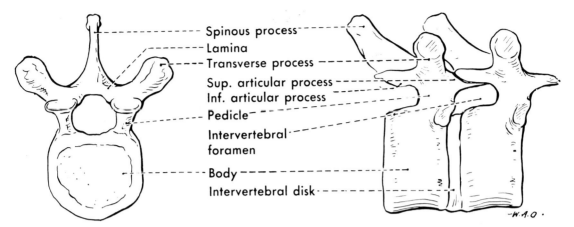

Figure 1–2. Anatomy of a typical vertebra. (From Hollinshead, WH, [41] p 304, with permission.)

nected to a pressure transducer, Nachemson[54] measured the lumbar intradiscal pressures of healthy and degenerated discs in individuals during different postures (Fig. 1–3). The intradiscal pressure increases as the individual moves from supine to standing to sitting. Furthermore, pressure rises when the trunk is flexed in a standing or sitting position. Pressures measured in degenerated lumbar discs were approximately 30 percent lower than those in healthy discs under identical conditions.

The weight-bearing, shock-absorbing capacity and mobility of the anterior segment of the spine depend on the deformable but incompressible nature of the nu-

cleus pulposus. As the water content of the nucleus pulposus declines with age, the individual discs lose height, which may contribute to spondylosis. The decline in water content of intervertebral discs now has been appreciated *in vivo* with magnetic resonance imaging, a technique very sensitive to water content.[53]

When the annulus fibrosus degenerates, conditions are set for herniation of the nucleus pulposus through the weakest portion of the annulus. In lumbar discs, the posterolateral region is most vulnerable because the annulus is thinnest posteriorly and the posterolateral region is not supported by the posterior longitudinal ligament. Intervertebral disc material may

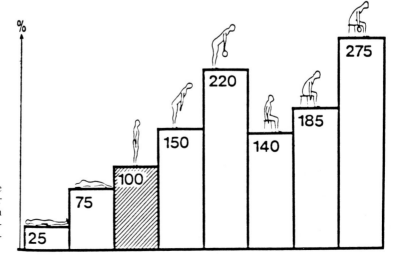

Figure 1–3. The relative change in pressure in the third lumbar disc during different positions in living subjects. (From Nachemson, AL, [55] p 61, with permission.)

also herniate into the adjacent vertebral body to form a Schmorl's node.

Posterior Segment

The posterior segment functions to protect the spinal cord as well as to set the direction and extent of spine mobility. The posterior segment consists of pedicles, lamina, transverse processes, posterior spinous processes, and the articulating facets (see Fig. 1–2). The pedicles and lamina form the lateral and posterior walls of the spinal canal.

Each posterior segment contains a superior and inferior articular facet, fused by a pars interarticularis. At the intervertebral level, each inferior articular facet articulates with the superior articular facet of its caudal neighbor. Unlike the intervertebral disc joint, facet joints are true synovial joints consisting of cartilage-covered apposing articular facets enclosed in a synovial capsule. The plane of the apposing articular facets determines the direction of movement of the spine. Whereas the intervertebral disc permits limited movement in all directions, the facet joints limit the direction to that governed by the plane of the apposing facets.

Like other synovial joints, the facet joints may be the seat of inflammation resulting in local pain. Each synovial joint is innervated by branches of the posterior division of two spinal nerves.[5] Since the facet joints are adjacent to the exiting spinal nerve roots at the intervertebral foramen, inflammation or spur formation may cause compression of the nerve root and resultant radicular pain.

Ligaments

The vertebral bodies and intervertebral discs are bordered anteriorly by the anterior longitudinal ligament, which extends from the atlas to the sacrum and limits hyperextension of the lumbar spine (Fig. 1–4). The posterior longitudinal ligament is on the posterior surface of the vertebral bodies and extends the entire length of the spine from the skull to the sacrum. The posterior longitudinal ligament limits flex-

ion of the spine. Two potential areas of weakness of the posterior longitudinal ligament are, first, in the lumbar region, where the ligament is thinnest along its lateral borders; and second, over the dorsal surface of the intervertebral disc, where a fascial cleft may be present. This configuration can permit a disc to herniate posterolaterally or to dissect beneath the ligament along the posterior aspect of a vertebral body.

The ligamenta flava are paired elastic structures that extend in a rostral-caudal direction, joining the lamina. Laterally, they extend to the facet joints and posterior border of the intervertebral foramina. Normal ligamenta flava are easily seen on CT scanning. The ligamenta flava stretch when the spine is flexed and buckle when it is hyperextended. This buckling can compress the spinal cord or cauda equina if the spinal canal is narrow or the ligamenta flava are hypertrophied.[33, 69]

Spinal Canal

The vertebral foramen, or spinal canal, is bordered by the posterior aspect of the vertebral body, paired pedicles, pars interarticularis, lamina, and spinous process. The shape of the spinal canal varies at different levels, which allows for considerable variation in the normal dimensions. Despite this fact, studies have determined the size of the canal that is associated with a greater risk of spinal cord or cauda equina compression. For the cervical spine, the anteroposterior dimension provides a reliable measurement.[80] The normal anteroposterior diameter of the canal is between 12 and 22 mm in the lower cervical spine as measured on lateral roentgenograms.[80] Because the anteroposterior diameter of the spinal cord is approximately 10 mm in the cervical spine, an anteroposterior dimension of the canal less than 11 or 12 mm usually signifies a risk of cord compression.

Measurements have been established for the normal dimensions of the lumbar canal with CT scanning.[74] The lower limit of normal of anteroposterior diameter is reported to be approximately 12 mm and that of the cross-sectional area greater

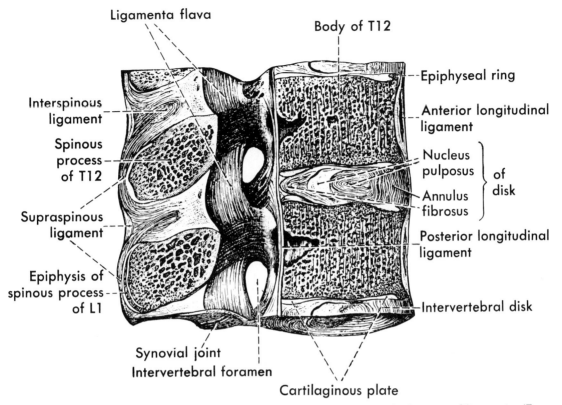

Ligamenta flava

Body of T12

Interspinous ligament

Spinous process of T12

Supraspinous ligament

Epiphysis of spinous process of L1

Epiphyseal ring

Anterior longitudinal ligament

Nucleus pulposus

Annulus fibrosus

} of disk

Posterior longitudinal ligament

Intervertebral disk

Synovial joint

Intervertebral foramen

Cartilaginous plate

Figure 1—4. Sagittal section through two vertebral levels demonstrating the location of ligaments. (From Hollinshead, WH,[41] p 315, with permission.)

than 1.45 square cm. Measurements less than these have been considered evidence for anatomical lumbar stenosis.[74] However, recent studies[33] have not consistently demonstrated that anatomical findings of lumbar stenosis, as demonstrated radiologically, accurately predict clinical evidence for neural compression (see Chapter 4, section entitled "Spinal Stenosis").

REGIONAL VARIATIONS

Cervical Spine

The atlantoaxial complex is the most mobile region of the vertebral column; it permits a considerable degree of nodding and rotational head movement. This mobility is associated with a relatively high degree of vulnerability, as the atlantoaxial complex resides between the less mobile atlanto-occipital joint above and C2—C3 joint below.

The atlas is the first vertebra and is essentially a ring structure that differs from other vertebrae in that it is devoid of a body. The occipital condyles of the skull rest on the superior articular facets of the atlas. In addition to the synovial articulations of the facets with the occipital condyles above and the facets of the second vertebral body below, the atlas also articulates with the odontoid process, which extends upward from the axis.

The most characteristic feature of the axis is the odontoid process, often called the dens (Fig. 1—5). The odontoid process arises from the C2 vertebral body and projects cephalad to be bordered anteriorly by the anterior ring of the atlas and posteriorly by the transverse atlantal ligament.[30,36] The odontoid process is bordered laterally by the lateral masses of the

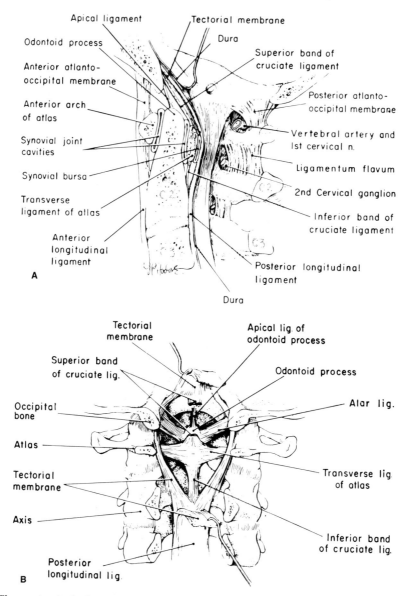

Apical ligament

Odontoid process

Anterior atlanto-
occipital membrane

Anterior arch
of atlas

Synovial joint
cavities

Synovial bursa

Transverse
ligament of atlas

Anterior
longitudinal
ligament

Tectorial membrane

Dura

Superior band of
cruciate ligament

Posterior atlanto-
occipital membrane

Vertebral artery and
Ist cervical n.

Ligamentum flavum

2nd Cervical ganglion

Inferior band of
cruciate ligament

Posterior longitudinal
ligament

A

Dura

Tectorial
membrane

Superior band
of cruciate lig.

Occipital
bone

Atlas

Tectorial
membrane

Axis

Posterior
longitudinal lig.

B

Apical lig. of
odontoid process

Odontoid process

Alar lig.

Transverse lig.
of atlas

Inferior band
of cruciate lig.

Figure 1–5. The anatomical relationships of the atlantoaxial complex are illustrated. (A) Midsagittal section. (B) Coronal section. (From Makela, A-L, Lang, H and Sillanpas, M, [50] p 489, with permission.)

atlas. In addition to its attachment to the atlas, the odontoid is attached to the skull base through the alar ligaments laterally and the apical ligament in the midline. The inferior articular facets of the atlas rotate on superior articular surfaces of the axis. This complex arrangement facilitates the nodding movements of the head. The anatomy of the atlantoaxial junction predisposes it to subluxation and dislocation.

There are other significant regional variations in the anatomy of the cervical spine. For example, the annulus fibrosus of the cervical spine is thicker posteriorly than anteriorly, unlike the situation in the lumbar spine.[13] Along the posterior lateral borders of the vertebral bodies of the cervical spine, there are bony protrusions, the uncovertebral joints, which are essentially pseudoarthroses between the edges of the vertebral bodies. These articulations, also referred to as joints of Luschka, lack articular cartilage, synovial fluid, and capsules and are not, therefore, considered synovial joints. The uncovertebral joints are adjacent to the intervertebral foramen and separate the latter from the intervertebral disc. The uncovertebral joints are often the site of osteophyte formation which may, as a result of proximity to the intervertebral foramen, cause spinal root compression.

Thoracic Spine

The vertebral bodies of the thoracic spine enlarge from the 1st through the 12th thoracic level. The pedicles arise from the superior portion of the vertebral body, creating a deep inferior vertebral incisura and shallow superior vertebral incisura. The laminae extend caudally below the inferior border of the vertebral bodies and overlap with the laminae of the vertebra below. At the thoracic levels, the spinal canal is relatively narrow compared with the spinal cord diameter, which becomes significant when mass lesions encroach on this space.[65] This may be one reason that the time of evolution of spinal compression is shorter in the upper and middle thoracic spine than in other regions.[65]

Lumbosacral Spine

The lumbar vertebral bodies are the largest, corresponding to their greater weight-bearing demands. The bodies of the lower lumbar vertebrae are wedge shaped, with the anterior height slightly greater than the posterior height. Unlike the cervical and thoracic spine, the laminae in the lumbar region do not overlap; this permits a lumbar puncture to be performed through the interspinous space.

The five sacral vertebrae are fused to form the triangular-shaped sacrum. The sacrum is tilted posteriorly and forms an articulation with the L5 vertebral body to form the lumbosacral angle. This is determined by measuring the angle formed by connecting a horizontal line with a line parallel to the superior border of the sacrum. When this angle is increased, an increased lordosis results and the shearing stress on the lumbosacral joint is also increased[14] as the L5 vertebral body tends to slip anteriorly on the sacrum. The posterior facet joints of L5 prevent this anterior movement and thereby function as weight-bearing joints. The abnormal stress on this joint may result in synovial inflammation and pain. According to Cailliet,[14] 75 percent of all postural low back pain is secondary to such an increase in lumbosacral angle and resulting lordosis.

EPIDURAL SPACE

The epidural space is the region located between the periosteum of the vertebrae and the dura mater. It therefore surrounds the spinal cord and cauda equina. It contains fat, connective tissue, and a venous plexus. The fat can be visualized by CT scanning, which can be helpful in determining whether lesions within the spinal canal are intradural or epidural.

The epidural venous plexus (discussed later in this chapter) is extensive and communicates with the dural venous sinuses within the cranium. According to Field and Brierley,[22] there are no lymph nodes in the epidural space; the regional lymph nodes of the spinal subarachnoid space are the prevertebral nodes.

MENINGES

The meninges consist of the dura mater, arachnoid, and pia mater (Fig. 1–6). The dura mater extends from the foramen magnum, where it is continuous with the cranial dura, to the level of the second sacral vertebra,[72] where it fuses with the sacral periosteum. The dura follows each nerve root to fuse with the epineurium and with the periosteum at each intervertebral foramen. Between the dura mater and the arachnoid is a potential space, the subdural space, which is important in the administration of anesthesia.

The arachnoid is a membrane continuous with the intracranial arachnoid that extends caudally with the dura to the second sacral vertebra. The term arach-

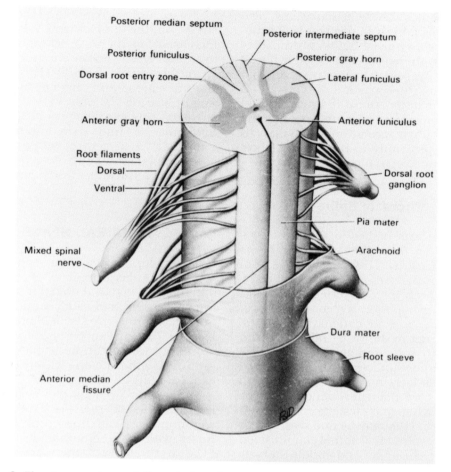

Figure 1—6. The gross anatomy of the spinal cord, gray matter, white matter, and nerve roots. (From Carpenter, MB, [15] p 215, with permission.)

noid arose due to the similarity between the numerous delicate trabeculae that course between the outer arachnoid membrane and the pia mater and the trabeculated pattern of a spider's web. These trabeculae course through the subarachnoid space, which contains the cerebrospinal fluid. The cross-sectional area of subarachnoid space is smallest in the thoracic spine and greatest in the lumbar region below the conus medullaris in the region of the cauda equina.

The pia mater is adherent to the spinal cord and follows penetrating blood vessels into the cord. Below the conus medullaris, the pia mater continues caudally as the filum terminale to attach to the dura at the level of second sacral vertebra. At the second sacral level, the filum merges with the dura to form the coccygeal ligament.

The denticulate ligaments arise from the pia along the lateral aspect of the spinal cord and pass through the arachnoid to attach to the dura mater. The 20 or 21 pairs of denticulate ligaments begin just above the first cervical root and are found between successive roots to approximately the first lumbar root. These ligaments suspend the spinal cord within the spinal canal.

SPINAL CORD

Gross Anatomy

The spinal cord begins at the level of the foramen magnum, which demarcates the caudal level of the medulla. Although early in fetal life the cord occupies the entire length of the spinal canal, the growth of the vertebral column exceeds that of the spinal cord so that by the ninth month of gestation, the spinal cord usually terminates at the level of the third lumbar vertebra. In the adult, the conus medullaris (conical termination of the cord) ends between the twelfth thoracic and third lumbar vertebrae, with the lower end of the first lumbar level being the most common site of termination.[3,62] The conus medullaris is anchored to the sacrum via the filum terminale.

The cervical and lumbar enlargements reflect the greater number of nerve cell bodies and synapses in the gray matter at these levels. These enlargements give rise to the brachial and lumbosacral plexuses, which innervate the upper and lower extremities. The anteroposterior and lateral dimensions of the spinal cord at the cervical enlargement are 9 and 13 mm; at the mid-thoracic region, the dimensions are 8 and 10 mm; at the lumbar enlargement, they are 8–9 and 12 mm.[15] Axial measurements are useful in the evaluation of the spinal cord using CT scanning and other imaging techniques.[34]

There are 31 paired nerve roots: 8 cervical, 12 thoracic, 5 lumbar, 5 sacral, and 1 rudimentary coccygeal. Each root is composed of ventral and dorsal filaments that carry motor and sensory axons, respectively, except for the first cervical and coccygeal nerves, which usually lack a sensory filament. In the cervical spine the numbered roots exit *above* the appropriately numbered vertebral body. The nerve root between C7 and T1 is numbered C8. This explains why there are 8 cervical roots and yet only 7 cervical vertebrae. In the remainder of the spine, the numbered roots exit below the appropriately numbered vertebral body (see Fig. 1–1).

Each spinal nerve root passes through its corresponding intervertebral foramen, occupying up to 50 percent of the cross-sectional area of the foramen.[71] The fit of the nerve root within the corresponding intervertebral foramen varies from level to level and may influence the effects of compressive lesions. For example, the fit is relatively tight at C5, possibly predisposing to pain in the C5 distribution when roots swell in disorders such as serum sickness.[43]

Below the conus medullaris is the cauda equina (horse's tail or collection of roots). As the spinal cord is shorter than the spinal canal, the length of spinal roots within the subarachnoid space progressively increases as the roots exit the spine more caudally. This is important in pathological conditions that affect the subarachnoid space, such as leptomeningeal carcinomatosis or arachnoiditis; those nerves with the longest courses within the subarachnoid space are most likely to be affected.

The surface of the spinal cord is demarcated by several topographical features. The cord is divided in the midsagittal plane by the anterior median fissure and the posterior median septum (see Fig. 1–6). The posterolateral and anterolateral sulci represent the location of entry and exit of the dorsal and ventral roots, respectively. In the cervical spinal cord, the posterior intermediate sulcus divides the fasciculus gracilis and fasciculus cuneatus.

The spinal cord gray matter is a butterfly-shaped structure surrounded by the white matter, which contains the axons of ascending and descending tracts (Fig. 1–7). The gray matter is divided into the anterior horn, posterior horn and, in the thoracic spine, the lateral horn. The central canal is a vestigial lumen lined by ependymal cells that lies within the gray commissure. The anterior and posterior white commissures are the sites of decussating fibers located adjacent to the gray commissure.

The white matter tracts of the spinal cord are divided into the posterior, lateral, and anterior funiculi. The posterior funiculus is located between the posterior horn and the posterior median septum. The lateral fasciculus is demarcated by the dorsal root entry zone and the exiting ventral filaments, and the anterior fasciculus lies between the ventral filaments and the anterior median fissure (see Fig. 1–7).

Gray Matter

The gray matter may be subdivided into an anterior horn, posterior horn, and intermediate zone (see Fig. 1–7). In studies on the cat spinal cord, Rexed[64] identified

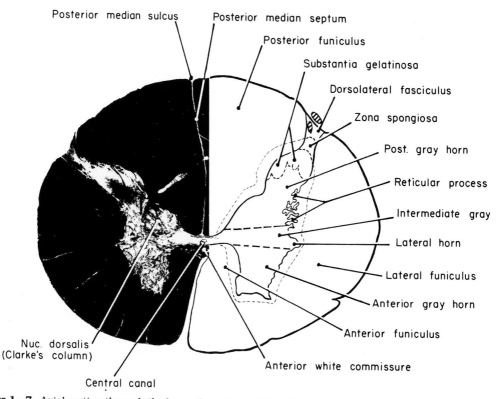

Posterior median sulcus   Posterior median septum

Posterior funiculus

Substantia gelatinosa

Dorsolateral fasciculus

Zona spongiosa

Post. gray horn

Reticular process

Intermediate gray

Lateral horn

Lateral funiculus

Anterior gray horn

Anterior funiculus

Anterior white commissure

Nuc. dorsalis
(Clarke's column)

Central canal

Figure 1–7. Axial section through the lower thoracic spinal cord. The left side is stained with Weigert's myelin stain and the right shows a schematic drawing of the tracts and gray matter subdivisions. The dotted area surrounding the gray matter contains short ascending and descending fibers of the fasciculus propius system. (From Carpenter, MB,[15] p 219, with permission.)

nine distinct cellular laminae within the spinal gray matter. The central gray substance within the gray commissure has been named area X. Studies in humans have shown a similar cytoarchitectonic organization.[73] The configuration and size of each of the nine laminae vary at different spinal levels. For example, lamina IX in the anterior horn, which consists of somatic motor neurons, is much larger in the cervical and lumbar regions than in the thoracic region.

The somatic efferent neurons are located within the anterior horn and give rise to the axons that traverse the ventral roots. These neurons may be divided into the larger (alpha) and smaller (gamma) motor neurons. The former innervate extrafusal muscle fibers and the latter innervate small intrafusal fibers of the muscle spindles. The alpha motor neurons are important in mediating individual muscle movements. The gamma efferent system is

important in setting the gain of the spindles and maintaining normal or abnormal muscle tone (e.g., spasticity or rigidity) through supraspinal influences.

The larger alpha motor neurons are functionally clustered in groups within the anterior horn. The motor neurons that innervate axial skeletal musculature are more medially placed and those innervating appendicular skeletal muscles are more laterally situated. In addition, the alpha motor neurons innervating flexor muscles are more dorsally located than those innervating extensors.

The visceral efferent fibers of the autonomic nervous system exit the spine with the somatic motor neurons in the ventral root. Within the spinal cord, the perikarya of the preganglionic sympathetic neurons are primarily located in the intermediolateral nucleus from the level of C8 through L3, with axons exiting in ventral roots T1–L3.[15,63] These axons terminate in the peripheral sympathetic ganglia. The parasympathetic neurons in the spinal cord are located at the S2, S3, and S4 levels in the lateral region of the gray matter. Preganglionic axons exit the spine through the ventral roots at these same levels to synapse in the peripheral ganglia located at or near the pelvic viscera, namely bladder, colon, rectum, and genitalia.

The posterior horn of the spinal gray matter receives afferent input from axons in the dorsal root; the cell bodies for these axons lie in the dorsal root ganglia. The dorsal root ganglia are located in the intervertebral foramina, along the dorsal roots. The dorsal root has two divisions;[61] the lateral division contains small-diameter fibers mediating sensation for pain and temperature, and the medial division contains large-diameter fibers mediating other sensory modalities such as proprioception.[15] The axons carrying different sensory modalities terminate and synapse in different locations within the posterior horn or pass through it to enter ascending tracts (e.g., posterior columns). Afferent fibers mediating the stretch reflex pass through the posterior horn to synapse on motor neurons and interneurons in the anterior horn. In the thoracic and upper lumbar region, the intermediate zone also contains the nucleus dorsalis, which receives input from the muscle spindles and joint receptors. This information is relayed ipsilaterally in the spinal white matter in the posterior spinocerebellar tract and may explain why patients with spinal cord compression can, though rarely, present with gait ataxia.[45]

MUSCLE STRETCH REFLEX

The muscle stretch, or myotatic, reflex is tested as a part of all neurological examinations. In its simplest form, the stretch reflex is a monosynaptic reflex where a sensory afferent neuron synapses directly onto a motor efferent neuron in the anterior horn of the gray matter. The sensory afferent (group 1a) is stimulated when the muscle spindle that it innervates is stretched, as occurs with percussion of a deep tendon. This 1a afferent makes direct excitatory monosynaptic connections with the alpha motor neurons of the same muscle and synergistic muscles, which are activated and cause muscle contraction.

The monosynaptic reflex depends on the temporal, as well as spatial, summation of impulses impinging on the motoneuron. Temporal summation requires the temporal synchrony of incoming impulses. Disease processes, such as demyelination of peripheral nerve, that interfere with this synchrony will result in loss of deep tendon reflexes.[76] In peripheral neuropathies, there can be temporal dispersion of impulses (due to unequal involvement of the axons within a nerve) even prior to slowing of nerve conduction below the lower limit of normal. This probably accounts for the early loss of deep tendon reflexes in peripheral neuropathies.[27] The loss of synchrony is greatest for those impulses that must be conducted over the largest distances, accounting for the early loss of distal reflexes such as ankle jerks.[77]

Integrated into this monosynaptic reflex are other interneurons and connections that can modulate it. For example, the 1a afferents also synapse with interneurons that inhibit the alpha motor neurons of antagonistic muscles. Furthermore, the threshold of the muscle spindles depends upon the degree of contraction of the intrafusal muscle fibers at the poles of the muscle spindle. The intrafusal muscle fibers are under the control of the gamma efferent motor neurons. The result is that descending supraspinal pathways are responsible for modulating muscle tone and the stretch reflex through the gamma motor system. Finally, the muscle tendon contains another sensory fiber, the Golgi tendon organ. This receptor measures the tension of the entire muscle; when excess muscle contraction occurs, it inhibits the alpha motor neurons via an inhibitory interneuron in the spinal gray matter.

White Matter

The white matter of the spinal cord, which surrounds the gray matter, is composed of well-defined myelinated tracts that are somatotopically organized. The white matter of the spinal cord is divided into three major regions: the posterior, lateral, and anterior funiculi. The funiculi, which contain ascending and descending axons, are sometimes referred to as columns.

Close to the gray matter, there are propriospinal tracts in which intraspinal axons run in a rostral-caudal direction and integrate information between segments into reflex patterns. These axons provide both crossed and uncrossed pathways linking neurons in one part of the spinal cord with those in others. They thus provide a basis for coordinated reflex activity, cyclic patterns of activity, and pattern generation within the spinal cord.[16,31] The remainder of the tracts that may be directly clinically evaluated are divided into ascending sensory and descending motor tracts.

ASCENDING PATHWAYS

Posterior Columns

The posterior columns, which consist of the medially located fasciculus gracilis and the laterally located fasciculus cuneatus, contain the centrally directed axons of a large proportion of the myelinated sensory fibers within the dorsal roots. The axons within the posterior columns are somatotopically organized so that the fibers from the more caudal regions of the body are located medial (fasciculus gracilis) to those representing the more rostral areas (fasciculus cuneatus) (Figs. 1–8 and 1–9). The cell bodies of these first-order sensory neurons are located in the dorsal root ganglia. The axons of these neurons, which ascend uncrossed in the posterior columns, synapse with second-order neurons in the gracile and cuneate nuclei in the medulla. Axons from these nuclei transmit sensory information rostrally via a pathway that decussates and ascends as the medial lemniscus and synapses in the ventral posterolateral (VPL) nucleus of the thalamus. Neurons in the VPL nucleus send their axons to the cortex.

The posterior columns represent a relatively new pathway phylogenetically and primarily conduct impulses concerned with position and movement of the extremities. Since these fibers mediate the discrimination of spatial and temporal cutaneous stimuli, their function is usually clinically tested by vibration, position, and two-point discrimination. However, there is a dispute over whether the posterior columns solely mediate these sensibilities.[17,29,59,75] In monkeys, lesions of the

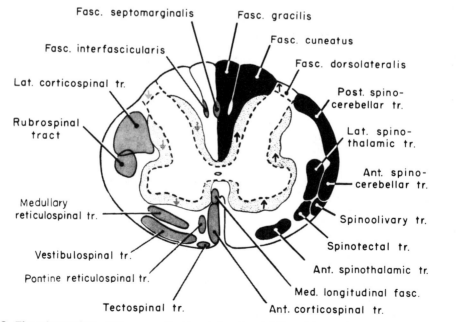

Figure 1–8. The relationships of the ascending tracts (on the right) and descending tracts (on the left). (From Carpenter, MB, [15] p 270, with permission.)

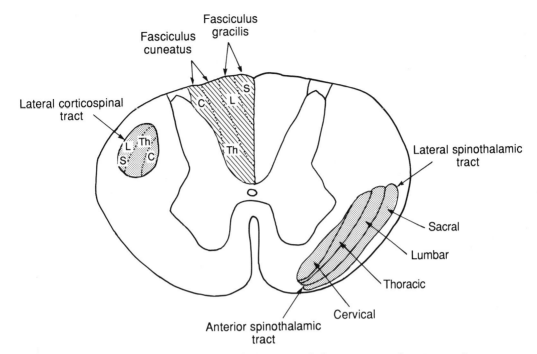

Figure 1—9. The lamination of the corticospinal tract, spinothalamic tract, and posterior columns.

posterior columns alone do not appreciably alter cutaneous sensation.[29,75]

Group 1a muscle spindle afferents, which innervate the neuromuscular spindle, also ascend in the posterior columns for a variable distance before synapsing in the dorsal nucleus of Clarke. The dorsal nucleus of Clarke is present in the gray matter from C8—L3 and projects ipsilaterally in the posterior spinocerebellar tract to the cerebellum.[60] Fibers from the group 1a afferents entering the spinal cord below L3 ascend in the fasciculus gracilis to the dorsal nucleus of Clarke. At upper thoracic and cervical levels, group 1a afferents do not synapse at the dorsal nucleus of Clarke but rather ascend in the fasciculus cuneatus to synapse in the accessory cuneate nucleus in the medulla. Like the neurons of Clarke's nucleus, the neurons of the accessory cuneate nucleus project to the cerebellum. The posterior spinocerebellar tract, located in the lateral funiculus, relays impulses from stretch receptors, muscle spindles, and Golgi tendon organs directly to the cerebellum. Lesions that interrupt these pathways at any level result in loss of the coordinated movements of gait and fine motor skills of ipsilateral extremities.[45]

The anterior spinocerebellar tract (see Fig. 1—8) conveys afferent impulses from Golgi tendon organs and other information related to muscle position and tone.[60]

Lateral Spinothalamic Tract

Cutaneous pain and temperature sensation is carried in the lateral spinothalamic tract, which ascends in the lateral funiculus. Evidence suggests that at least some of the fibers in the lateral spinothalamic tract carry information related to bowel and bladder fullness and pain from the lower urinary tract (lower ureter, urethra, and bladder) and mediate the desire to micturate.[57]

Axons mediating pain and temperature sensation enter the spinal cord at the posterior horn and synapse, either at the level of entry into the cord or after ascending or descending for one or two segments, with second-order neurons in the deep layers of the posterior horn (laminae VI, VII and VIII of Rexed).[15] The axons of the second-order neurons decussate in gray matter just anterior to the spinal canal to form the spinothalamic tract. Within the brain, the lateral spinothalamic tract axons synapse in the VPL nucleus and the posterior intralaminar nuclei of the thalamus.[7,8,52]

The spinothalamic tracts are somatotopically organized such that the sacral dermatomes run most laterally and the cervical dermatomes are ultimately represented most medially in the upper cervical spine (see Fig. 1–9). Thus, impulses associated with sensibility for the lower parts of the body are carried laterally within the tract and those associated with sensibility for the upper trunk and arms are located medially.

Unilateral complete lesions of the lateral spinothalamic tract produce a contralateral loss of somatic pain and temperature sensibility that often (as a result of the pattern of decussation of the fibers) extends 1–2 segments below the level of the lesion. In some cases after the lateral spinothalamic tract is transected, there is some return of sensibility to pain, possibly reflecting the presense of a small uncrossed spinothalamic pathway.[15]

Evidence suggests that fibers associated with pain and temperature are segregated within the lateral spinothalamic tract, the latter being located more posteriorly.[15] However, since the tract is relatively small, it is unusual for one component to be damaged selectively; pain and temperature sensibility are usually impaired together.

Anterior Spinothalamic Tract

The anterior spinothalamic tracts arise from the axons of second-order neurons in the spinal gray matter which, like those of the lateral spinothalamic tract, decussate over several segments. The fibers ascending in the anterior spinothalamic tract are somatotopically arranged; fibers originating in caudal spinal segments run in the most lateral parts of the tract, whereas those from more rostral levels are located more medially (see Fig. 1–9). Most fibers in this tract ascend without interruption to the thalamus, where they synapse in the VPL nucleus. Some fibers give off collaterals, en route, to the brain-stem reticular formation or other medullary nuclei.

Impulses traveling in the anterior spinothalamic tract are associated with sensibility for light touch. However, the posterior columns also relay this sensory modality to the brain, so that loss of light touch sensibility has little value in localization in the transverse plane of the spinal cord.

Knowledge of the anatomy of the anterior and lateral spinothalamic tracts has been important in performing cordotomies in an attempt to control pain, especially that arising from cancer. This procedure is performed via a percutaneous stereotaxic approach or as an open surgical procedure. It is most commonly performed in the cervical or thoracic regions and, is most effective in controlling unilateral pain below the waist.[23] It is more effective in controlling somatic pain than visceral pain because the latter pain pathways ascend the cord bilaterally.[79]

DESCENDING PATHWAYS

Corticospinal Tract

The descending pathways are divided into the corticospinal tract (generally corresponding to the pyramidal tract) and nonpyramidal pathways. The corticospinal neurons are located in the cerebral cortex and their axons descend to terminate within the spinal cord, directly on lower motor neurons or on other interposed neurons within the gray matter. This pathway is responsible for the ability of humans to perform discrete and fine movements of the distal extremities.

Corticospinal axons pass through the medullary pyramids where they largely decussate en route to the spinal cord. There are corticobulbar axons that also pass through the medullary pyramids en route to the brain-stem nuclei. The pyramids are not, therefore, entirely synonymous with corticospinal tracts but the terms are often used synonymously.

The corticospinal tracts originate in cerebral cortex and phylogenetically first appeared in mammals. The great majority of fibers in the corticospinal tract arise from pyramidal neurons (mostly the large Betz cells in cortical layer IV) in the precentral gyrus, and to a lesser extent, from the premotor area and the parietal lobe (especially the somatosensory cortex). In primitive mammals, the majority of corticospinal neurons project to the posterior horn,[24] whereas in primates there is a large projection directly to those alpha motor neurons innervating the distal extremities,[46,49] which subserve discrete appendicular movements.

Each corticospinal tract is composed of approximately 1 million fibers, most of them myelinated. After passing into the medullary pyramids, 75 to 90 percent of the corticospinal fibers decussate to form the lateral corticospinal tract, which is in the posterior portion of the lateral funiculus (see Fig. 1—9). Nondecussation of the pyramidal tract has been associated with mirror movements seen in cases of Klippel-Feil syndrome.[32] Fibers within the lateral corticospinal tract exhibit a distinct lamination, with important clinical implications. Fibers controlling lumbar- and sacral-innervated musculature run in the posterolateral part of the tracts and fibers controlling cervical-innervated musculature are located anteromedially, closer to the central gray. As a result of this lamination, in the central cervical cord syndrome, one often finds impairment of the upper extremities with relative sparing of the legs.

Usually 10 to 25 percent of the corticospinal fibers do not decussate, but descend in the spinal cord ipsilateral to the cerebral hemisphere of origin. Most of these fibers descend in the anterior corticospinal tract within the anterior funiculus of the spinal cord white matter. These fibers, after descending, either cross the midline in the anterior white commissure to terminate in the centromedial portion of the contralateral anterior horn or, less commonly, terminate in the same area of the ipsilateral anterior horn[58,66] to synapse with neurons innervating neck and trunk musculature. Although few in number, other corticospinal fibers may descend as an uncrossed pathway within the anterolateral funiculus.[2,19,78]

There is also evidence for the existence of some recrossed fibers in the lateral corticospinal tract. Evidence from postmortem examination of patients who had undergone spinal cordotomies for relief of intractable pain suggests that recovery of motility of the leg after damage to the ipsilateral corticospinal tracts is due to activity of descending fibers in the contralateral lateral corticospinal tract.[56] According to this view, most corticospinal fibers innervate motor neurons contralateral to the cerebral hemisphere where they originate, but a small proportion descend from the cortex in the contralateral lateral corticospinal tract and subsequently re-cross at spinal levels to activate ipsilateral leg motoneurons controlling proximal musculature, possibly via interneuronal chains within the spinal gray matter. These proximal muscles, while not mediating fine or discrete motor activity, appear sufficient for some aspects of stance and, in some patients, gait. This re-crossing of a small number of fibers from the lateral corticospinal tract could provide a neuroanatomical basis for the recovery of motility seen after cord hemisections in experimental animals[44,48] and after damage to the cerebral peduncle in humans.[10] There is a considerable degree of variation between individuals, which may account for some of the unexpected findings in occasional patients[58] such as may be seen in Klippel-Feil syndrome.[32] The important point here is that there can be some recovery of motor function even after a cord hemisection. This recovery involves gross postural movements, not discrete activity of distal limb muscles, suggesting that the more medially located motoneuron pools may receive bilateral innervation from the cerebral cortex.

The hallmark of corticospinal function is the movement of individual muscle groups to perform skilled movements of the distal extremities. This clinical observation is reflected in the pattern of distribution of corticospinal fibers. Weil and Lassek[78] estimated that 55 percent of corticospinal fibers project to the cervical region, 20 percent to the thoracic spine, and 25 percent to the lumbosacral area. The disproportionately large number of fibers projecting to the upper extremity, and to a lesser extent the lower extremity, compared with the thoracic spine, is due to the large contribution of fibers mediating discriminative movements of the distal extremity. In testing corticospinal function in patients with spinal cord disease, therefore, there is usually a loss of individual toe or finger movement long before there is loss of proximal muscle strength and control.

Corticospinal tract dysfunction also results in release phenomena such as the

Babinski response, which is a withdrawal response. The Babinski sign is observed more often with the loss of skilled movements of the foot than with hyperreflexia.[25] Gijn[25] has described the Babinski sign as due to a disturbance of direct pyramidal tract projections to distal motoneurons.

Spasticity is generally considered a sign of corticospinal disturbance; however, experiments in monkeys[11] and observations in humans[10] have shown that sectioning of the corticospinal tracts at the level of the medullary pyramids or cerebral peduncles results in decreased muscle tone and reduced or normal reflexes. Spasticity, therefore, appears to result from disturbance of pathways to the spinal cord that have been termed parapyramidal.[47] Nevertheless, because pure lesions of the corticospinal tract occur only rarely in clinical practice,[12] in practical terms, spasticity suggests corticospinal damage.

Nonpyramidal Tracts

Nonpyramidal pathways are phylogenetically older than the pyramidal pathways. These pathways originate in the brain stem and project to spinal gray matter. The major nonpyramidal pathways located in the anterior funiculus of the spinal cord are the reticulospinal tracts, the vestibulospinal tract, and the tectospinal tract (see Fig. 1–8). These pathways project to spinal gray matter innervating axial musculature and control muscle tone, reflex activity, posture, and balance.

Autonomic   Pathways. Descending pathways for autonomic control of breathing, blood pressure, sweating, and urinary bladder control are located primarily in the anterolateral quadrant of white matter in the spinal cord. Segmental innervation of the diaphragm most commonly occurs at levels C3–C5. Sympathetic fibers arising in the upper lumbar segments, parasympathetic fibers from S2–4, and somatic efferents originating at S2–4 innervate the urinary bladder. The anal sphincter and genitalia share similar pathways to those of the urinary bladder. The clinical anatomy and pathophysiology of these pathways are discussed in greater detail in Chapter 2.

VASCULAR ANATOMY

The detailed studies of Adamkiewicz in the late 19th century form the basis of our understanding of the vascular anatomy of the human spinal cord. These findings have been extended by more recent injection studies.[6, 39, 70] The arterial supply to the spinal cord is provided by the unpaired anterior spinal artery and the paired posterior spinal arteries (Fig. 1–10). Rostrally, the anterior spinal artery is most commonly formed in the region of the foramen magnum or upper cervical spine from branches of the vertebral arteries. Although radicular arteries accompany each spinal nerve root, only a few (usually fewer than 10) serve as tributaries to the anterior spinal artery.[28]

Individuals vary considerably in the contribution of different anterior radicular arteries to perfusion of the anterior spinal artery, especially in the cervical and thoracic regions.[28] Despite this variability, the artery of Adamkiewicz has come to be recognized as the largest and most constant in the lumbar region. It is an unpaired vessel and is located on the left side in two thirds of cases. It usually accompanies the spinal root of L1 or L2 but may accompany any root from T7 to L3.[18] The artery of Adamkiewicz is the major source of blood flow to the anterior spinal artery region for 50 percent of the spinal cord in 50 percent of individuals.[35]

The anterior spinal artery gives rise to a number of sulcal branches that enter the anterior median fissure and then divide into left and right branches to perfuse the gray matter and central white matter (see Fig. 1–10).[28] The sulcal branches are least numerous in the thoracic region; this arrangement may contribute to the already tenuous blood supply to this region. In addition to the vascular supply arising from the sulcal branches, the arterial vasocorona surrounding the spinal cord supplies another source of blood flow. Through these two arterial systems, the anterior spinal artery perfuses the anterior and lateral horns, the base of the posterior horn and the central gray matter, and the anterior and lateral funiculi. The remaining portion of the posterior horn and the

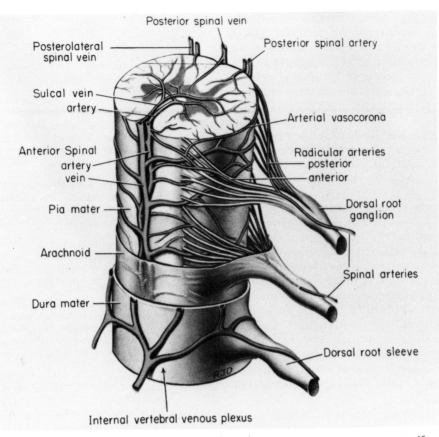

Posterior spinal vein

Posterolateral spinal vein

Posterior spinal artery

Sulcal vein artery

Arterial vasocorona

Anterior Spinal artery vein

Radicular arteries posterior anterior

Pia mater

Dorsal root ganglion

Arachnoid

Spinal arteries

Dura mater

Dorsal root sleeve

Internal vertebral venous plexus

Figure 1—10. The arterial and venous anatomy of the spinal cord. (From Carpenter, MB, [15] p 603, with permission)

posterior funiculi are perfused by the posterior spinal arteries.

The cervical and lumbar regions are the locations of the most copious blood flow from radicular arteries, making the anterior spinal artery supply of the thoracic spinal cord a watershed region. Interruption of blood flow to the cord will, therefore, often be clinically manifest in this region, resulting in an anterior spinal artery syndrome in the thoracic region near the level of T4.[21, 38] This syndrome is manifest by paraplegia and a middle-to-upper thoracic pin and temperature sensory level, with preservation of posterior column function due to perfusion by the posterior spinal arteries. As will be discussed in Chapter 8, spinal cord ischemia has been considered to be a rare phenomenon in the past but is increasingly

reported.[9] Some causes of spinal cord infarction include cardiac arrest, aortic dissection, aortic surgery, coarctation operation, and intra-aortic balloon pump counterpulsation.[1,4,9,26,40,42,68]

The posterior spinal arteries are paired structures and often form a network of blood vessels in which none is dominant. Rostrally, the posterior spinal arteries arise from the vertebral or the posterior inferior cerebellar arteries.[38] Caudally, they are fed by the radicular arteries. In the cervical region the blood flow is caudally directed, but in the thoracic and lumbar spine, blood flows rostrally.[6] The posterior spinal arteries perfuse the posterior columns and lateral aspects of the posterior horns.

In general, the draining venous system follows a similar pattern to that of the arterial system, although there are more individual variations. An anterior spinal vein is fed by sulcal veins and accompanies the anterior spinal artery. A single prominent median posterior draining vein is usually found near the posterior median septum. The anterior and posterior median veins are drained by radicular veins. As is the case with radicular arteries, some of these veins are more prominent than others; in the lumbar region the most prominent vein is the vena radicularis magna.[70]

A network of veins termed the internal vertebral venous plexus or Batson's plexus courses in the epidural space. Batson's plexus forms a collateral valveless route for venous return from intra-abdominal and intrathoracic organs to the heart. Venous effluent from these organs enters the valveless system when intrathoracic and intra-abdominal pressure is increased, such as occurs during straining, coughing, and sneezing. Neoplasms and infections in the viscera of these locations may thus metastasize to the spine through this collateral circulation.

REFERENCES

1. Albert, ML, Greer, WER, and Kantrowitz, W: Paraplegia secondary to hypotension and cardiac arrest in a patient who has had previous thoracic surgery. Neurology 19:915–918, 1969.
2. Barnes, S: Degeneration in hemiplegia, with special reference to a ventrolateral pyramidal tract. Brain 24:463–501, 1901.
3. Barson, AJ: The vertebral level of termination of the spinal cord during normal and abnormal development. J Anat 106:489–497, 1970.
4. Blackwood, W: Discussion on the vascular disease of the spinal cord. Proc R Soc Med 51:543–547, 1958.
5. Bogduk, N: The innervation of the lumbar spine. Spine 8:286–293, 1983.
6. Bolton, B: Blood supply of the human spinal cord. J Neurol Neurosurg Psychiatry 2:137–148, 1939.
7. Bowsher, D: Termination of the central pain pathway: The conscious appreciation of pain. Brain 80:606–622, 1957.
8. Bowsher, D: The termination of secondary somatosensory neurons within the thalamus of Macaca mulatta: An experimental degeneration study. J Comp Neurol 177:213–227, 1961.
9. Buchan, AM and Barnett, HJM: Infarction of the spinal cord. In Barnett, HJM, Mohr, JP, Stein, BM, and Yatsu, FM (eds): Stroke: Pathophysiology, Diagnosis and Management. Churchill Livingstone, New York, 1986, pp 707–719.
10. Bucy, PC, Keplinger, JE, and Siqueira, EB: Destruction of the pyramidal tract in man. J Neurosurg 21:385–398, 1964.
11. Bucy, PC, Ladpli, R, and Ehrlich, A: Destruction of the pyramidal tract in the monkey: The effects of bilateral destruction of the cerebral peduncles. J Neurosurg 25:1–20, 1966.
12. Burke, D: Spasticity as an adaptation to pyramidal tract injury. In Waxman, SG (ed): Functional Recovery in Neurological Disease. Raven Press, New York, 1988.
13. Cailliet, R: Neck and Arm Pain, ed 2. FA Davis, Philadelphia, 1981.
14. Cailliet, R: Low Back Pain Syndrome, ed 4. FA Davis, Philadelphia, 1988.
15. Carpenter, MB: Human Neuroanatomy, ed 7. Williams & Wilkins, Baltimore, 1976, pp 213–384.
16. Coghill, GE: Anatomy and the Problem of Behavior. Oxford University Press, London, 1929.
17. Cook, AW and Browder, EJ: Function of the posterior column. Transactions of the American Neurological Association 89:193–194, 1964.
18. Craige, EH: Vascular supply of the spinal cord. In Austin, GM (ed): The Spinal Cord: Basic Aspects and Surgical Considerations. Charles C Thomas, Springfield, Ill, 1961, pp 217–243.
19. Dejerine, J: Anatomie des centres nerveux. Reuff, Paris, 1901.
20. DeJong, RN: The Neurologic Examination, ed 4. Harper & Row, Hagerstown, 1979.
21. Domisse, GF: The blood supply of the spinal cord: A critical vascular zone in spinal surgery. J Bone Joint Surg 56B:225–235, 1974.
22. Field, EJ and Brierley, JB: The lymphatic connexions of the subarachnoid space: An experimental study of the dispersion of particulate matter in the cerebrospinal fluid, with special reference to the pathogenesis of poliomyelitis. Br Med J 1:1167–1171, 1948.
23. Foley, KM and Sundaresan, N: Management of cancer pain. In DeVita, VT, Hellman, S, and Rosenberg, SA (eds): Cancer Principles and Practice of Oncology. JB Lippincott, Philadelphia, 1985, pp 1940–1961.
24. Ghez, C: Introduction to the motor systems. In Kandel, ER and Schwartz, JH (eds): Principles of Neural Science. Elsevier, New York, 1985, pp 429–442.
25. Gijn, J van: The Babinski response and the pyramidal syndrome. J Neurol Neurosurg Psychiatry 41:865–873, 1978.
26. Gilles, FH and Nag, D: Vulnerability of human spinal cord in transient cardiac arrest. Neurology 21:833–839, 1971.
27. Gilliatt, RW and Willison, RG: Peripheral nerve conduction in diabetic neuropathy. J Neurol Neurosurg Psychiatry 25:11–18, 1962.

28. Gillilan, LA: The arterial supply of the human spinal cord. J Comp Neurol 110:75–103, 1958.

29. Gilman, S and Denny-Brown, D: Disorders of movement and behavior following dorsal column lesions. Brain 89:397–418, 1966.

30. Greenberg, AD: Atlanto-axial dislocations. Brain 91:655–684, 1968.

31. Grillner, S: Locomotion in vertebrates: Central mechanisms and reflex interaction. Physiol Rev 55:247–304, 1975.

32. Gunderson, C and Solitaire, G: Mirror movements in patients with Klippel-Feil syndrome. Arch Neurol 18:675–679, 1968.

33. Hall, SH, Bartleson, JD, Onofrio, BM, et al: Lumbar spinal stenosis: Clinical features, diagnostic procedures, and results of surgical treatment in 68 patients. Ann Intern Med 103:271–275, 1985.

34. Haughton, VM and Williams, AL: Computed Tomography of the Spine. CV Mosby, St Louis, 1982.

35. Haymaker, W: Bing's Local Diagnosis in Neurological Disease, ed 15. CV Mosby, St Louis, 1969, pp 57–59.

36. Hensinger, RN and MacEwen, GD: Congenital anomalies of the spine. In Rothman, RH and Simeone, FA (eds): The Spine. WB Saunders, Philadelphia, 1982, pp 189–239.

37. Hensinger, RN and MacEwen, GD: Congenital anomalies of the spine. In Rothman, RH and Simeone, FA (eds): The Spine. WB Saunders, Philadelphia, 1982, pp 188–315.

38. Henson, RA and Parsons, M: Ischaemic lesions of the spinal cord: An illustrated review. Q J Med 36:205–222, 1967.

39. Herren, TY and Alexander, I: Sulcal and intrinsic blood vessels of human spinal cord. Archives Neurology and Psychiatry 41:678–687, 1939.

40. Hogan, EL and Romanul, FCA: Spinal cord infarction occurring during insertion of aortic graft. Neurology 16:67–74, 1966.

41. Hollinshead, WH: Textbook of Anatomy. ed 2. Hoeber Medical Division, Harper & Row, New York, 1967, pp 303–326.

42. Hughes, JT and MacIntyre, AG: Spinal cord infarction occurring during thoracolumbar sympathectomy. J Neurol Neurosurg Psychiatry 26:418–421, 1963.

43. Iqbal, A and Arnason, BGW: Neuropathy in serum sickness. In Dyck, PJ, Thomas, PK, Lambert, EH and Bunge, R (eds): Peripheral Neuropathy, ed 2. WB Saunders, Philadelphia, 1984, pp 2044–2049.

44. Jane, JA, Evans, JP, and Fisher, LE: An investigation concerning the restitution of motor function following injury to the spinal cord. J Neurosurg 21:167–171, 1964.

45. Karp, SJ and Ho, RTK: Gait ataxia as a presenting symptom of malignant epidural spinal cord compression. Postgrad Med J 62:745–747, 1986.

46. Kuypers, HGJM: Central cortical projections to motor and somato-sensory cell groups. Brain 83:161–184, 1960.

47. Lance, JW: The control of muscle tone, reflexes and movement: Robert Wartenberg Lecture. Neurology 30:1303–1313, 1980.

48. Lassek, AM and Anderson, P: Motor function after spaced contralateral hemisections in the spinal cord. Neurology 11: 362–365, 1961.

49. Liu, CN and Chambers, WW: An experimental study of the corticospinal system in the monkey (Macaca mulatta). The spinal pathways and preterminal distribution of degenerating fibers following discrete lesions of the pre- and postcentral gyri and bulbar pyramid. J Comp Neurol 123:257–284, 1964.

50. Makela, A-L, Lang, H, and Sillinpas, M: Neurological manifestations of rheumatoid arthritis. In Vinken, PJ and Bruyn, GW (eds): Handbook of Clinical Neurology, Vol 38. North-Holland Publishing, Amsterdam, 1979, pp 479–503.

51. McRae, DL: Bony abnormalities in the region of the foramen magnum: Correlation of the anatomic and neurologic findings. Acta Radiol 40:335–354, 1953.

52. Mehler, WR, Feferman, ME, and Nauta, WJ: Ascending axon degeneration following anterolateral cordotomy. An experimental study in the monkey. Brain 83:718–750, 1960.

53. Modic, MT, Masaryk, T, and Paushter, D: Magnetic resonance imaging of the spine. Radiol Clin North Amer 24:229–245, 1986.

54. Nachemson, A: In vivo discometry in lumbar discs with irregular nucleograms. Acta Orthop Scand 36:418–434, 1965.

55. Nachemson, AL: The lumbar spine: An orthopaedic challenge. Spine 1:59–71, 1976.

56. Nathan, PW and Smith, M: Effects of two unilateral cordotomies on motility of the lower limb. Brain 96:471–494, 1973.

57. Nathan, PW and Smith, MC: The centripetal pathway from the bladder and urethra within the spinal cord. J Neurol Neurosurg Psychiatry 14:262–280, 1951.

58. Nathan, PW and Smith, MC: Long descending tracts in man: Review of present knowledge. Brain 78:248–303, 1955.

59. Netsky, M: Syringomyelia: A clinicopathologic study. AMA Archives of Neurology and Psychiatry 70:741–777, 1953.

60. Oscarsson, O: Functional organization of the spino- and cuneocerebellar tract in the cat. Physiol Rev 45:495–522, 1965.

61. Ranson, SW: The tract of Lissauer and the substantia gelatinosa Rolandi. Am J Anat 16:97–126, 1914.

62. Reiman, A and Anson, B: Vertebral level of the termination of the spinal cord with a report of a case of sacral cord. Anat Rec 88:127–138, 1944.

63. Rethelyi, M: Cell and neuropil architecture of the intermediolateral (sympathetic) nucleus of cat spinal cord. Brain Res 46:203–213, 1972.

64. Rexed, B: The cytoarchitectonic atlas of the spinal cord in the cat. J Comp Neurol 100:297–379, 1954.

65. Schliack, H and Stille, D: Clinical symptomatology of intraspinal tumors. In Vinken, PJ and

Bruyn, GW (eds): Handbook of Clinical Neurology, Vol 19. North-Holland Publishing, Amsterdam, 1975, pp 23–49.

66. Schoen, JHR: Comparative aspects of the descending fibre systems in the spinal cord. Prog Brain Res 11:203–222, 1964.

67. Sherrington, CS: The Integrative Action of the Nervous System. Yale University Press, New Haven, 1923.

68. Silver, JR and Buxton, PH: Spinal stroke. Brain 97:539–550, 1974.

69. Stoltman, HF and Blackwood, W: The role of ligamenta flava in the pathogenesis of myelopathy in cervical spondylosis. Brain 87:45–50, 1964.

70. Suh, TH and Alexander, L: Vascular system of the human spinal cord. Archives of Neurology and Psychiatry 41:659–677, 1939.

71. Sunderland, S: Anatomical perivertebral influences on the intervertebral foramen. In The Research Status of Manipulative Therapy, NINCDS Monograph 15. US Dept of Health, Education, and Welfare, Washington, DC, 1975, pp 129–140.

72. Trotter, M: Variations of the sacral canal: Their significance in the administration of caudal analgesia. Anesth Analg 26:192, 1947.

73. Truex, RC and Taylor, M: Gray matter lamination of the human spinal cord. Anat Rec 160:502, 1968.

74. Ullrich, CG: Quantitative assessment of the lumbar spinal canal by computerized tomography. Radiology 134:137–143, 1980.

75. Wall, P: The sensory and motor role of impulses traveling in the dorsal columns towards the cerebral cortex. Brain 93:505–524, 1970.

76. Waxman, SG: Pathophysiology of nerve conduction: Relation to diabetic neuropathy. Ann Intern Med 92:297–301 (part 2), 1981.

77. Waxman, SG, Brill, M, Geschwind, N, et al: Probability of conduction deficit as related to fiber length in random-distribution models of peripheral neuropathies. J Neurol Sci 29:39–53, 1976.

78. Weil, A and Lassek, A: Quantitative distribution of pyramidal tract in man. Archives of Neurology and Psychiatry 22:495–510, 1929.

79. White, J and Sweet, W: Pain: Its Mechanisms and Neurosurgical Control. Charles C Thomas, Springfield, Ill, 1955.

80. Wolfe, BS, Kilnani, M, and Malis, L: The sagittal diameter of the bony cervical spinal canal and its significance in cervical spondylosis. J Mt Sinai Hosp (NY) 23:283–292, 1965.

Chapter 2

CLINICAL PATHOPHYSIOLOGY OF SPINAL SIGNS AND SYMPTOMS

The first task of the physician examining a patient with suspected spinal cord disease is to establish the presence or absence of such disease and, if present, then the location(s) of the lesion(s). The anatomical coordinates are the "level" in the rostrocaudal axis, and the extent in the transverse plane of spinal cord involvement. These coordinates are determined by clinically testing specific functions originating in myotomes and dermatomes served by both nerve roots and tracts that may be involved. A third coordinate is the time-course of evolution of spinal cord compression, this often being important in predicting the etiology and the physiological response of the cord to compression, and in determining prognosis. For example, a patient showing a complete block on myelography from a longstanding lesion such as a benign meningioma may manifest few signs, whereas a patient with a comparable myelographic block from a rapidly enlarging malignancy may be paraplegic. The purpose of this chapter is to provide an understanding of the clinical pathophysiology of the spinal cord and to demonstrate the methods of history-taking and physical examination that are helpful in assessing the patient suspected of harboring spinal cord disease.

SEGMENTAL INNERVATION

As indicated in Chapter 1, the spinal cord is divided into 31 segments, with a spinal nerve root representing each segmental level. A segment is defined as the entire region innervated by a single nerve root. Segments are further generally characterized by dermatomes, myotomes, and angiotomes.[143] A *dermatome* is the cutaneous area innervated by the sensory nerves of a single nerve root and a *myotome* refers to the skeletal musculature innervated by the motor nerves of one spinal root. An *angiotome* refers to the blood vessels innervated via the autonomic efferents in a spinal nerve. Autonomic efferents also supply other autonomic functions such as sudomotor and pilomotor activity. As discussed below, the distribution of segmental autonomic innervation differs significantly from that of dermatomal innervation.

Traversing the ventral roots of spinal nerves along with motor axons are unmyelinated axons that are probably sensory.[31] At levels from C7 to L2 and S2 to S4, autonomic fibers also traverse the ventral root. The dorsal roots convey myelinated and unmyelinated sensory fibers.

Ventral Root Dysfunction

A disturbance of ventral root function usually results in characteristic motor disturbances distinct from those arising from corticospinal tract disease or from plexus or peripheral nerve dysfunction. Although there may be a variety of signs and symptoms, in most cases the presenting chief complaint is that of weakness. The localization of this complaint to the ventral root is determined by the pattern of weakness and the associated physical findings.

Those aspects of physical examination that are most helpful are the assessment of muscle strength, bulk, and tone. The discussion below begins with a brief review of these physical signs and then focuses on features of the examination important in differentiating ventral root disturbance from the other causes of weakness.

MUSCLE STRENGTH

Muscle strength may be determined by individual muscle testing or by functional assessment. Three methods of muscle strength testing are described below.

Individual muscle strength is commonly graded according to the British Medical Research Council[109] classification as shown in Table 2–1. This classification is helpful but it is insufficiently sensitive to describe accurately the many grades of weakness commonly seen. It is often necessary to assign a plus (+) or minus sign (−) to these grades. For example, a supine patient who could maintain an extended leg at the knee with the thigh supported off the bed but is unable to elevate the leg independently would be assigned a grade 3 for quadriceps strength. If the individual could elevate the leg against gravity but could not resist any further force, a grade 3+ might be assigned. We have found this modification to be helpful in following the clinical evolution of patients as well as in comparing patients.

Another potentially useful scale of strength is the modified scheme of Vignos and Archibald[166] shown in Table 2–2. Like the Karnofsky index,[81] it is a measure

Table 2–2 SCALE OF MUSCLE STRENGTH*

Grade 0:	Preclinical. All activities normal.
Grade 1:	Walks normally. Unable to freely run.
Grade 2:	Detectable defect in posture or gait. Climbs stairs without using bannister.
Grade 3:	Climbs stairs only with bannister.
Grade 4:	Walks without assistance. Unable to climb stairs.
Grade 5:	Walks without assistance. Unable to rise from a chair.
Grade 6:	Walks only with calipers or other aids.
Grade 7:	Unable to walk. Sits erect in a chair. Able to roll a wheelchair and eat and drink normally.
Grade 8:	Sits unsupported in a chair. Unable to roll a wheelchair or unable to drink from a glass unassisted.
Grade 9:	Unable to sit erect without support or unable to eat or drink without assistance.
Grade 10:	Confined to bed. Requires help for all activities.

*From Walton, J,[168] p 452, with permission.

of overall performance but it may be particularly valuable in evaluating patients with spinal cord disease because it is sensitive to disturbances in ambulation.

Finally, a recently reported assessment of motor strength of the lower extremities measures the time required for an individual to rise from a standard chair 10 times.[32] Although this may not be helpful in patients suffering from pain or marked weakness, it is often useful in following patients longitudinally and is particularly helpful in measuring proximal muscle strength, which is often diminished by corticosteroids or chronic disease.

Table 2–1 BRITISH MEDICAL RESEARCH COUNCIL SCALE OF MUSCLE STRENGTH[109]

0:	No muscular contraction
1:	A flicker of contraction, either seen or palpated, but insufficient to move joint
2:	Muscular contraction sufficient to move joint horizontally but not against the force of gravity
3:	Muscular contraction sufficient to maintain a position against the force of gravity
4:	Muscular contraction sufficient to resist the force of gravity plus additional force
5:	Normal motor power

MUSCLE BULK

Causes of muscular atrophy include disuse, endocrinological disturbance, malnutrition, and loss of innervation (neurogenic atrophy). Neurogenic atrophy is present in cases of radiculopathy. In cases of monoradiculopathy, however, the atrophy is not prominent since most muscles receive innervation from multiple nerve roots. In cases of chronic radiculopathy such as cervical spondylosis, atrophy may precede weakness. Alternatively, weakness may precede atrophy in cases of acute radiculopathy such as acute disc herniation.

Neurogenic atrophy may be associated with fasciculations, which represent spontaneous contraction of a group of muscle fibers innervated by a single motor neuron. The movements are not sufficiently strong to move a joint, and are usually seen as a rippling movement just beneath the skin. They may be difficult to see if the period of observation is brief or if the lighting is poor. It is generally best to observe the muscle obliquely rather than perpendicularly, to take advantage of the shadows created by the rippling movement of the skin. Fatigue, cold, medications, and metabolic derangements often cause similar movements.

Fasciculations are commonly seen in anterior horn cell disease. In cases of compressive root lesions, fasciculations may occur in the myotomal distribution of the compressed root. These fasciculations are different from those seen in anterior horn cell disease, however, in that they occur repetitively in the same fasciculus during minimal contraction and are absent during complete rest.[168] Spontaneous benign fasciculations occasionally are seen in healthy individuals. Typically, they occur only after contraction of the muscle and are not associated with weakness or atrophy.[168]

MUSCLE TONE

Muscle tone, the resistance that a muscle presents to passive limb movement, is often a very valuable sign in distinguishing the site of a lesion causing weakness. When measuring muscle tone, it is imperative that the muscles be relaxed, and it is often helpful to distract the patient's attention.

Spasticity and rigidity refer to common forms of increased muscle tone due to central nervous system disease. In spasticity, the increased tone is due to an exaggeration of the stretch reflex. If the muscle is slowly stretched, increased tone may not be found. However, if the muscle is stretched more rapidly, increasing amounts of resistance are found. Spasticity has been referred to as rate-sensitive for this reason. When due to cortical disease, spasticity preferentially involves the flexors in the upper extremities and extensors in the lower extremities.

Rigidity refers to increased muscle tone that is not rate-sensitive—that is, not dependent on the rate of movement. Unlike spasticity, it is found equally in both extensors and flexors. Rigidity is commonly seen in Parkinson's disease.

Spasticity usually results from dysfunction of the descending tracts, including the corticospinal tract.[22–24,88,164] Alternatively, spinal shock is one very important condition in which interruption of descending motor tracts results in flaccid weakness.

SPINAL SHOCK

When patients present with weakness associated with reduced muscle tone or flaccidity, the examiner is usually directed to diseases of the peripheral nerves or multiple nerve roots (although other causes such as cerebellar lesions are known). A critically important diagnostic error, however, may be made in the situation of spinal shock, a state in which all spinal reflexes caudal to an acute transection are lost.

The clinical manifestation of spinal shock is flaccid paralysis with loss of deep tendon reflexes below the level of the lesion. When this occurs in the cervical spine, it may resemble the clinical picture of an acute polyneuropathy or polyradiculopathy, such as Guillain-Barré syndrome. If the lesion is in the thoracic spine, it may give the appearance of a cauda equina syndrome or peripheral neuropathy. These errors will delay the correct diagnosis and appropriate intervention, which in many cases may require surgical decompression of the cord. The clinical differentiation of spinal shock from peripheral nerve or root disease can usually be made on the basis of a sensory level, which will not be present in the latter but is present in spinal cord transection. Severe bowel and bladder dysfunction early in such a course also suggests cord involvement rather than peripheral nerve disease. A more detailed discussion of spinal shock appears on page 41.

DIFFERENTIATION FROM OTHER CAUSES OF WEAKNESS

As indicated above, the pattern of weakness and associated neurological findings is of considerable localizing value. Individual nerve roots generally project to several different muscles and individual skeletal muscles usually receive their innervation from multiple roots. An important clinical corollary is that muscle paresis is common after injury to a single nerve root but frank paralysis is unusual. Also, corticospinal and peripheral nerve dysfunction often present with paralysis of several muscles or muscle groups.

Atrophy, often severe, develops in peripheral nerve lesions as well. Atrophy is generally less prominent in isolated root lesions because multiple nerve roots innervate single muscles and there is usually reinnervation of chronically denervated muscle fibers from adjacent roots. In some cases of radiculopathy, denervation may only be seen with electrodiagnostic studies. The one very sensitive clinical finding in root lesions, however, is a depressed deep tendon reflex of the muscle that receives much of its innervation from the injured root.

"SEGMENT-POINTER" MUSCLES

Although most muscles receive multiple innervation from multiple roots, in many cases a single muscle suffers the greatest dysfunction from a monoradiculopathy. Schliack has termed such muscles segment-pointer muscles.[143] Table 2–3 lists a group of muscles that may point the examiner to a specific nerve root. Because some individuals have prefixed and some have postfixed innervation, this listing, although very helpful as a screening examination of nerve roots, should not be considered infallible. A more detailed review is found in the Appendix.

PAIN

Pain is not often considered to be a manifestation of ventral root dysfunction. However, recent clinical reports suggest that irritation of the ventral root may result in pain that is distinct in character

Table 2–3 SEGMENT-POINTER MUSCLES*

Root	Muscle	Primary Function
C3	Diaphragm	Respiration
C4	Diaphragm	Respiration
C5	Deltoid	Arm abduction
C5	Biceps	Forearm flexion
C6	Brachioradialis	Forearm flexion
C7	Triceps	Forearm extension
L3	Quadriceps femoris	Knee extension
L4	Quadriceps femoris	Knee extension
L4	Tibialis anterior	Foot dorsiflexion
L5	Ext. hal. longus	Great toe dorsiflexion
S1	Gastrocnemius	Plantar flexion

*Adapted from Schliack, H,[143] p 172.

from the pain experienced from dorsal root irritation.[13, 17] According to the theory advanced by Sir Charles Bell,[20] the ventral roots are responsible for conveying impulses controlling muscular contraction and the dorsal roots conduct those for sensation. Magendie[19] provided the most extensive experimental support for this doctrine, which has come to be called the law of Bell and Magendie.

A fact often forgotten, however, is that pain can be induced in experimental animals through the stimulation of the ventral root. Using modern techniques, investigators have confirmed the presence of sensory afferents in the ventral roots and have suggested that some of these sensory fibers may enter the spinal cord directly via the ventral root.[101,175]

In a series of patients undergoing operation for cervical ventral root compression, Frykholm[51] found that with mechanical stimulation of the ventral roots, the patient experienced deep, boring, and diffuse pain, whereas stimulation of the dorsal root caused a rapid electric-like shock sensation. The pain arising from the ventral roots was termed myalgic and that from the dorsal root, neuralgic. Ventral roots that had been pathologically compressed chronically were more susceptible to elicitation of pain than those which had not been pathologically compressed prior to stimulation. Furthermore, if the dorsal roots were anesthetized, the pain was not experienced.

These experimental findings in animals and humans may explain some of the myalgic type pain that some patients report. For example, several publications have cited the cervical spine as the source for pain that may be difficult to differentiate from angina pectoris.[13, 17, 110, 123] Because the lower cervical myotomes extend to the chest wall (see Chapter 3), and the pain arising from ventral root irritation may be similar to that arising from coronary ischemia, the designation cervical angina has been applied.[13,17] There is little doubt that pain, perhaps of a myalgic character, may result from compression of the ventral roots elsewhere. In such cases, other signs of nerve root dysfunction such as motor, sensory, and reflex loss are often present.[13]

AUTONOMIC FIBERS

Preganglionic autonomic projections within the ventral root contain fibers that project to ganglia outside the spine. Lesions of individual roots may not disturb sweating or vasomotor control but more extensive lesions may cause such abnormalities including hypohydrosis and hyperhydrosis. Sympathetic innervation exits the spine from C8 to L2. Therefore lesions in this region may have distant effects. For example, the trigeminal region and C2−C4 receive sympathetic innervation from C8−T3. For this reason, a lesion in the paravertebral region of the upper thoracic spine, such as a superior sulcus tumor, may present with a Horner's syndrome.[120] Table 2−4 lists the dermatomal distribution of sympathetic (sudomotor) efferents.

The parasympathetic efferents in the spine exit with the sacral roots 2−4 to innervate the pelvic viscera, genitalia, and bladder. Within the spinal cord, the nerve cell bodies for these efferents are located within the conus medullaris. Disease processes involving the conus or cauda equina may therefore present with disturbances of these functions.

Dorsal Root Dysfunction

The dorsal roots convey sensory information to the spinal cord and disturbance of their function is most commonly manifest

Table 2−4 CUTANEOUS DISTRIBUTION OF SYMPATHETIC EFFERENTS (SUDOMOTOR FIBERS)*

Ventral Spinal Root	Corresponding Dermatomal Areas Receiving Sweat Gland Innervation
C8	C2−C4
T1−T3	Trigeminal area and C2−C4
T4	C5−C6
T5−T7	C5−T9
T8	T5−T11
T9	T6−L1
T10	T7−L5
T11	T9−S5
T12	T10−S5
L1	T11−S5
L2	T12−S5

*From Schliack, H,[143] p 164, with permission.

by pain and, to a lesser extent, by sensory impairment. The pain may be local, referred in a radicular or nonradicular distribution, and/or secondary to muscle spasm. Back symptoms are often caused by mechanical disease of the spine, such as the common problem of spondylosis.

Low back pain is the second most common cause for absenteeism in industrial settings.[138] This pain is usually self-limited and often responds to bed rest.[37] However, it may be the first symptom of a much more serious underlying disease. For example, as will be seen in the chapter on metastatic epidural spinal cord compression, back pain and/or radicular pain is reported in approximately 95 percent of such patients at the time of diagnosis of cord compression.[58,125] Pain may also be a sign of serious visceral disease referred to the spine or elsewhere. In some cases this pain may be confused with benign regional pain, resulting in a delay in diagnosis. Clinical clues discussed below and in Chapter 3 suggest those cases where pain is more likely to be due to a serious pathology.

PAIN

Local Pain

Local or regional back or neck pain is secondary to irritation or damage of innervated structures of the spine. The periosteum, ligaments, dura, and apophyseal joints are innervated structures. However, the central regions of the vertebral body and nucleus pulposus are not innervated and cannot, therefore, be a source of pain. For this reason, one may often see the central region of a vertebral body replaced by tumor on CT scanning and yet the patient does not complain of pain. If the tumor invades the periosteum, however, pain will be reported.

The clinical characteristics of local pain are that it is appreciated in the region of the spine and that it is deep, aching, and exacerbated by activity that places an increased load on the diseased structures. Patients suffering from pain due to epidural tumor generally report that their pain is made worse by the supine position,[115,128] whereas those suffering from spondylosis and musculoligamentous strain generally favor bed rest. The reason for pain exacerbation in the reclining position in patients with epidural tumor is uncertain, although Rodriguez and Dinapoli[135] suggest that recumbency is associated with lengthening of the spine, which presumably would cause increased traction of compressed nerve roots and spinal cord.

Palpation of the involved structures may exacerbate the local pain regardless of the cause. Surprisingly, however, percussion tenderness may not always be elicited in patients with metastatic disease. This has been shown in a study using CT scanning to identify spine metastases and epidural disease;[117] of 43 patients with spine metastases demonstrated by CT, only 20 (46 percent) had spinal percussion tenderness. Furthermore, of 20 patients with extension of tumor into the epidural space, only 13 (65 percent) had spinal percussion tenderness. *The absence of percussion tenderness should not reassure the examiner that metastatic disease is unlikely.*

In addition to irritation of local innervated structures, muscle spasm often causes local pain. Such pain is usually diffuse and aching, and spasm is often found on examination. Myofascial pain syndromes[152,153] may cause both local and referred pain.

Projected Pain

Projected pain arises from one anatomical site but is projected or referred to a site some distance from the site of pathology. Projected pain arising from irritation of dorsal nerve roots is of a radicular type, whereas that due to irritation of other spinal structures is usually of a nonradicular type. Although these forms of pain are not always easy to differentiate, it is important to distinguish between them because radicular pain has strong localizing value but nonradicular pain does not. Radicular pain will be used to describe pain arising from irritation of nerve roots with projection in that root distribution. Nonradicular referred pain (called simply referred pain in the interest of brevity) will be discussed separately.

Referred Pain

Referred pain arising from disease of the spine has been studied by several investigators.[84, 104, 154] After injecting hypertonic saline in the region of the interspinous ligament, Kellgren concluded that pain arising from pathology of this region was referred in a segmental distribution. These studies were criticized by Sinclair and associates,[154] who concluded that the pattern of segmental pain referral was, in fact, due to nerve root irritation.

McCall and associates[104] studied the pattern of pain referral in normal volunteers after injection of 6 percent saline into the apophyseal joints of L1–2 and L4–5. The pain was cramping and aching in quality. As shown in Figure 2–1, there was overlap in the regions of pain referral from upper and lower lumbar injections, with most of the pain being referred to the flanks, buttocks, groin, and thighs. It is of clinical interest that referred pain did not project below the knee despite the fact that the L4–5 level was stimulated. These authors, therefore, concluded that unlike radicular pain, referred pain does not follow segmental dermatomes and is not helpful in localization.

Although there may be paresthesias in the cutaneous area of pain referral as well as tenderness to deep palpation of the muscles, there are no neurologic abnormalities found in cases of referred pain of nonradicular origin. (This situation is unlike cases of radicular pain, where disturbance of the nerve root may often be

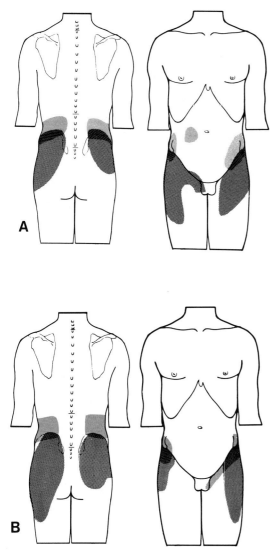

Figure 2–1. Patterns of referred pain. The distribution of pain referral from L1–2 (diagonal lines) and L4–5 (cross-hatching) are superimposed following intracapsular (A) and pericapsular (B) injections. Overlap of the patterns is shown in the region of the iliac crest and the groin. (From McCall et al, [104] p 18, with permission.)

Table 2–5 PATTERNS OF VISCERAL PAIN REFERRAL*

Visceral Source of Pain	Roots	Pain Referred to
Heart	T1–5	Chest and arm
Stomach	T5–9	Region of xiphoid
Duodenum	T6–10	Xiphoid to umbilicus
Pancreas	T7–9	Upper abdomen or back
Gallbladder	T6–10	Rt. upper abdomen
Appendix	T11–12	Rt. lower quadrant
Kidney, glans	T9–L2	Costovertebral angle, penis
Prostate region	S2–4	Glans penis, lumbar

*Adapted from Haymaker, W, [17] p. 67.

afferent innervation of the viscera. Up to 10 percent of all dorsal root afferents are visceral in origin.[49] Visceral pain may thus be referred in segmental distributions. The skin in these areas of referral may be hypersensitive. Head's zones and muscles may be tender in the region of pain referral.[73] Table 2–5 lists patterns of pain referral from common causes of visceral disease, which often create diagnostic problems.

Radicular Pain

Radicular pain arises from irritation of dorsal roots, with the resultant pain being projected to the region of segmental innervation of the respective nerve. As noted above, unlike other forms of referred pain, radicular pain has great specificity for localizing disease causing irritation of a nerve root. Since it is diagnostically so valuable, it is important to recognize and accurately diagnose the level of radicular involvement. Table 2–6 lists the common sites to which pain of radicular origin is projected.

Radicular pain is often a sharp stabbing pain in association with a chronic ache that radiates from the spine to the distribution of the involved nerve root. Maneuvers that stretch or further compress the nerve root, such as coughing, sneezing, straight leg raising and neck flexion, generally aggravate the pain. The patient may avoid certain activities and postures that place further stretch on the nerve. For example, in the case of sciatica, the patient may prefer to maintain the leg in a flexed

present in the form of sensory loss, hyporeflexia, and/or ventral root dysfunction.) Referred pain is generally aggravated and relieved by the same maneuvers that alter local pain.

Referred pain arising from disease of visceral structures may mimic referred pain from the spine. The autonomic nervous system provides both efferent and

Table 2—6 DIFFERENTIAL DIAGNOSIS OF LESIONS OF NERVE ROOTS*

Roots	C5	C6	C7	C8	D1
Sensory supply	Lateral border upper arm	Lateral forearm including thumb	Over triceps, mid-forearm and middle finger	Medial forearm to include little finger	Axilla down to the olecranon
Sensory loss	As above	As above	Middle fingers	As above	As above
Area of pain	As above and medial scapula border	As above esp. thumb and index finger	As above and medial scapula border	As above	Deep aching in shoulder and axilla to olecranon
Reflex arc	Biceps jerk	Supinator jerk	Triceps jerk	Finger jerk	None
Motor deficit	Deltoid Supraspinatus Infraspinatus Rhomboids	Biceps Brachioradialis Brachialis (Pronators and supinators of forearm)	Latissimus dorsi Pectoralis major Triceps Wrist extensors Wrist flexors	Finger flexors Finger extensors Flexor carpi ulnaris (thenar muscles in some patients)	*All* small hand muscles (in some thenar muscles via C8)
Some causative lesions	Brachial neuritis Cervical spondylosis Upper plexus avulsion	Cervical spondylosis Acute disc lesions	Acute disc lesions Cervical spondylosis	Rare in disc lesions or spondylosis	Cervical rib Outlet syndromes Pancoast tumour Metastatic carcinoma in deep cervical nodes

Roots	L2	L3	L4	L5	S1
Sensory supply	Across upper thigh	Across lower thigh	Across knee to medial malleolus	Side of leg to dorsum and sole of foot	Behind lateral malleolus to lateral foot
Sensory loss	Often none	Often none	Medial leg	Dorsum of foot	Behind lateral malleolus
Area of pain	Across thigh	Across thigh	Down to medial malleolus	Back of thigh, lateral calf—dorsum of foot	Back of thigh, back of calf lateral foot
Reflex arc	None	Adductor reflex	Knee jerk	None	Ankle jerk
Motor deficit	Hip flexion	Knee extension Adduction of thigh	Inversion of the foot	Dorsiflexion of toes and foot (latter L4 also)	Plantar flexion and eversion of foot
Some causative lesions		Neurofibroma Meningioma Neoplastic disease Disc lesions very rare (except L4 <5 percent *all*)			Disc lesions Metastatic malignancy Neurofibromas Meningioma

*From Patten, J, [121] p 195 and 211, with permission.

posture at the hip and knee and to plantar flex the foot. Such a posture results in a rather characteristic gait in these patients. Cutaneous paresthesias and tenderness of tissues in the region of pain projection, as in referred pain, are common. However, in cases of radicular pain there may also be sensory disturbances and, at times, reflex and motor abnormalities corresponding to the injured nerve root. The motor disturbances are those described in the section on ventral root disorders.

Case Illustration

A 62-year-old man with lymphoma was referred for neurological evaluation of pain. The pain was present in the right buttock and radiated down the lateral aspect of the thigh to the region of the patella. The pain was provoked by neck flexion and occasionally was present in the recumbent position. Neurological examination was remarkable for an equivocal reduction of the right patellar reflex and positive reverse straight leg raising that provoked the leg pain. Plain films of the spine were unrevealing but a

CT scan with intravenous contrast enhancement demonstrated a small mass lesion in the region of the L3–L4 foramen compressing the L3 nerve root. This was considered to be lymphoma and radiation therapy was commenced. Following radiation therapy, the pain resolved entirely and the knee reflex returned to normal.

Comment. This case illustrates the sensitivity and specificity of radicular pain in localizing an epidural neoplasm. The pain, which was primarily present on neck flexion, convinced the examiner that the lesion was most probably in the spinal axis and not in the pelvis, hip, or elsewhere. The work-up, therefore, was immediately directed to the spine despite the fact that there were only equivocal reflex findings.

SENSORY DISTURBANCES

Just as referred pain from the spine or from visceral sources may mimic radicular pain, so may irritation of peripheral nerves cause diagnostic confusion. For example, carpal tunnel syndrome may commonly cause pseudoradicular symptoms in the proximal arm. Similarly, the piriformis muscle in the pelvis may compress the sciatic nerve, causing sciatica that may be difficult to differentiate from radicular syndromes. In cases of nerve root injury and peripheral nerve injury, pain may be associated with sensory loss, unlike other forms of referred pain in which true sensory loss is not found. Careful attention to the sensory exam may help distinguish between these various causes of radicular and nonradicular projected pain and pain arising from peripheral nerve injury.

Although there is sensory loss in cases of both radicular pain and pain secondary to peripheral nerve injury, the type and pattern of sensory loss is different in the two situations. A knowledge of dermatomal and peripheral nerve cutaneous innervation is, of course, helpful in distinguishing the two causes. Furthermore, it is important to recognize that since there is considerable overlap in dermatomal areas of tactile sensation, loss of touch does not generally occur as a result of monoradiculopathy. However, since the dermatomal representation of pain sensation has less overlap, monoradiculopathies result in a greater area of pinprick analgesia than of tactile anesthesia. Alternatively, in the case of a peripheral nerve lesion, one will often find an area of tactile anesthesia due to lack of overlap of peripheral nerve cutaneous distribution. However, individual variations in cutaneous innervation occur frequently.

Dermatomes

A knowledge of the dermatomal map is valuable in recognizing and localizing radicular syndromes. As in many other areas of neurophysiology, Sherrington laid the groundwork for our current anatomical knowledge of dermatomes.[148] Using the method of residual sensibility, he mapped the dermatomes in primates by sectioning the adjacent dorsal roots above and below a single dorsal root. The remaining area of sensibility was considered to be the dermatome of the intact dorsal root.

Modern knowledge of dermatomal maps in humans dates back to Foerster's work,[50] which utilized the strategy noted above by Sherrington in monkeys. Foerster demonstrated that there is significant overlap in dermatomal representations in humans.

More recent physiological studies in monkeys have demonstrated even greater variability in the dermatomal maps than previous studies had suggested.[41] Recent studies suggest that the axons of each dorsal root innervate the cutaneous region of up to five adjacent dermatomes.[36] This would mean that each area of skin may be innervated by several adjacent dorsal root ganglia. Thus, our current definition of a dermatome may need to be reformulated.[171]

Although these newer findings are expected to lead to changes in our concepts and definitions of dermatomes, Figure 2–2 illustrates a currently recognized dermatomal map that has considerable clinical value. A few points deserve emphasis:

1. There is no C1 dermatome.
2. On the trunk the C4 and T2 dermatomes are contiguous.
3. The thumb, middle finger, and fifth digits are innervated by C6, C7, and C8 respectively.
4. The nipple is at the level of T4.
5. The umbilicus is at the T10 level.

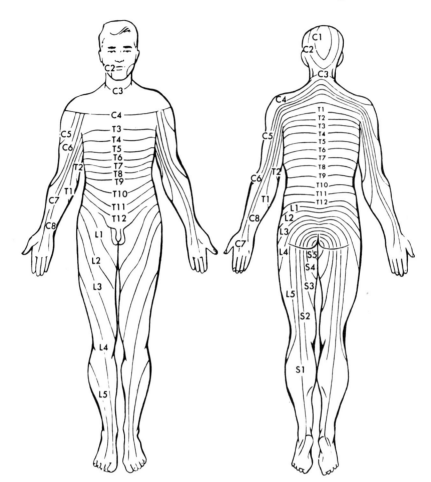

Figure 2–2. A dermatomal map. (From Haymaker, [71] p 62, with permission.)

6. In the posterior axial line of the leg (medial thigh), the lumbar and sacral dermatomes are contiguous.

Finally, there are variations in dermatomal maps between individuals that may make clinical conclusions based upon sensory testing alone problematic.

Deep Tendon Reflexes

In addition to motor and sensory disturbances, deep tendon reflex abnormalities can be of precise localizing value in spine disease. As demonstrated in Figure 2–3, the stretch, or myotatic reflex, is a monosynaptic reflex that requires both ventral and dorsal roots to function normally. When deep tendon reflexes are focally hy-poactive, they can be sensitive indicators of specific root disturbance. When they are hyperactive below a specific level (or acutely hypoactive or absent in spinal shock), they may indicate a myelopathy at some more rostral level.

The combination of hypoactive reflexes at a segmental level with hyperactive reflexes caudal to this level is commonly found with cervical spine disease. For example, although a variety of diseases may be responsible, cervical spondylosis in the lower cervical spine may result in the combination of hyporeflexia of the brachioradialis, due to impingement on C5 and C6 roots, and hyperreflexia below this level secondary to an associated myelopathy. When the brachioradialis reflex is stimulated in this case, one paradoxically finds

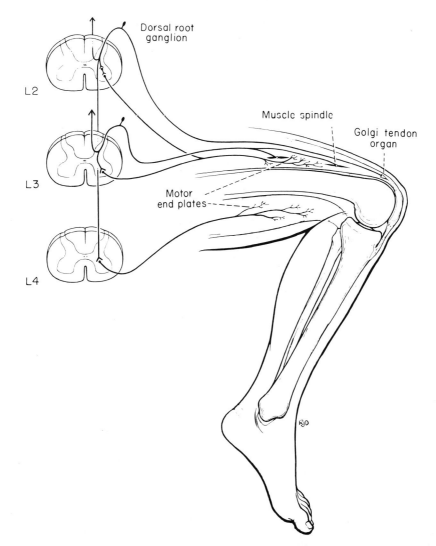

Figure 2−3. The motor and sensory pathways in the femoral nerve and L2, L3, and L4 which mediate the patellar myotatic reflex. The muscle spindles, which respond to a brisk stretching of the muscle as occurs with tapping the patella, are shown entering the L3 spinal segment. These afferent nerves synapse with anterior horn cells at the same levels to complete the reflex arc. Excessive stretching stimulates the Golgi tendon organs which are shown entering the L2 spinal segment and which inhibit the extrafusal muscle fibers via an interneuron. A pathway for reciprocal inhibition of the antagonistic muscle, the hamstring, is also shown. (From Carpenter,[26] p 236, with permission.)

contraction of the finger flexors rather than flexion and supination of the hand.[35] Such a response is called inversion of the radial reflex. Table 2−6 identifies nerve roots and their associated deep tendon reflexes.

The superficial reflexes also require intact spinal roots as well as intact descend-

ing tracts from the brain through the spinal cord. The most commonly tested superficial reflexes are shown in Table 2−7. Diminution or absence of the abdominal, cremasteric, or anal reflexes may occur due to lesions interrupting the nerve roots subserving such reflexes or following lesions of pyramidal and/or other descend-

**Table 2−7 COMMONLY TESTED
SUPERFICIAL REFLEXES AND
CORRESPONDING SPINAL ROOTS**

Abdominal, T7−T12
Cremasteric, L1−L2
Anal, S2−S4
Plantar, S1−S2

ing tracts. When there is a reduction in these superficial reflexes and an increase in deep tendon reflexes, the lesion is generally found in the descending tracts within the brain or spinal cord. A pathological plantar response, the Babinski sign, indicates corticospinal tract dysfunction and is discussed below.

Nerve Root vs. Peripheral Nerve Lesion

As indicated above, monoradiculopathies rarely cause frank paralysis of a single muscle or muscle group, whereas such paralysis is quite common in cases of peripheral nerve damage. A knowledge of innervation of muscle groups is important in making the distinction (Table 2−8; see Table 2−6).

The sensory examination may be helpful in distinguishing peripheral nerve lesions from radiculopathies. Knowledge of the peripheral nerve sensory distributions and of dermatomal anatomy is important. In addition, as already discussed, cutaneous tactile loss is more frequent in peripheral nerve lesions than in monoradiculopathies; in radiculopathies, loss of tactile sensation is unusual due to overlap of dermatomes.[143]

Finally, whereas peripheral nerve injuries frequently are associated with autonomic complaints, monoradiculopathies ordinarily are not. This distinction is due to the fact that the sympathetic ganglia are located peripheral to the spine and receive their preganglionic input from several segmental levels. The postganglionic efferents then join the peripheral nerves, so that injuries to peripheral nerves generally are associated with loss of sweating.[143]

LOCALIZATION OF LESIONS IN THE TRANSVERSE PLANE

Motor Disorders

Following pain, the most common symptom of patients suffering from neoplastic spinal cord compression is weakness.[58] Weakness, particularly of the legs, must always be viewed as a possible early manifestation of spinal cord disease. The pattern of weakness as well as the associated reflex findings and muscle tone can direct the physician to the anatomical localization and may suggest the etiology as well. In spinal cord disease, weakness is classified as either due to lower motor neuron or corticospinal tract dysfunction.

As mentioned above, the findings of lower motor neuron dysfunction are weakness associated with atrophy, hypotonia, fasciculations, and depressed reflexes of a single extremity (myotome). Upper motor neuron disease often manifests with spasticity, hyperreflexia, and Babinski sign (note the exception of spinal shock) as well as weakness involving more than a single extremity. In the case of cervical spine disease, one may find a combination of lower motor neuron disturbance involving the upper extremity and upper motor neuron findings in one or both lower extremities.

Perhaps the most important clue in suggesting a spinal origin to weakness is the pattern of weakness. In individuals with hemiparesis involving the face, arm, and leg, there is usually no confusion that the site of localization is in the brain. Similarly in patients with definite paraparesis or quadriparesis, the examiner is usually directed to the spinal cord. The occurrence of monoparesis creates the most diagnostic confusion. Early in spinal cord tumors, the patient may present with unilateral leg weakness, and examination may not reveal findings in the contralateral leg or the arms. In such cases, the physician may erroneously attribute the disorder to an anterior cerebral artery stroke, especially if the patient indicates that it was acute in onset. In our experience, anterior cerebral artery strokes are a relatively uncommon cause of unilateral leg

Table 2–8 DIFFERENTIAL DIAGNOSIS OF LESIONS OF PERIPHERAL NERVES*

Nerves	Axillary	Musculocutaneous	Radial	Median	Ulnar
Sensory supply	Over deltoid	Lateral forearm to wrist	Lateral dorsal forearm and back of thumb and index finger	Lateral palm and lateral fingers	Medial palm and 5th and medial half ring finger
Sensory loss	Small area over deltoid	Lateral forearm	Dorsum of thumb and index (if any)	As above	As above but often none at all
Area of pain	Across shoulder tip	Lateral forearm	Dorsum of thumb and index	Thumb, index and middle finger. Often spreads up forearm	Ulnar supplied fingers and palm distal to wrist. Pain occasionally along course of nerve
Reflex arc	Nil	Biceps jerk	Triceps jerk and supinator jerk	Finger jerks (flexor digitorum sublimis)	Nil
Motor deficit	Deltoid (teres minor cannot be evaluated)	Biceps Brachialis (coracobrachialis weakness not detectable)	Triceps Wrist extensors Finger extensors Brachioradialis Supinator of forearm	Wrist flexors Long finger flexors (thumb, index and middle finger) Pronators of forearm. Abductor pollicis brevis	All small hand muscles excluding abductor pollicis brevis. Flexor carpi ulnaris. Long flexors of ring and little finger
Some causative lesions	Fractured neck of humerus. Dislocated shoulder Deep I.M. injections	Very rarely damaged	Crutch palsy. Saturday night palsy. Fractured humerus. In supinator muscle	Carpal tunnel syndrome Direct trauma to wrist	Elbow: trauma, bed rest, fractured olecranon. Wrist: local trauma, ganglion of wrist joint

Nerves	Obturator	Femoral	Sciatic Nerve	
			Peroneal Division	Tibial Division
Sensory supply	Medial surface of thigh	Anteromedial surface of thigh and leg to medial malleolus	Anterior leg, dorsum of ankle and foot	Posterior leg, sole and lateral border of foot
Sensory loss	Often none	Usually anatomical	Often just dorsum of foot	Sole of foot
Area of pain	Medial thigh	Anterior thigh and medial leg	Often painless	Often painless
Reflex arc	Adductor reflex	Knee jerk	None	Ankle jerk
Motor deficit	Adduction of thigh	Extension of knee	Dorsiflexion, inversion and eversion of the foot (+lateral hamstrings)	Plantar flexion and inversion of foot (+medial hamstrings)
Some causative lesions	Pelvic neoplasm Pregnancy	Diabetes Femoral hernia Femoral artery aneurysm Posterior abdominal neoplasm Psoas abscess	Pressure palsy at fibula neck Hip fracture/dislocation Penetrating trauma to buttock Misplaced injection	Very rarely injured even in buttock Peroneal division more sensitive to damage

*From Patten, J,[121] p 195 and 211, with permission.

weakness in comparison with the frequency of cases due to spinal pathology.

Lesions of the craniocervical junction and cervical spine often present with a pattern of unilateral arm weakness before progressing to ipsilateral leg weakness, then contralateral involvement.[46, 161] However, although weakness involving an ipsilateral arm and leg with sparing of the face suggests a high cervical lesion, cerebral disturbances or pyramidal infarction[136] may account for this localization. Finally, not all cases of apparent lower extremity weakness are due to spinal cord disease. Many patients treated with corticosteroids or with generalized cachexia appear to present with leg weakness because their chief complaint is often gait difficulty.

Case Illustration

A 75-year-old man, with a history of lymphoma for several years, was referred for progressive gait difficulty over a two-month period. The patient had a history of bone marrow involvement with lymphoma and had received multiple courses of chemotherapy. His most recent course of chemotherapy was completed three months earlier and had included vinca alkaloids and corticosteroids. His extent of disease evaluation just prior to neurological referral had included no evidence of lymphoma on physical examination and a negative chest-abdominal CT scan, negative bone marrow and negative CSF cytology, although the CSF protein was mildly elevated at 75 mg per dl. The patient denied any pain but complained of leg weakness out of proportion to weakness elsewhere.

His neurological examination revealed a normal mental status and cranial nerves. Leg weakness was out of proportion to upper extremity weakness; his motor examination was judged as a grade 6 (Vignos Archibald scale[166]) with only apparent mild to moderate weakness of the upper extremities. He had no deep tendon reflexes (due to vinca alkaloids) and had only minimal sensory loss distally in the upper and lower extremities. Sphincters were intact. There was no evidence of spinal tenderness or Lhermitte's sign and straight leg raising provoked no pain. Total spine films were unrevealing. The patient died within a few days of referral.

Autopsy demonstrated a pulmonary embolus as the proximate cause of death. There was no evidence of brain or spinal involvement by lymphoma. There was no evidence of motor neuronopathy on histological examination of the spinal cord.[146] Muscle histological examination revealed no sign of polymyositis. The patient had a massive amount of lymphoma in the mesentery and retroperitoneal space that was not evident on a CT scan or ultrasound three weeks before death.

Comment. This case illustrates apparent paraparesis due to advanced malignancy without spinal cord involvement. The absence of

back or radicular pain made a diagnosis of cord compression less likely but, of course, did not exclude it. The pathophysiological basis for such cases of severe gait difficulty is not usually satisfactorily explained, although they are often attributed to a paraneoplastic syndrome without further pathological or physiological definition. The important lesson is that without definitive imaging of the spine (MRI or myelography) one could not be confident that the cause of weakness was not cord compression from lymphoma. The following companion case further illustrates this point.

Case Illustration

A 35-year-old man with a diagnosis of diffuse, poorly differentiated lymphoma for six years was referred for Lhermitte's sign and interscapular discomfort. He had not received any therapy for his lymphoma but was being following closely by his oncologist. Five months prior to referral he noted vague interscapular discomfort after playing basketball, which he attributed to muscle strain. The pain remitted with rest. Two months later he noted recurrence of the symptoms with less strenuous activity. His oncologist found no evidence for progression of his minimal cervical and axillary adenopathy and a chest roentgenogram and thoracic spine films revealed no abnormality.

At the time of neurological referral he reported that neck flexion caused paresthesias beginning in the interscapular area, radiating down his back into his legs. He had increasing interscapular discomfort, especially on lying supine. His neurological examination revealed no signs of myelopathy, but he did have subjective complaint of tightness in his chest and abdomen. He had spine tenderness in the midthoracic spine.

Plain films of the spine were negative. An MRI of the entire spine, performed on a 1.5 Tesla unit, showed no evidence of bone pathology and there was no definite evidence for intraspinal pathology; the study was technically limited, however, due to patient movement artifact because the patient had discomfort during the procedure. A myelogram was performed by lumbar and then C1−2 approach followed by CT scanning (Figure 2−4). An epidural block was found extending from T4 to L2. The CT scan demonstrated that paravertebral lymphoma had invaded the epidural space through intervertebral foramina. The patient was given high-dose corticosteroids and radiation therapy

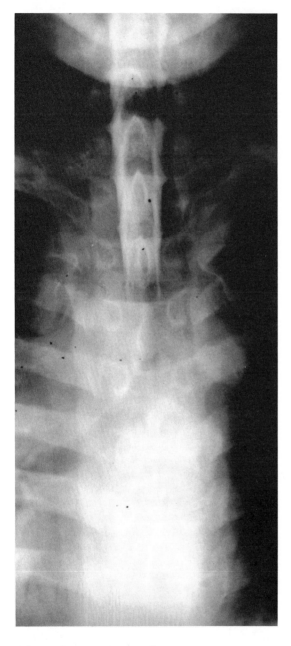

Figure 2–4. Myelogram following C1–2 puncture demonstrates an epidural block from lymphoma at the T3 level.

was administered to the involved parts of the spine. He had complete resolution of his complaint.

Comment. This case illustrates the need to evaluate patients carefully who complain of pain and are harboring malignancy. Although the patient had no signs of myelopathy and was

able to run without difficulty, he had a complete block on myelography. The symptoms were so suggestive of an intraspinal mass lesion that a myelogram was requested when the MRI did not reveal the cause of his symptoms. This case and the previous one demonstrate the limitations of the physical examination in evaluating patients with epidural spinal cord compression, and they emphasize the need to proceed with imaging studies when the cause of symptoms is not definitely understood.

Case Illustration

A 30-year-old woman was referred for evaluation of Lhermitte's sign. She had been well until one year previously, when she noted a mass above the right elbow. Biopsy of the lesion revealed a fibrosarcoma. She underwent amputation of the arm at the level of the shoulder. There was no evidence of disease elsewhere. She received adjuvant chemotherapy consisting of several cycles of doxorubicin and cisplatin.

Although she denied any pain, she reported that on neck flexion she had experienced electric-like sensations into her trunk and legs during the three weeks prior to referral. She denied any history suggestive of prior demyelinating disease. Physical examination revealed no evidence of recurrent cancer. Neurological examination was entirely within normal limits except for the elicitation of Lhermitte's sign on neck flexion. Plain films of the spine were normal, as were bone scan, chest roentgenogram, and screening chemistries.

The examining physician's impression, given the presence of Lhermitte's sign, was that the patient was suffering from spinal cord disease. Malignant epidural spinal cord compression was considered the most ominous etiology. However, the absence of pain and a negative extent of disease evaluation did not strongly argue for this diagnosis. Furthermore, the cisplatin was considered a possible etiology to her complaint. On the basis of her prior history, it was apparent that the patient was reliable and close clinical follow-up would be possible. Rather than proceed directly to myelography, it was elected to follow the patient carefully, after explaining to her the symptoms of spinal cord compression and urging her to contact her physician if these symptoms or *any* pain developed. During the 18 months of follow-up, her Lhermitte's sign abated after chemotherapy was discontinued.

Comment. This case underscores the advantage in performing a meticulous history and physical examination, being able to follow a patient clinically, and having a detailed knowledge of the literature. The examining physician knew that pain was usually the first manifestation of malignant epidural spinal cord compression, present in over 90 percent of patients in some series.[28, 58] Although the patient had a normal neurological examination, many published reports indicate that the absence of a clinically demonstrable myelopathy does not exclude epidural spinal cord compression.[95,133] In one recent study of cancer patients with back pain, 55 of 75 (73 percent) patients with no signs of myelopathy had epidural spinal cord compression on myelograms.[134] A normal neurological examination was not a factor in the decision to defer myelography in the above case. The cooperation of the patient and the ability to perform longitudinal follow-up was very important in deciding to defer a myelogram, which would have been the definitive test to exclude spinal metastasis. (This patient was seen prior to the availability of MRI.)

Lhermitte's sign, a commonly encountered neurologic complaint, is thought to be due to demyelinated ascending tracts of the spinal cord that discharge spontaneously when mechanically stimulated.[156] Although Lhermitte[92] recognized its common occurrence in patients with multiple sclerosis,[85] it is now recognized to occur in a variety of clinical settings of spinal cord disease, including cervical spondylosis and disc herniation,[34] head injuries,[30] following radiation injury,[80, 173] and in subacute combined degeneration.[8, 55, 140] Furthermore, cisplatin has been reported to cause Lhermitte's sign in two patients.[167] Given the rarity of this clinical occurrence, this diagnosis could only be tentative. If, however, at any time this patient developed pain or symptoms or signs of radiculopathy or myelopathy, a myelogram or MRI (if available) would have been performed.

Superficial Reflexes

Superficial reflexes, those that occur in response to stimulation of the skin or mucous membranes, are often abnormal in patients suffering from spinal cord or cauda equina disease. The most commonly tested superficial reflexes in the patient suspected of spine disease are the superficial abdominal, anal, cremasteric, and Babinski reflexes. The superficial abdominal reflexes are tested by stimulating the abdominal wall with a blunt or sharp object unilaterally and observing for contraction of the ipsilateral abdominal muscles. The normal response is contraction of the underlying abdominal muscles resulting in deviation of the umbilicus or linea alba to the ipsilateral side. Each of the four quadrants of the abdominal wall is stimulated independently. The upper abdominal, or supraumbilical, reflex is innervated by nerve roots T7—T9. The umbilical reflex is innervated by nerve roots T9—11 and the lower abdominal, or infraumbilical, is innervated by the lower thoracic and upper lumbar roots.

As in the case of deep tendon reflexes, if there is injury or compression of the spinal roots subserving the reflex, then there may be selective diminution of that specific abdominal reflex. There is a pathway that facilitates the superficial abdominal reflexes. This pathway ascends the spinal cord to the brain, where it synapses with neurons, giving rise to descending fibers that course within or adjacent to the pyramidal tracts. If this cerebral loop is interrupted, then the superficial abdominal reflex is diminished or abolished. If the lesion is above the decussation of the pyramidal tract, then the absent abdominal reflexes will be contralateral to the lesion. If the lesion is within the spinal cord, then the reflex loss will be ipsilateral to the pathology. Such damage to the pyramidal pathways may give rise to dissociation of reflexes, that is, absent superficial abdominal reflexes with exaggerated deep tendon reflexes.

Superficial abdominal reflexes may, however, be absent for a number of reasons other than neurological disease, such as cases of deep sleep, anesthesia, coma, obesity, multiparous females, the acute abdomen, postsurgical abdominal incisions, childhood, advanced age, and others. It is important to recognize that the reflex may fatigue easily after a few stimuli. When there is *unilateral* loss of the reflex in the absence of local cause such as abdominal incision, neurological etiologies are usually responsible.

The superficial abdominal reflexes are often lost in cases of intrinsic cord disease such as demyelination, as well as in cases of cord compression from extramedullary disease. Although considered a sign of pyramidal tract disease, they are not involved in most cases of amyotrophic lateral sclerosis, suggesting that the pathways subserving the superficial abdominal reflex are not dependent on the upper motor neuron pathways.

The cremasteric reflex is elicited by stimulating the skin of the upper, inner thigh from proximal to distal and observing for ipsilateral elevation of the testicle as a result of contraction of the cremasteric muscle. The nerve roots innervating the reflex are L1 and L2 via the ilioinguinal and genitofemoral nerves. The cremasteric reflex may be absent in the elderly man or in the presence of a varicocele, epididymitis, or other urological diseases. As above, one may find a loss of the cremasteric reflex in association with exaggeration of the deep tendon reflexes. This finding also suggests disturbance in the ascending or descending tracts of spine or brain.

The cutaneous anal reflex is the contraction of the external anal sphincter upon stimulation of the perianal tissues. This reflex is innervated by nerve roots S2−4(5) via the inferior hemorrhoidal nerve. The cutaneous anal reflex is to be distinguished from the internal anal sphincter reflex, which is elicited by introduction of a finger into the anus.

BABINSKI SIGN

The Babinski response, or upgoing toe, is recognized as a very useful sign of corticospinal tract disease. Plantar stimulation is, therefore, tested in patients with leg weakness in an attempt to differentiate upper motor neuron causes from other etiologies. Landau, Gijn, and others have studied the pathophysiological basis of the plantar response extensively.[57, 89, 113]

There are many pitfalls in the method of testing. If the stimulus is applied to the medial or tender palm of the sole, then a flexor response may falsely be elicited.[122] Alternatively, if the flexor creases of the toes are stimulated directly, then an extensor response with no diagnostic value can generally be expected. The examiner should stimulate the lateral aspect of the foot from the heel towards the toes and then move the stimulating object across the ball of the foot in order to avoid false-positive or false-negative results.

The Babinski sign may be found in otherwise asymptomatic patients with no neurological complaints. For example, a Babinski sign was reported in approximately 4 percent of a series of 2500 non-neurological hospitalized patients.[141] In addition, a Babinski reflex developed in over 7 percent of normal individuals after a 14-mile march.[174]

Sensory Disturbances

The sensory examination is generally recognized as the most difficult part of the neurological examination for two reasons: First, it is often difficult to know whether the slight alterations in sensation that the patient reports are clinically significant. The second, and perhaps more important, reason is that subjective sensory complaints generally precede objective sensory signs and therefore may be the first sign of serious underlying neurological disease. One corollary is that in the absence of sensory complaints, the sensory examination is usually normal. Thus in the patient with no sensory complaints, a survey of sensory function by testing position and vibration sense in the toes and fingers and pin sensation of the face, trunk, and extremities is usually sufficient. If abnormalities are found or there is evidence of spinal root or peripheral nerve dysfunction, then a more detailed examination is, of course, required.

Some techniques are helpful in performing the sensory exam: (1) test pinprick *from* the area of reduced sensation *to* the normal area; (2) test pinprick sensation over the entire limb, from distal to proximal, in the patient who does not report decreased sensation; (3) watch the patient's facial expression (i.e., look for a wince) when testing pinprick sensation, especially in the encephalopathic or demented patient; (4) ask the patient to use his or her own index finger to outline the area of subjectively reduced sensation.

As already discussed, radicular sensory complaints may be the first manifestation of spinal root pathology. Dysfunction of the posterior columns or lateral spinothalamic pathways also may first present with characteristic symptoms. Tingling paresthesias that may be vibratory in nature are sometimes reported below the level of a posterior column lesion.[122] Subjective reports of the skin being too tight or an extremity or trunk being wrapped in bandages also may be due to posterior column disturbances.[122]

Spinothalamic tract disturbance is often first manifest, especially in chronic cases such as intramedullary lesions, by poorly characterized and localized pain. We have seen one patient with an intramedullary neoplasm involving the lateral spinothalamic tracts who complained of burning, searing pain of the arms and trunk. Convinced that she had visceral disease, she underwent bone scans, mammography, ECGs, and other imaging studies until it was clear that her pain was spinal in origin. Many complaints of patients with intramedullary lesions are not associated with any abnormal signs early in their course, so that the complaints may be inappropriately dismissed after what is considered a negative work-up of the suspected organ. Since the descriptions of the sensation often seem atypical, they may incorrectly be ignored by the physician when the physical examination is normal.

When signs of sensory disturbance are present, the cause of sensory symptoms is more readily recognized. Pain sensation, usually measured by pinprick and temperature, is conveyed via the lateral spinothalamic tract. As noted in Chapter 1, these pathways are somatotopically organized so that the sacral fibers are most peripheral and the cervical fibers are most central. Since a laterally placed extramedullary lesion will compress the peripheral fibers before the more centrally located fibers, a lesion in the rostral spine may give rise to an apparently ascending myelopathy. The pin and temperature sensory disturbance is, of course, contralateral to the involved spinothalamic tract.[19]

Infrequently, a centrally placed anterior epidural lesion such as central cervical disc herniation may result in a sensory level several segments below the level of the spinal cord compression. A recent report[151] describes five cases of radiographically proven painless, central cervical disc herniations between C3 and C6 with the clinical examination demonstrating thoracic levels of hypalgesia between T5 and T7 (Table 2–9). Some patients had other signs of myelopathy such as spasticity, leg weakness, and hyperreflexia. The progressive neurological complaints of numbness and, when present, weakness, resolved with surgical excision of the offending disc material. The pathophysiology of this discrepancy could not be confidently explained, nor could the authors attribute the discrepancy in the level of cord compression from the sensory level on the basis of the lamination of the tracts, since each mass was anterior, not lateral. These findings, and similar falsely localizing sensory levels with laterally placed extramedullary lesions, underscore the importance of recognizing that *a rostral lesion may give rise to a sensory level far below the site of the compression.* In practical terms, therefore, one may need to image the entire spine rostral to the sensory level in order to exclude a higher lesion with certainty. This principle will be discussed further in later chapters.

Position and vibration sensation, transmitted through the posterior columns, are generally easily evaluated. Ataxia due to spinal lesions is not as readily recognized. A bizarre ataxic gait may result from disturbances of posterior columns or possibly the spinocerebellar tracts,[82] and may be particularly evident in combined systems disease. Light touch is conveyed by both

Table 2–9 PAINLESS CERVICAL MYELOPATHY: CORRELATION OF CLINICAL PRESENTATION WITH THE LEVEL OF DISC PATHOLOGY*

Case	Sensory Level	Level of Cord Compression
1	T5–T12 bilaterally	C3–C4
2	T5 bilaterally	C5–C6
3	T7 left	C5–C6
4	T6 right	C3–C4
5	T6 right	C5–C6

*From Simmon, Z et al,[151] p 871, with permission.

lateral columns and posterior columns and usually is not impaired as early in spinal cord disease as the more specific modalities.

Immediately after complete transverse lesions of the spinal cord, a sensory level with loss of all sensation caudal to the lesion is found (Fig. 2−5A). In time, however, the area of analgesia extends higher than the area of complete anesthesia,[68] owing to the wider distribution of tactile sensibility than pain sensibility of nerve roots.

Several incomplete lesions of the spinal cord result in characteristic sensory signs. A hemisection of the spinal cord results in the so-called Brown-Séquard syndrome, in which there is loss of pain and temperature sense contralateral to the lesion and loss of position and vibration senses

and paralysis ipsilateral to the lesion (Fig. 2−5B).

An early intramedullary lesion of the cord may give rise to a dissociated sensory loss in which the decussating fibers at the level, mediating sensation of pin and temperature, are lost or decreased, whereas the position and vibratory sensibilities remain unimpaired (Fig. 2−5C). In the cervical spine, such a clinical presentation may be caused by a syrinx, or by a neoplasm or central contusion of the cord. Central cord lesions may also result in a suspended sensory level (Fig. 2−5D). In such cases, sacral sensation is preserved until late in the course because these fibers are most peripheral in the lateral spinothalamic tracts and tend to be involved later. Similarly, a lateral brain-stem lesion may rarely give rise to a rostral sensory level

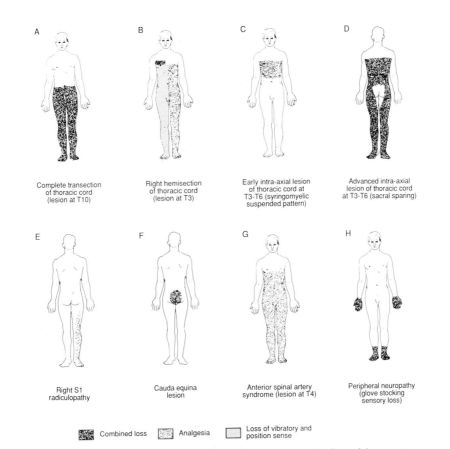

Figure 2−5. Characteristic sensory disturbances found in various spinal cord lesions in comparison to peripheral neuropathy.

over the contralateral trunk or a suspended sensory level with the lower border
over the trunk.[99]

Autonomic Disorders

Disturbances of spinal cord and caudal
equina function are often manifested as
symptoms and signs of bladder, bowel, and
sexual dysfunction and, less commonly, as
respiratory compromise. The anatomy and
pathophysiology of these pathways are discussed in this section.

Although the diaphragm, intercostal
muscles, and abdominal muscles all are
used for normal respiration, individuals
may ventilate adequately with only the
diaphragm intact. This massive muscle is
usually innervated by nerve roots C3–C5
(though it may be prefixed, innervated by
nerve roots C2–C4, or postfixed, innervated by nerve roots C4–C6). With complete transection of the cord between the
cervicomedullary junction and C3, respiration cannot be maintained. In partial
transections involving bilateral anterolateral quadrants, a condition referred to as
Ondine's curse occurs.[18, 62, 124] Since the
pathways for voluntary control of respira-
tions in the lateral quadrant of the spinal
cord are intact but the pathways for automatic control in the anterior quadrant are
lost, the patient must remain awake in
order to avoid apnea, which occurs upon
falling asleep.[9] Foramen magnum tumors,
atlantoaxial dislocation,[63] and congenital
disturbances of the craniocervical junction
are frequent causes of upper cervical spine
compression.

The urinary bladder is innervated by: (1)
sympathetic nerves beginning in the intermediolateral cell column at the lumbar
level (primarily L1 and L2 with some contribution from L3 and L4); (2) parasympathetic nerves exiting at S2–S4; and (3) the
somatic efferent nerves to the skeletal
muscles of the external urethral sphincter,
exiting at S2–S4 to form the pudendal
nerves. In complete transverse lesions of
the cord, an immediate flaccid bladder
ensues. In unilateral lesions, as demonstrated by anterolateral cordotomy,[112] voluntary control of micturition is not lost.

Thus it is unusual to have sphincter function disturbed early in spinal cord compression when there is only unilateral or
equivocal bilateral lower extremity weakness or sensory disturbance. The most
common exception to this rule is when the
conus medullaris or sacral nerve roots
alone are compressed.

In infancy and early development, bladder contraction occurs as a reflex mediated
largely via S2–S4. Voluntary bladder control involves the development of inhibition
of the bladder evacuation reflex. Micturition is initiated by voluntary modulation of
this inhibition and requires the integrity
of descending axons. The majority of these
fibers run in the lateral columns near the
equatorial plane, lateral to the central
canal and just anterior to the corticospinal
tract.[112] The descending micturition pathways are just posterolateral to the descending pathways for automatic breathing in
the cervical spine and just medial to the
ascending spinothalamic pathways.[112]
When the cord is injured above the spinal
segment S1, descending inhibition is lost
and the sacral (S2–S4) reflex arc for bladder emptying reverts to a reflexic mode of
functioning. As a result, after the initial
period of spinal shock, which is often
accompanied by urinary retention and
overflow incontinence, a reflex (neurogenic) bladder develops. If the disturbance
of upper motor neuron function evolves
slowly, then the reflex bladder may develop
without a preceding period of spinal shock
and flaccid bladder.

The reflex or spastic bladder is characterized by overactivity of both the detrusor
muscle and the external sphincter, causing incontinence of urine or precipitant
micturition. In addition, the bladder capacity is diminished due to the detrusor
contraction. The sensation of bladder dis-
tention may be lost if ascending tracts are
also involved. The anal reflex is often intact
in cases of reflex bladder. On cystometrogram testing, the detrusor muscle demonstrates excessive contraction to small in-
crements of fluid volume.

In contrast to the reflex bladder, when
the damage occurs in the region of the
conus medullaris or the cauda equina, a
decentralized or autonomous flaccid blad-

der ensues. Voluntary control over bladder function is impaired or abolished. Detrusor tone is lost and the bladder distends so that overflow incontinence occurs. Bladder sensation is impaired. Control over the anal sphincter and the anal reflex are usually lost. A region of saddle anesthesia may be present. The cystometrogram usually demonstrates diminished or absent contractions of the detrusor muscle.

The anatomical pathways subserving bowel function are similar to those controlling the urinary bladder. Spinal shock is generally associated with ileus and a neurogenic megacolon may develop. The anal reflex is usually lost. In slowly evolving lesions above the sacral level, voluntary control of the sphincter ani may be lost, but the anal reflex remains intact unless complete cord transection occurs, in which case it may be absent. In disturbances of the conus medullaris and cauda equina (nerve roots S3–5), fecal incontinence and a flaccid anal sphincter with loss of the anal reflex may be a presenting manifestation. Saddle anesthesia is often seen in such cases. Partial impairment may be present in any of these syndromes before frank paralysis and a flaccid sphincter ensues.

Disturbances of sexual function are common in spinal cord disease, especially in men. The descending pathways from the neocortex, limbic system, and hypothalamus course adjacent to the corticospinal tracts in the lateral funiculi. Penile erection occurs through the sacral parasympathetics (S3 and S4), the pudendal nerves, and nervi erigentes, and by inhibition of the sympathetic vasoconstrictor center located in the intermediolateral cell column at L1–2 and then through the superior hypogastric plexus.[71] Vascular channels in the penis dilate in response to parasympathetic innervation and tumescence occurs. Ejaculation is performed via the reflex arc beginning with the afferent limb arising in the genital epithelium and passing centrally via the dorsal nerve of the penis and pudendal nerve to the S3 and S4 dorsal roots. These afferent impulses synapse with two centers: a sympathetic center from T6 to L3 and a parasympathetic center at S3–4, which together form the

efferent limb of the reflex arc. The perineal branch of the pudendal nerve is an important peripheral efferent pathway.[71]

COMMON SPINAL CORD SYNDROMES

Spinal Shock

A complete transverse lesion of the spinal cord results in total loss of motor and sensory functions below the level of the lesion. If the lesion is slow in development, as may occur with a benign tumor or cervical spondylosis, or incomplete, then spinal reflexes such as hyperactive deep tendon reflexes and Babinski signs generally are present. Alternatively, as mentioned earlier in the chapter, if the lesion is acute in development, spinal shock ensues, with loss of all spinal reflex activity below the level of the lesion. Spinal shock is characterized by flaccid, areflexic paralysis of skeletal and smooth muscles. There is a complete loss of autonomic functions below the level of the lesion, resulting in a loss of urinary bladder tone and paralytic ileus. Sweating and piloerection are also diminished or absent below the lesion. Since vasomotor tone is lost, dependent lower extremities may become edematous and temperature regulation may be a major problem. Genital reflexes are lost. Sensation below the level of the lesion is completely absent.

In a series of experiments, Sherrington performed initial transections of the spinal cord of animals.[149] He then waited for the animal to recover spinal reflex activity, before sectioning the cord again, this time below the initial level of injury. Following the second transection, he found that no spinal shock ensued, showing that it was the acute loss of facilitatory supraspinal influences rather than trauma itself that was responsible for spinal shock. The specific pathways responsible for providing this facilitatory influence on spinal neurons are as yet unknown. Sherrington's studies showed that the duration of spinal shock is longer in primates than in more primitive mammals. In humans, the duration is quite variable. In the majority of cases, spinal reflex activity begins to return after 1–6 weeks. In one series, spinal shock was reported to be permanent in 5 out of 29 patients.[87]

Evolution of Spinal Shock

The period of spinal shock typically evolves into a stage of heightened reflex activity.[131] Thus the Babinski response, which usually involves only dorsiflexion of the great toe and fanning of the remaining toes, may develop into a triple flexion response involving the hip, knee, and foot after only minimal tactile stimulation. Simple withdrawal reflexes may develop into flexor spasms.

When these reflexes occur together in response to various stimuli such as touch or a distended or infected bladder, the resulting flexor spasms, hyperhydrosis, and piloerection form the mass reflex. In addition to a reduction in the threshold of stimulation that will evoke a spinal reflex, there is an enlargement of the reflexogenic zone to a level just caudal to the transection of the cord. The deep tendon reflexes below the lesion also become hyperactive.

The mechanism of this heightened reflex response after spinal shock is not understood. One hypothesis is that hyperreflexia is secondary to sprouting of afferent neurons below the level of transection.[29] It is thought that after degeneration of the descending supraspinal tracts, spinal motor neurons and interneurons are left with many postsynaptic vacancies, which presumably are innervated by sprouting of intact afferent neurons. Based on this hypothesis, the heightened reflex activity is not, therefore, an exaggeration of a normal reflex but rather a new, abnormal reflex.

In the evolution of spinal shock, thermoregulatory sweating is impaired below the lesion but it may be exaggerated, resulting in hyperhydrosis, above the lesion. In fact, autonomic disturbances above the level of the lesion are common. Bradycardia, hypertension resulting in headache, and flushing of the skin are often seen in these patients and are thought to be due to release of norepinephrine from disinhibited sympathetic neu-

rons caudal to the lesion and epinephrine from the adrenal medulla.

Riddoch's studies[131] during World War I led to the belief that, following spinal shock, complete transverse lesions of the spinal cord ultimately developed into paraplegia-in-flexion, while incomplete lesions developed into paraplegia-in-extension. Thus one could determine the extent of the transection on such a clinical basis. Although this view was supported by some experimental work,[52] Sherrington[68,149] had earlier shown in experimental animals that following complete transections of the cord a preponderance of extensor tone was sometimes found, and Kuhn[87] demonstrated that 18 of 22 patients with complete cord transection eventually developed extensor reflexes after they had fully developed flexor reflexes.

The experience of World War II demonstrated that, with the avoidance of decubiti and urinary tract infections (which provoke flexor spasms) and with other forms of improved medical care, paraplegia-in-extension often ultimately evolves after complete transection of the cord.[44,66] Guttmann[67,68] found other factors important in determining the ultimate posture, such as the posture of individuals in the early period following cord transection. He found that if the lower extremities of patients were maintained in an adducted and flexed position (as with a pillow beneath the knees), paraplegia-in-flexion would more commonly develop. Alternatively, if the legs were maintained in an abducted and extended position, then paraplegia-in-extension was more common. The extensor posture is also favored if the patient is maintained in a prone position. These observations and the changes in medical care for spinal-cord-injured patients that derived from them have had an important impact on the outcome of patients with spinal cord injuries.

The level of the lesion also is important in determining the ultimate posture of the legs. Higher lesions, such as at the level of the cervical spine, are much more likely to result in paraplegia-in-flexion than more caudal lesions. Intermittent extensor posturing is much more likely in patients with incomplete cord transections than in those with complete transverse lesions.[1]

Incomplete Lesions of the Spinal Cord

There is an extremely broad variety of clinical presentations of incomplete spinal cord syndromes. This variability is due both to the specific anatomical regions of the cord involved and to the dramatic ability, at times, of the spinal cord to adapt to chronic pathology. The characteristic incomplete spinal cord syndromes are presented later in this section. Many cases of incomplete spinal cord dysfunction, however, do not fit a classic pattern. The following case provides an example of the fact that the time of evolution of spinal cord compression can be of great importance in determining the clinical presentation.

Case Illustration

In November, a 19-year-old college student complained of vague right upper quadrant pain. Physical examination was unremarkable and she underwent a negative GI laboratory work-up including abdominal ultrasound. The pain seemed to remit and there was no follow-up. The following September she complained of difficulty ascending the stairs to the third-floor dormitory room she had occupied the previous year because her right knee gave way. She noted that she had injured her knee while skiing the previous winter. Her internist again noted some vague upper abdominal discomfort and possibly even tenderness in this area but otherwise found no abnormalities. The patient was referred to an orthopedist for suspected knee injury. One month later an orthopedic examination was unremarkable but the orthopedist was concerned that the patient had equivocal right leg weakness and brisk reflexes in the lower extremities but down-going toes.

In November, a neurological consultant confirmed the brisk lower extremity reflexes, right greater than left. At this time the patient seemed to have definite right leg weakness (4/5), equivocal left leg weakness, and an equivocal right plantar reflex. Sensory examination was unremarkable except for an area of hypesthesia over the right upper quadrant. Neck flexion provoked right upper quadrant pain, suggesting a radicular cause. There were no sphincter disturbances.

Plain thoracic spine films demonstrated an enlarged intervertebral foramen on the right at T8–9. A neurosurgical consultation was obtained and the patient was admitted to the hospital for myelography. The myelogram, performed by a lumbar approach, confirmed the presence of an intradural extramedullary mass on the right causing a complete block at the T8–9 level. With CT scanning after the myelogram, the mass could be seen to be localized to the T8–9 level on the right, displacing the cord to the left. The patient was placed on corticosteroids and surgery was scheduled for the following day.

During the evening following the myelogram, routine neurological checks revealed rapidly evolving bilateral leg weakness. The right leg had deteriorated to 2+/5 and the left to 3+/5. A sensory disturbance to pin stimulus was found in both legs and position sense was impaired at the toes, but preserved at the ankles. The patient was taken on an emergency basis to the operating room and an intradural neurofibroma at the T8–9 level was resected. The compressed cord was found to be significantly thinned at this level. Following surgery, the patient was able to ambulate within a week and all the signs of myelopathy resolved over a few months, as did the right upper quadrant pain. There was only a minimal area of residual hypalgesia in the distribution of the right T8 dermatome.

Comment. This case illustrates several important clinical points. First, the patient was suspected of having visceral disease since her original pain was referred and not localized to the spine. This confusion was compounded by the fact that she had tenderness in the distribution of the projected pain. As noted earlier, *both referred and radicular pain may be associated with tenderness at the site of pain projection.*

Second, in cases in which spinal cord compression evolves slowly over months or years, the spinal cord may adapt to the compression so that there may be only minimal or equivocal clinical signs of myelopathy although there is atrophy of the cord. Studies in experimental animals[12] and humans[38] indicate that impulse conduction may persist, with a decreased safety factor, in spinal cord compression, possibly as a result of continuous conduction in fibers demyelinated as a result of compression.[170] Alternatively, previously unused pathways may be used to transmit information following conduction block of normal pathways. *The clinician should, therefore, never assume that a patient could not have a complete block on myelography because the patient does not display signs of myelopathy.*

Third, *patients with complete subarachnoid block may rapidly deteriorate after lumbar puncture or myelography.*[43,76] Clinicians must, therefore, be extremely vigilant in monitoring such patients for signs of spinal coning following these procedures. The mechanism of deterioration has been considered to be a vascular insult, either arterial or even venous infarction.[76] If surgery had been delayed in this case, the patient probably would not have had such an excellent outcome.

This case, therefore, demonstrates that the signs of an incomplete transverse myelopathy may be variable and poorly localizing in cases of chronic cord compression. The clinical manifestations can be different in cases where the anatomical mass is identical but the effects are acute and possibly mediated through, or complicated by, vascular insufficiency. Also, the prognosis and management of cord compression depends in large measure on the etiology and expected evolution of the offending lesion.

Despite these protean clinical manifestations of spinal cord compression, there are a group of characteristic incomplete cord syndromes which may be recognized and are described below.

UNILATERAL TRANSVERSE LESION

As mentioned, a unilateral lesion or hemisection of the spinal cord produces a Brown-Séquard syndrome.[19] In reality, such pure unilateral lesions are rare (except in pure stab injuries), and most clinical cases are described as a modified Brown-Séquard syndrome.

The clinical presentation of a pure Brown-Séquard syndrome is that of ipsilateral weakness and loss of position and vibration below the lesion, with contralateral loss of pain and temperature. The loss of pain and temperature is usually manifest a few segments below the level of the lesion because the decussating fibers enter the spinothalamic tract a few segments rostral to the level of entry of the nerve root. At the level of the insult, there may be a small ipsilateral area of anesthesia, analgesia, and lower motor neuron weakness because the segmental afferent and effer-

ent pathways are disrupted (see Fig. 2–5B).

There are many known causes of the pure syndrome, with trauma probably the most common.[71,158] Radiation necrosis has also been reported as a cause.[42] Spinal metastases rarely present with a Brown-Séquard syndrome. In one large series of spinal metastases,[159] of 106 patients with signs of myelopathy, only 2 had a pure Brown-Séquard syndrome. An additional 8 had greater weakness ipsilateral to the lesion and more marked pain and temperature loss contralateral to the lesion, but no dorsal column signs. This group would be considered to have "modified Brown-Séquard syndromes."

CENTRAL CORD SYNDROME

The central cord syndrome is due to an intra-axial lesion disturbing the normal structures of the central or paracentral region of the spinal cord. Such disturbances may be acute, usually due to hemorrhage or contusion following trauma,[145] or chronic, due to tumor or syringomyelia. Although a demyelinating process may occasionally cause a similar syndrome, it is usually not confused with the more typical causes. The clinical presentations of these disorders share some common features. Contusions following trauma and syringomyelia frequently occur in the cervical spine and cervicothoracic junction. Spontaneous hematomyelia generally presents with the acute onset of severe back or neck pain, followed by paralysis. It can occur at any level of the cord and may be due to an arteriovenous malformation or coagulopathy.

When the cervical spine or cervicothoracic junction is the site of a central cord syndrome, the upper extremities show weakness of a lower motor neuron type. Characteristically, there is loss of sensation in the upper extremities of a dissociated type, that is, loss of pin and temperature with preservation of position and vibration, because the decussating fibers destined for the spinothalamic tracts are interrupted while those projecting within the posterior columns are spared. As a result of the laminated structure of the spinothalamic tract, sensation from the more caudal regions is preserved, with sacral sparing of pin and temperature sensation being the rule (see Fig. 2–5D).

In slowly developing lesions, the lower extremities ultimately exhibit signs of weakness of an upper motor neuron type. In acute lesions, there is usually initial spinal shock. Bowel, bladder, and sexual function are generally impaired immediately in acute lesions and later in chronic lesions. In cases involving the cervical and cervicothoracic spine, there may also be a Horner's syndrome unilaterally or bilaterally.

ANTERIOR SPINAL ARTERY SYNDROME

Although first described in 1904[127] as syphilitic paraplegia with dissociated sensibility, spinal cord infarction had been considered a clinical rarity. In a series of over 3700 postmortem examinations at a London hospital between 1909 and 1958, no cases of arterial infarction of the spinal cord were found.[11] More recently, however, it has been recognized much more frequently, in part due to an increased number of invasive procedures such as vascular[39, 75] and thoraco-abdominal surgery,[77] and improved survival after cardiac arrest and hypotention.[3, 59, 60, 150] (See Chapter 8.)

The anterior horns and anterolateral tracts are involved in this syndrome (Fig. 2–6). Initially spinal shock is expected. Subsequently, the motor examination shows lower motor neuron weakness in the region of ischemia and corticospinal deficits below the level of the infarction. The autonomic pathways are also involved, so there is loss of bowel, bladder, and sexual functions. The sensory disturbance is dissociated in that posterior column function is intact but the spinothalamic tracts are disrupted.

Anterior spinal artery syndrome is differentiated from acute central cord syndrome[145] by the sacral sensory sparing that tends to occur in the latter. Moreover, the intact posterior column function seen

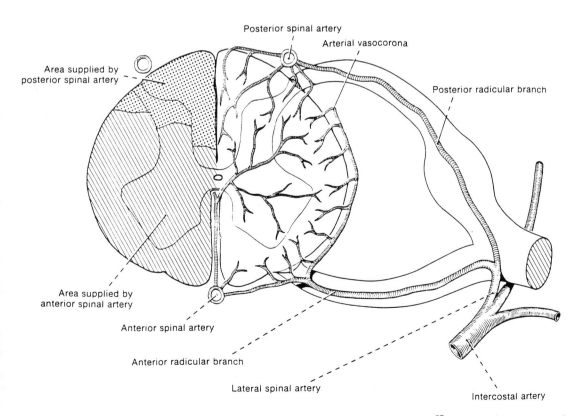

Figure 2–6. The arterial supply of the spinal cord. (From DeJong,[35] p 580, with permission.)

in the anterior spinal artery syndrome differentiates it from the syndrome of acute complete transverse myelopathy.[137]

ANTERIOR HORN SYNDROME

Prior to development of the polio vaccine, the acute anterior horn syndrome was commonly encountered due to invasion of the spinal cord by poliomyelitis virus. Rarely, other enteroviruses may cause the acute syndrome. The chronic anterior horn syndrome in the adult population is commonly seen in the setting of degenerative diseases such as amyotrophic lateral sclerosis or in the post-polio syndrome. Paraneoplastic syndromes may also present as an anterior horn syndrome, such as the subacute motor neuronopathy that has been reported as a remote effect of lymphoma.[146] Finally, there are several forms of inherited spinal muscular atrophy that may present as an anterior horn syndrome.

These patients present clinically with lower motor neuron weakness that may be asymmetric, especially in the acquired forms. The muscles become areflexic and flaccid. Fasciculations may occur. Sensory and autonomic disturbances are not generally seen. A similar clinical syndrome may, of course, be due to intramedullary lesions such as syringomyelia or tumors but must be differentiated from ventral root disturbances such as those due to spondylosis.

ANTERIOR HORN AND PYRAMIDAL TRACT SYNDROME

Disturbances of the anterior horns and pyramidal tracts with sparing of the sensory functions and autonomic nervous system are seen in motor neuron disease. Clinically, one typically finds a combination of lower motor neuron weakness with its attendant atrophy and fasciculations (and fibrillations on EMG) and upper motor weakness with spasticity, hyperreflexia, and Babinski signs. However, either the lower motor neuron or upper motor neuron disturbance may predominate for months or years. Ultimately, as the lower motor neuron disease progresses, there is

increasingly severe atrophy and evolution from hyperreflexia to hyporeflexia.

COMBINED POSTERIOR AND LATERAL COLUMN DISEASE

The clinical presentation of loss of posterior column and lateral column (pyramidal) function is that of spastic ataxic gait. Although Friedreich's ataxia may cause such a syndrome, the classic cause is subacute combined degeneration [139] associated with pernicious anemia. When symptoms such as paranoia or megaloblastic madness accompany a gait that appears nonorganic or hysterical, the patient often is referred for psychiatric evaluation. The following illustrates a case of combined systems disease.

Case Illustration

A 52-year-old woman presented with a three-month history of distal extremity paresthesias and weakness manifested by difficulty walking. Her internist found her depressed and suspicious. Her gait was unsteady and she had depressed reflexes and she was uncooperative for the remainder of the examination. She believed that she had injured both knees but could not relate any specific injury. When her knee roentgenograms were reported as negative, she refused a further work-up and was lost to follow-up. Several months later she was seen by a psychiatrist who recognized the need for neurological assessment. On mental status examination, the patient manifested agitation and suspiciousness. Her gait was both ataxic and spastic; each step was associated with choreoathetoid arm movements as though she was walking a tight rope. She could not tandem walk, had poor foot position sense and a positive Romberg. Her deep tendon reflexes were diminished but her lower extremity muscle tone was increased. Babinski signs were present and vibration sensation was impaired in both legs.

A CBC showed a mild anemia and an MCV of 110 (82–92, normal range). A serum vitamin B_{12} level was 13 micrograms per ml (200–800, normal range). A diagnosis of subacute combined degeneration of the spinal cord was made. The Schilling test was positive and confirmed the clinical impression. Intramuscular injections of vitamin B_{12} were begun. The patient's neurological status did not significantly change after one month, although she had a hematological response. She remained insistent that her problem was due either to a knee disturbance or to a lumbar spine problem because she had had a long history of back pain. She sought the care of other physicians unfamiliar with her medical history and underwent knee arthroscopy and a lumbar myelogram. When these studies were reported normal, she returned for her vitamin B_{12} injections. Her gait and mental status improved but she continued to have mild gait ataxia and depression, and required psychiatric counseling and physical therapy.

Comment. This case illustrates the predominance of neuropsychiatric as well as sensorimotor findings in patients with subacute combined degeneration.[93] The patient's persistent delusion that she had back and knee disease, despite evidence to the contrary, was a manifestation of suspiciousness and paranoia secondary to the vitamin B_{12} deficiency. This delayed her work-up and treatment. Subacute combined degeneration is a treatable disorder that can be diagnosed noninvasively. It should be considered in all patients with signs of posterior column and pyramidal tract dysfunction.

CHARACTERISTIC CLINICAL FEATURES OF LESIONS AT DIFFERENT LEVELS

Spinal tumors at different levels often present with characteristic symptoms and signs referable to the segmental levels involved. In cases of extramedullary tumors, disturbances at the segmental level usually herald the presentation of the neoplasm. Intramedullary tumors frequently do not present with segmental disturbances but rather with tract dysfunction.[144]

Foramen Magnum

Lesions of the foramen magnum, which include tumors, syringomyelia, multiple sclerosis, Arnold-Chiari malformation, atlantoaxial dislocation and other bony abnormalities of the craniocervical junction, present one of the most challenging diagnostic problems for the clinician because the symptoms are often vague or may be distant from the foramen magnum. For example, although patients with Arnold-Chiari malformation, Type 1 (without meningocele), often present with progressive cerebellar dysfunction, increased intracranial pressure, or lower cranial nerve dysfunction, they may present with a syndrome of syringomyelia.

Since many foramen magnum lesions such as benign tumors, neurofibromas or meningiomas, or atlanto-axial dislocation are surgically treatable, there is a high premium on early diagnosis and treatment.[63] Congenital bony abnormalities in the region of the foramen magnum may be entirely asymptomatic, but when found, often lead to difficult clinical decision making.[105, 106]

FORAMEN MAGNUM TUMORS

When the foramen magnum lesion is a tumor, occipital or neck pain, often increased by neck movement, is the most common initial manifestation.[161] The pain may also radiate into the shoulders or the ipsilateral arm. In the latter situation, the pain may be difficult to differentiate from that secondary to cervical spondylosis. In many such cases the latter diagnosis may be suspected clinically, only to be confirmed by plain films of the cervical spine. As documented elsewhere,[119] cervical spondylosis as diagnosed on plain radiographs is found in 50 percent of individuals over 50 years of age and 75 percent of those over 65 years old, many of whom are asymptomatic. This high prevalence of spondylosis in the general population may result in the delay of diagnosis of a rare condition such as a foramen magnum tumor, which constitutes only approximately 1 percent of intracranial and intraspinal tumors.[2] In other cases of foramen magnum tumors, the pain may also radiate into the lower back.[2]

The neurological signs associated with foramen magnum tumors may also be perplexing. Cranial nerve symptoms and signs are inconstant; nystagmus, impaired sensation over the face (due to involvement of the descending tract of cranial nerve V), and dysarthria, dysphonia, and dysphagia are present in some patients.[161]

Motor system involvement characteristically presents itself by spastic weakness. The corticospinal tracts are compressed by the extramedullary intradural neurofibroma or meningioma so that weakness typically begins in the ipsilateral arm, followed in order by weakness of the ipsilateral leg, and the contralateral leg and arm.[161]

It has been long recognized, however, that foramen magnum tumors may cause signs of lower motor neuron weakness, atrophy, and depressed reflexes in the arms and hands.[161] The mechanism of this lower motor neuron disturbance well below the level of the tumor has never been fully elucidated but may be secondary to circulatory disturbances affecting the distribution of the anterior spinal artery. It is important to recognize that atrophy of the hand muscles may arise from tumors above C4, since the findings could be mistaken for a syrinx, motor neuron disease, or pathology at the level of the lower cervical spine.[161]

Sensory disturbances consisting of pain and numbness are early manifestations of foramen magnum tumors. Remarkably, the paresthesias are often reported along the ulnar aspect of the forearm and hand despite the fact that the lesion is several segments above the C8–T1 dermatomes. In one series,[161] pain and paresthesias affecting the same upper extremity first involved by spastic weakness were an early finding. The mechanism whereby the upper motor neuron weakness and sensory loss occur in the same upper extremity has not been explained but is thought to be secondary to a disturbance of an intramedullary pathway.[161]

The sensory disturbances found in these patients are often of the dissociated type, so that patients suffer from loss of pin and temperature but have preserved tactile sensation. A suspended sensory loss also has been reported in some cases. This pattern often leads to the mistaken clinical impression that the patient has an intramedullary lesion such as a syrinx. Lhermitte's sign is frequently reported and some patients exhibit loss of vibration sensibility over the clavicle or acromion

process.[161] In the past, myelography was the imaging modality of choice. CT scanning has been helpful in defining lesions of this region, especially if bone such as the skull base is being imaged. With the advent of MRI, this area may be readily and noninvasively visualized.[14, 102]

ATLANTOAXIAL DISLOCATION

Atlantoaxial dislocation is another important craniocervical abnormality that may result in spinal cord compression. It may be caused by incompetence of either the odontoid process or of the transverse atlantal ligament. Greenberg[63] has classified incompetence of the odontoid process into four major categories: congenital (types I–V); traumatic; infectious; and neoplastic. Similarly, he has classified incompetence of the transverse ligament into the following causes: congenital (e.g., idiopathic and Down's syndrome); traumatic; and hyperemic (e.g., infectious and rheumatoid).

When posterior atlantoaxial subluxation is due to congenital and developmental causes there also may be a variety of anomalies of the spine and craniocervical junction. Some of the disorders associated with atlantoaxial instability and dislocation include craniocervical junction anomalies, basilar impression, neurofibromatosis, congenital scoliosis, and others.[74]

Metastatic cancer to the dens is becoming a more frequently recognized cause of atlantoaxial dislocation, especially in patients harboring malignancy.[70] Rheumatoid involvement of the transatlantal ligament is another acquired cause, seen in patients with rheumatoid arthritis.[94]

With atlantoaxial subluxation, the spinal cord may be compressed. Compression is reported to occur regularly when the sagittal diameter of the spinal canal at this level is 14 mm or less and may occur at 15–17 mm.[63] This measurement is considerably greater than that at which compression occurs in the lower cervical spine (10–13 mm).[172] As the sagittal diameter of the spinal cord varies by only 1 mm from C1 to C7, this difference probably is due to the sagittal diameter of the transverse atlantal ligament (4–5 mm), which is interposed between the odontoid process and spinal cord.

The mechanism of neural injury in many cases of atlantoaxial subluxation is reported to be compression of the medullocervical junction by the odontoid process.[10] The clinical presentation of atlantoaxial instability and subluxation may be perplexing. Symptoms are often intermittent and may include weakness of an upper motor neuron type or muscle wasting of the upper extremities, ataxia, dizziness, lower cranial nerve symptoms, and pain. Priapism is seen in some patients. Patients are often considered to have demyelinating disease or motor neuron disease before the correct diagnosis is made. Patients with atlantoaxial instability, especially if not recognized, are at risk for deterioration when undergoing general anesthesia.[74] There is a great deal of literature devoted to atlantoaxial instability and subluxation.[10,63,74,105,157]

Case Illustration

A 16-year-old, mildly retarded young man was brought to the emergency room after suddenly falling to the ground, not losing consciousness but unable to move, while at a dance. The emergency room physician noted a sustained penile erection but could find no other abnormalities on examination. The neurological consultant was called to rule out a hysterical pseudoseizure.

Examination revealed an alert young man with dulled mental capacities. When questioned, he stated he had lost control of his arms and legs after hyperextending his neck while dancing. The weakness resolved over several hours. Examination revealed no cranial nerve abnormalities. Motor examination was normal except for decreased muscle tone in all extremities. Sensory examination revealed inconsistent results, but a spinal level could not be appreciated. Deep tendon reflexes were moderately brisk bilaterally and the plantar responses were mute. Abdominal reflexes were absent. There was a sustained penile erection.

Because of the suspicion of an atlantoaxial dislocation, the patient's neck was immobilized and cervical spine x-rays were performed. These roentgenograms showed nonfusion of the dens, which was minimally displaced.

Comment. This case illustrates several points. First, in atlantoaxial dislocation, neuro-

logical dysfunction can be transient, presumably reflecting the variable anatomy of the unstable atlantoaxial junction. Thus, in the patient with a history of transient tetraparesis, pathology of this crucial region must be sought. The absence of signs of spinal cord compression on examination does not rule out atlantoaxial pathology. Second, this case illustrates the importance of priapism as a localizing sign in disorders of the high cervical spine. This sign was well known to professional hangmen, who in the past were paid by the families of convicted criminals to hang their victims privately, so as to avoid the embarrassment of the penile erection reflex in response to the hangman's fracture at C1–2.

Upper Cervical Spine

Neoplasms involving the upper cervical spine have similar clinical characteristics to those arising at the foramen magnum. Pain in the neck, occipital region, or shoulder is a very common presenting complaint. The first cervical root does not have a sensory dermatomal distribution, but the second cervical root innervates the posterior aspect of the scalp, explaining the pattern of radicular pain to this location. If the tumor is at the third or fourth cervical level, radicular pain may be projected to the neck or top of the shoulder. When pain occurs, it is usually provoked by neck movements, resulting in marked limitation of spontaneous head turning and nodding. This may be apparent on casual inspection.

Furthermore, since the descending tract of the trigeminal nerve may be irritated, sensory disturbances and funicular pain in the face may occur. Sensory disturbances in the face are rare presenting manifestations of spinal tumors; when they are the initial complaint of such a patient, they are much more likely to be secondary to an intramedullary rather than an extramedullary tumor. For example, Elsberg[46] described a patient harboring a high cervical intramedullary tumor who had an early symptom of numbness and shooting pain on the side of the face. In the absence of numbness, one might consider a diagnosis of tic douloureux in such a patient.

Usually following the initial complaint of pain, upper extremity weakness becomes apparent on the same side. The weakness may be of an upper or lower motor neuron type. Some patients, therefore, may have spasticity and hyperreflexia, whereas others may have atrophy and hyporeflexia of a portion or of the entire upper extremity including the hand.[46] The cause of lower motor neuron findings in patients with foramen magnum and upper cervical lesions several segments above the disturbed segmental levels is unknown. It has been attributed to circulatory disturbances, although this has not been proven. When upper motor neuron findings develop in the ipsilateral leg, a spinal hemiplegia is present. Weakness may progress to the contralateral lower extremity and then to the contralateral upper extremity. The weakness in both lower extremities may be of the upper motor neuron type and that of the upper extremities may be either of the lower motor neuron variety or a combination of both upper and lower motor neuron. If attention is limited to the lower cervical spine using CT scanning or other imaging procedures, an upper cervical mass lesion may be missed.

Frequently, sensory disturbances do occur. Sensory loss may appear initially in the same upper extremity as the weakness, and may be quite variable in distribution and type. Cases have been reported[144] that presented with upper extremity astereognosis that was interpreted as suggesting a parietal lesion. Lhermitte's sign also often occurs.

Cranial nerve symptoms and signs are infrequent in upper cervical spine disease.[46] Reference to involvement of the descending trigeminal tract has already been made. In addition, atrophy and weakness involving the trapezius and sternocleidomastoid may occur owing to the spinal component to the eleventh cranial nerve. Nystagmus may be present. Other cranial neuropathies such as facial and tongue weakness have also rarely been reported. Unequal pupils may occur, secondary to a central Horner's syndrome if the descending pathways are injured en route to the neurons involved in ciliospinal reflexes, situated at the intermediolateral horn at C8, T1, and T2. The Horner's

syndrome may be incomplete, in which case loss of sweat and vasodilatation due to vasoconstrictor paralysis, and enophthalmos may not uniformly be present.

Weakness or paralysis of the diaphragm may occur at lesions at or above the C4 level. Complete transverse lesions at the C4 level may not be associated with paralysis of the diaphragm if the innervation of the phrenic nerve at the C3 level is adequate.[68] The weakness may of course be unilateral or bilateral. Emphasizing that diaphragmatic paralysis is the most life threatening of complications of lesions of the spine, Ely[47] concluded that the symptoms of injury to the first, second, and third cervical vertebrae are death.

Lower Cervical and Upper Thoracic Spine

Extramedullary neoplasms at the levels of C5–T1 frequently cause radicular symptoms at the affected level in the shoulder or upper extremity in the form of pain and later reflex, motor, and sensory disturbances. With lesions at the C4–C6 level, pain and sensory disturbances are frequently reported along the radial aspect of the arm, forearm, and thumb (see dermatomal map, Fig. 2–2, and Table 2–6). Pain is also frequent with intramedullary growths at these levels but the localization is usually more diffuse and less typically radicular in nature.

Pain and sensory symptoms at the C7–T1 levels frequently are localized to the ulnar aspect of the arm, forearm, and hand. As demonstrated in the dermatomal map, the C7 dermatome usually includes the middle finger and the T1, T2 dermatomes are located at the ulnar border of the hand and forearm. Tumors at the T1 and T2 levels often cause pain to radiate into the elbow and hand along with sensory complaints along the ulnar border of the hand. Such complaints are often attributed to an ulnar neuropathy at the elbow or to orthopedic problems. As at other locations, intramedullary growths usually give rise to more diffuse symptoms that are often bilateral, while extramedullary neoplasms frequently present with exquisite localizing symptoms.

Weakness usually follows pain in extramedullary tumors, with a preponderance of weakness often present at the affected segmental level. As might be expected based on the myotomal map of the upper extremity, intramedullary and extramedullary lesions at C4–C6 tend to involve the muscles in the shoulder and upper arm (see Table 2–6). As with foramen magnum and upper cervical spine tumors, atrophy and weakness of the hand are also seen occasionally with lesions at C4–C6, possibly due to vascular factors affecting the lower cervical segments. Such a pattern of weakness and atrophy may lead the examiner to consider a lesion at the C7–T2 level instead, for tumors at these levels typically cause muscle symptoms and signs in the forearm and hand.

The pattern of extremity weakness may be a guide in distinguishing intramedullary from extramedullary disorders. Although there are exceptions, extramedullary lesions tend to affect the ipsilateral upper and lower extremity before involving the contralateral side. In contrast, intramedullary lesions may involve both upper extremities before the lower extremities, or show bilateral arm and leg involvement from the onset.[46]

The deep tendon reflexes are very helpful in localizing the segmental level of involvement in the cervical spine. Disease at the C5–6 levels often is associated with depressed biceps (C5) and/or brachioradialis reflex (C6) (see Table 2–6). One may encounter cases of a depressed biceps reflex associated with a hyperactive brachioradialis reflex if there is a compressive myelopathy at the C5 level. Although not specific for cervical spondylosis, a depressed brachioradialis (C6) reflex with hyperactive finger flexors (C8–T1) is often seen in individuals who have a C6 radiculopathy with myelopathy; neoplasms or other diseases at the C6 level may cause a similar clinical presentation. When the lesion is at the C7 level, the triceps reflex may be affected.

With lesions at C8 and T1, the finger flexor response, the Hoffmann sign, may be impaired. The Hoffmann sign is performed by dorsiflexing the patient's wrist and then flicking the distal phalanx of the middle finger with the examiner's thumb.[35] The patient's middle finger is thus flexed and suddenly extended. When the Hoffmann sign is present, this maneuver is followed by sudden flexion of the patient's thumb and other fingers. When present bilaterally, it usually indicates hyperactive deep tendon reflexes. Although there may be disease of the pyramidal pathways, healthy individuals may have bilateral Hoffmann signs in conditions such as anxiety, hyperthyroidism, and use of CNS-stimulating drugs. When unilaterally present, it usually signifies disease of the nervous system, and the examiner must distinguish between disease of the pyramidal tract and disease of the peripheral nervous system, such as of the C8–T1 nerve roots or the lower brachial plexus (e.g., Pancoast tumor), resulting in loss of a Hoffmann reflex in an individual with diffuse hyperreflexia. The associated physical findings and history are usually helpful.

Although a Horner's syndrome may develop with neoplasm at any level of the cervical spine, it is most commonly seen as an early manifestation of tumors near the intermediolateral cell column at the C7–T2 segmental levels.[71] In addition, the close anatomical relationship with the sympathetic ganglion near the T1 level makes a Horner's syndrome an early hallmark of epidural tumors in this region. For example, among cancer patients with brachial plexus lesions, the presence of a Horner's syndrome is a risk factor for the extension of paravertebral tumor into the epidural space.[86]

Thoracic Levels

As with neoplasms at other levels of the cord, pain is the most frequent presenting manifestation. The pain may be local, radicular, or both. The thoracic dermatomal landmarks that guide the examiner to the level of involvement are the nipple (T4), the umbilicus (T10), and the inguinal ligament (L1). Pain or sensory alterations in a radicular distribution are localized to a specific dermatome using these levels as points of reference. Pain in the upper thoracic level may be mistaken for pleural disease, whereas in the right upper abdominal quadrant, attacks of radicular pain may be considered symptoms of cholelithiasis. Other abdominal or thoracic viscera might be suspected as the source of pain at other levels. Radicular pain may also be bilateral, creating a girdle sensation.

When the lesion is in the lower thoracic spine, the segmental level of involvement sometimes may be determined by the presence of Beevor's sign. Since tensing the abdominal musculature (as in elevating the head off the bed in the supine position) requires the supraumbilical and infraumbilical muscles, a lesion at or adjacent to the level of T10 may be associated with upward movement of the umbilicus with such a maneuver.

The relatively small vertebral canal and the vascular watershed area of the spinal cord in the thoracic region make the thoracic spinal cord extremely vulnerable to injury from compression.[64] Consequently, the temporal course of symptoms of cord compression is often shorter in this region than elsewhere.[64,144] Pain often evolves rapidly into weakness, sensory loss, and reflex abnormalities caudal to the lesion. Sphincter disturbances ultimately develop.

Lesions in the region of the thoracolumbar junction may present with clinical manifestations of a myelopathy, conus medullaris syndrome, or a cauda equina syndrome. For example, diastematomyelia is a congenital abnormality of the spine in which a bony spicule or fibrous band from a thoracic or upper lumbar vertebra protrudes into the spinal canal, dividing the spinal cord. The resulting duplication of the spinal cord is referred to as diplomyelia. Diastematomyelia is often associated with other congenital abnormalities such as spina bifida or meningomyelocele. Clinical manifestations include progressive spastic lower extremity weakness, an acute or progressive cauda equina syndrome, or syringomyelia. When patients with diastematomyelia present in adult life, there is typically a cutaneous abnormality such as hypertrichosis over the buttocks.

Conus Medullaris and Cauda Equina

Lesions of the cauda equina and conus medullaris cause similar symptoms and signs including local, referred, and radicular pain; sphincter disturbances; loss of buttock and leg sensation; and leg weakness. It may be relatively easy to establish the level of a single radiculopathy, but it is much more difficult to assign the cause and localization when there are several lumbosacral levels involved. In such situations one must consider the possibility of a lower spinal cord lesion or a cauda equina syndrome. There has been a long effort to differentiate conus medullaris lesions from those of the cauda equina,[37, 169] but some authors conclude that it usually is not possible to discriminate between neoplasms arising from the lower spinal cord and those arising from the cauda equina[91, 116] because in most cases, both anatomical regions are involved. This section describes features traditionally considered valuable in differentiating these lesions.

The conus medullaris is comprised of levels S3−C1 and the epiconus, levels L4−S2.[71] Disturbances of epiconus function involve weakness, sensory loss and reflex loss in the lower extremities subserved by L4−S1 roots, along with sphincter disturbances. Patients, therefore, experience difficulty with external rotation and extension of the thigh at the hip, flexion of the knee, and weakness of all muscles below the knee. Although rare in its pure form, the conus medullaris syndrome presents with sphincter disturbances, saddle anesthesia (S3−5), impotence, and absence of lower extremity abnormalities. The pure conus medullaris syndrome is usually due to an intramedullary lesion such as tumor, cyst, or infarct.[71, 111] The following case illustrates a nearly pure conus lesion.

Case Illustration

A 68-year-old woman complained of burning numbness in her posterior thighs and distal lower extremities. Her physician found reduced ankle reflexes and diminished sensation in her feet to pinprick, and diagnosed peripheral neuropathy. These sensory symptoms progressed to painful dysesthesias and she was referred for neurological consultation when she developed incontinence of both urine and stool 6 weeks later. Neurological examination revealed flaccid rectal tone, saddle anesthesia, reduced sensation in the legs in the S1−S2 dermatome, and absent ankle jerks. There was no lower extremity weakness and no spine tenderness or paravertebral spasm. A conus medullaris tumor was suspected.

After plain spine films were reported as unremarkable, the patient underwent a thoracolumbar myelogram with water-soluble dye. The neuroradiologist saw no abnormality and the patient immediately underwent CT scanning of the region of the lower spinal cord and conus medullaris. The conus was significantly enlarged as compared with an image at the T10 vertebral level (Fig. 2–7), confirming the impression of a conus medullaris neoplasm. The

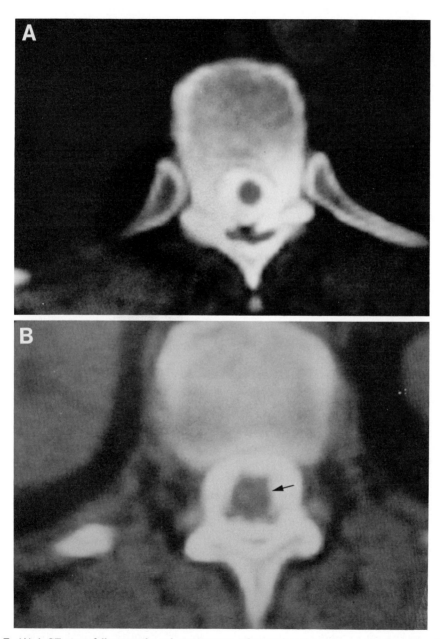

Figure 2–7. (A) A CT scan following the administration of intrathecal contrast material at the level of T10 demonstrating the spinal cord of normal size. (B) At the level of T12, the spinal cord is abnormally enlarged (arrow) due to an intramedullary metastasis from breast cancer.

spinal fluid obtained at the time of the myelogram demonstrated a slightly elevated protein but no pleocytosis and a negative cytology.

The remainder of the patient's work-up revealed an unsuspected breast mass and lung metastases. A breast biopsy revealed poorly differentiated adenocarcinoma. A metastasis to the conus medullaris was considered the most likely cause for the patient's clinical and radiographic findings and she underwent radiation therapy to the conus and chemotherapy. She showed symptomatic improvement of her painful dysesthesias but no improvement of her sphincter function. She died six months later due to metastatic cancer.

Comment   Although a rare clinical presentation, this case illustrates the major clinical findings in conus medullaris syndrome. As in the Brown-Séquard syndrome, these cases are usually not pure but rather modified conus medullaris syndromes. The clinical constellation for the conus syndrome merges with the epiconus syndrome and the cauda equina syndrome. As mentioned above, these distinctions are not strict because lesions often involve more than one structure of the caudal cord and cauda equina. Table 2–10 attempts to identify the clinical features that may help in differentiating conus and epiconus lesions from cauda equina lesions.

DISTINGUISHING INTRAMEDULLARY FROM EXTRAMEDULLARY TUMORS

Neoplasms of the spine may be classified on the basis of location (Fig. 2–8, Table 2–11). Intramedullary tumors consist of neoplasms arising from neuroectodermal tissues, such as ependymoma, astrocytoma, or glioblastoma. Extramedullary-intradural growths are usually the histologically benign meningiomas and nerve sheath tumors, although metastatic neoplasms to the leptomeninges also occur. Epidural tumors are usually metastatic deposits to the vertebral column with extension into the spinal canal and secondary cord/cauda compression, or, less frequently, epidural tumors may be primary tumors of the skeletal tissues such as multiple myeloma, or osteogenic sarcoma.

The relative frequency of epidural, extramedullary-intradural, and intramedullary tumors is difficult to ascertain. This problem arises from the selection of patients inherent in the neurosurgical literature in which primary spinal tumors are much more common than metastatic lesions; the converse is true in oncologic series. Since the majority of metastatic spinal neoplasms occur in the epidural space, whereas primary spinal tumors are more frequently intradural lesions, some estimate of the relative frequency of these locations for neoplastic growth may be

Table 2–10 DIFFERENTIATION OF CONUS/EPICONUS FROM CAUDA EQUINA LESIONS*

	Conus Medullaris/ Epiconus	Cauda Equina
Spontaneous pain	Unusual and not severe; bilateral and symmetric in perineum or thighs	Often very prominent and severe, asymmetric, radicular
Motor findings	Not severe, symmetric Fibrillary twitches are rare	May be severe, asymmetric, fibrillary twitches of paralyzed muscles are common
Sensory findings	Saddle distribution, bilateral, symmetric, dissociated sensory loss (impaired pin and temperature sensibility with sparing of tactile sensibility)	Saddle distribution, may be asymmetric, no dissociation of sensory loss
Reflex changes	Epiconus: Only Achilles absent Conus: Achilles and patellar present	Patellar and Achilles may be absent
Sphincter disturbance	Early and marked (both urinary and fecal incontinence)	Late and less severe
Male sexual function	Impaired early	Impairment less severe
Onset	Sudden and bilateral	Gradual and unilateral

*Adapted from DeJong, RN[35] and Haymaker, W.[71]

determined by histological type. Based on population studies, metastatic cancer to the spine is much more common than primary spinal tumors. For example, Alter[4] has reported that primary spinal tumors occur at an annual incidence rate of 0.9–2.5 per 100,000. For a population of 250 million in the United States, this would mean a maximum annual incidence of 6250 in the United States. The annual mortality for cancer in 1980 was 184 per 100,000 in the United States (data from Center for Environmental Health, CDC). With approximately 5 percent of patients dying from cancer developing spinal cord compression,[7] the annual incidence of metastatic spinal cord compression is approximately 9 per 100,000. For a population of 250 million, this corresponds to an annual incidence of 22,500 in the United States. Therefore, it appears, based on available epidemiological data, that metastatic spinal tumors are 3 to 4 times more common than primary spinal tumors. This calculation is very similar to other reports of relative frequency.[118]

Distinguishing among intramedullary, extramedullary-intradural, and epidural tumors of the spinal cord may be a vexing clinical problem that ultimately requires radiographic confirmation. The explanation for this clinical experience has been provided by a clinicopathological study of ex-

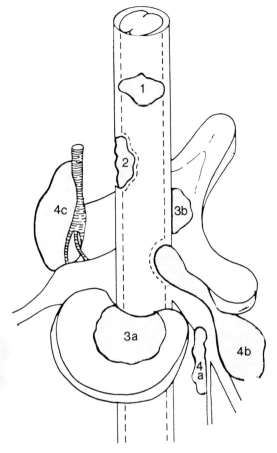

Figure 2–8. The potential sites of neoplasms which may cause myelopathy. (1) The neoplasm may arise in or metastasize to the spinal cord (intramedullary). (2) The neoplasm may be extramedullary but intradural. (3) The neoplasm may be extradural, extending from the vertebral body (3a) or from a spinous process (3b) or pedicle. (4) The neoplasm may originate in or spread to the paravertebral space and become clinically manifest either by invading nerve roots (4a), or by invading the epidural or subdural space through intervertebral foramina (4b), or by compressing radicular blood vessels and thereby causing cord ischemia (4c). (From Andreoli, TE et al (eds): Cecil's Essentials of Medicine, WB Saunders, Philadelphia 1986, p 719, Fig. 119–4, with permission.)

Table 2–11 CLASSIFICATION OF SPINAL NEOPLASMS ACCORDING TO LOCATION WITH SOME EXAMPLES OF HISTOLOGICAL TYPES

Intramedullary neoplasms
    Ependymoma
    Astrocytoma
    Glioblastoma
    Vascular neoplasm
    Metastasis
Extramedullary-intradural neoplasms
    Meningioma
    Nerve sheath tumor
    Vascular neoplasm
    Metastasis
Epidural neoplasms
    Metastasis
    Multiple myeloma
    Osteogenic sarcoma (osteoma)
    Chondrosarcoma (chondroma)
    Lipomas
    Teratoma

tramedullary spinal neoplasms,[103] which demonstrated that extramedullary tumors can cause ischemia and demyelination in the posterior and lateral column with relative sparing of the anterior columns regardless of the location of the extramedullary tumor. Both coup and contrecoup injuries occurred in the spinal cord. The areas of infarction and demyelination were

Table 2–12 CHARACTERISTICS THAT CAN HELP IN
DIFFERENTIATION BETWEEN EXTRAMEDULLARY AND
INTRAMEDULLARY TUMORS OF THE SPINAL CORD*

	Extramedullary Tumors	Intramedullary Tumors
Spontaneous pain	Radicular or regional (local) in type and distribution; an early and important symptom	Funicular; burning in type; poorly localized
Sensory changes	Contralateral loss of pain and temperature; ipsilateral loss of proprioception; (Brown-Séquard type)	Dissociation of sensation; spotty changes
Changes in pain and temperature sensations in saddle area	More marked than at level of lesion. Sensory level may be located *below* site of lesion.	Less marked than at level of lesion. Sensory loss can be suspended
Lower motor neuron involvement	Segmental	Can be marked and widespread with atrophy and fasciculations
Upper motor neuron paresis and hyperreflexia	Prominent	Can be late and less prominent
Trophic changes	Usually not marked	Can be marked
Spinal subarachnoid block and changes in spinal fluid	Early and marked	Late and less marked

*Adapted from DeJong, RN.[35]

often deep and did not follow a specific pattern. In some instances the pathological findings were more marked ipsilateral to the tumor; in other cases, they were primarily contralateral. Therefore, definite clinical patterns of evolution would not be expected. Nevertheless, at times the clinical presentations may be helpful in evaluating patients (Table 2–12).

Pain

Pain is a common initial symptom of all types of spinal tumors. Although the pain is usually progressive, it has been reported to remit transiently in some cases.[46] Guidetti and Fortuna state, "It is pointless to try to predict the type of growth from the presence or absence of pain,"[64] but there are some characteristics of pain that may be helpful in the evaluation.

As already mentioned, approximately 90 percent of patients with metastatic epidural tumors complain of vertebral or radicular pain at the time of diagnosis.[126] In cases of extramedullary-intradural tumors, radicular pain is often a prominent complaint and may be present for months or years prior to diagnosis.[15, 79] With neurofibromas, the pain is usually unilateral,

whereas it may be bilateral in meningiomas.

Typical radicular pain is much less common in cases of intramedullary tumor.[65] Individuals with intramedullary tumors rarely present with root symptoms or signs alone.[144] The projected pain is usually burning, biting, and pinching.[25, 46] Funicular pain is much more common than radicular pain in these patients and it is often bilateral.[147] It is typically poorly localized, diffuse, and burning, and often involves large areas of the body. Funicular pain may be triggered by tactile stimulation or movement of the spine.

Funicular pain is rare in cases of epidural tumors, having been found in only 3 percent of Torma's series.[163] However, in Guidetti's series,[64] funicular pain was the initial symptom in 22 percent and appeared later in 45 percent. Lhermitte's sign has been reported in patients with both extramedullary and intramedullary tumors and is not, therefore, helpful in distinguishing between them.[64]

Motor Disorders

Motor disorders are second only to pain as the most common presenting manifestation of spinal cord tumors, perhaps because the pyramidal pathways may be more sensitive to the compressive and ischemic effects of neoplasms than the sensory pathways.[64] The rate of evolution of weakness is not helpful in distinguishing between intramedullary and extramedullary tumors. Slow progressive weakness is frequently seen in both types of neoplasms. Similarly, rapid deterioration in motor function has been reported in cases of intramedullary tumors, extramedullary-intradural tumors, and extradural tumors.[58, 64] Hemorrhage into the tumor has been found in some cases of intramedullary tumors such as glioblastoma.[64, 155] Vasogenic edema and circulatory disturbances have been reported to occur experimentally in epidural tumors[83, 165] and probably also play a role in intramedullary and extramedullary-intradural tumors. Although progressive weakness is the rule in all spinal neoplasms, transient remissions may occur,[64] reflecting secondary mechanical and vascular factors.

Weakness has been found in 13–60 percent of cases of intramedullary tumors at the time of diagnosis.[64] Weakness due to intramedullary tumors may characteristically spread in the limbs from a proximal to a distal location.[46, 147] This pattern is due to the lamination of the corticospinal tract. Intramedullary lesions in the cervical spine, such as gliomas or syringomyelia, may cause unilateral or bilateral arm paresis with sparing of the lower extremity strength early in their course[147] (suspended area of weakness). Except for foramen magnum tumors, extramedullary cervical neoplasms infrequently give a clinical picture of bilateral arm weakness with preservation of leg strength. As discussed earlier, neoplasms of the foramen magnum often present with unilateral arm weakness before progressing to leg weakness.[64, 96, 160]

Unlike the case in intramedullary tumors, in cases of extramedullary-intradural tumors of the cervical spine such as neurofibromas and meningiomas, lower extremity strength is usually impaired to a comparable degree with the arms.[33, 54] In addition, the weakness at the level of the neoplasm may be radicular as well. In epidural tumors, signs of weakness are frequently seen at the time of diagnosis, the prevalence being approximately 85 percent in one series.[58] Other series of epidural metastases have reported a lower incidence of weakness,[95] but only pain is a more frequent complaint in patients with metastatic spinal cord compression.[58, 64]

Sensory Disturbances

Sensory disturbances may begin with subjective complaints of paresthesias. For unknown reasons, paresthesias are unusual presenting manifestations in most patients with spinal tumors. Frequencies of less than 10 percent have been reported in cases of epidural tumors, nerve sheath tumors, and intramedullary tumors.[15,64,163] In cases of meningiomas, though, the complaint of paresthesia appears to be common, with frequencies of 23–37 percent reported.[33, 64, 163]

Isolated sensory loss in the absence of other complaints and signs on examination is a rare presenting manifestation of either intramedullary or extramedullary spinal tumors. The cutaneous pattern and evolution of sensory loss may be helpful in distinguishing between these tumors. Dissociated sensory loss, preservation of posterior column function with loss of spinothalamic functions, is considered characteristic of intramedullary lesions; however, extramedullary tumors also have been reported to cause this pattern.[46, 64] Extramedullary neoplasms may present with an ascending sensory level and intramedullary growths may cause a suspended sensory level, most prominent at the level of the tumor.[162] This difference is due to the lamination of the spinothalamic tracts. Because the fibers conducting the caudal dermatomes are most posterolateral and those mediating rostral regions are more anteromedial, extramedullary compressive lesions tend to injure the fibers representing the caudal locations initially. Conversely, intramedullary growths tend to involve the more medial fibers initially and later invade the more laterally placed pathways. Thus, intramedullary tumors may appear to cause a descending sensory loss.

The evolution of sensory loss does not necessarily follow the classical patterns. For example, an eccentric intramedullary growth may give rise to an ascending sensory level rather than a suspended sensory loss. Exceptions to the ascending sensory levels are frequently found with epidural growths. Benign extramedullary tumors in the region of the foramen magnum frequently cause position sense loss more marked in the upper extremity than in the lower extremity ipsilateral to the tumor.[40, 160] These examples of variability are probably explained on the basis of the tracts affected by ipsilateral and contralateral injuries. In a clinicopathological study of extramedullary spinal tumors, McAlhany and Netsky[103] found that regions of spinal ischemia and demyelination cannot be predicted on the basis of the location of the tumor in relationship to the cord.

Autonomic Disorders

Sphincter disturbances are considered unusual early manifestations of extramedullary and intramedullary tumors, unless the conus or cauda equina is the site of involvement.[64, 130, 163] In one large series of intramedullary tumors,[155] only 3 percent of patients presented with sphincter disturbances as their first symptom. Of 130 patients with epidural tumor reported by Gilbert and associates[58] none had sphincter disturbances as an initial complaint. However, sphincter disturbances were present in 57 percent of these cases by the time patients were seen in neurological consultation. Most authors report that sphincter disturbance occurs after motor and sensory disturbances are already manifest[147, 155] unless the lesion is in the region of the conus or cauda equina.[64] Thus with either intramedullary or extramedullary mass lesions of the conus or mass lesions compressing the cauda equina, sphincter disturbances may be the initial manifestation.[116, 130]

Other autonomic disorders generally do not help distinguish between intramedullary and extramedullary disorders, as they are found in both instances. For example, Horner's syndrome has been found in both types of growths.[64] The superior sulcus tumor as described by Pancoast is a common cause of a Horner's syndrome.[120] Both primary tumors of the lung and metastases to this region commonly cause a combination of lower brachial plexopathy and Horner's syndrome.[27, 86, 90] In this setting, the tumor can extend into the epidural space by invading through the intervertebral foramina; thus, the radionuclide bone scan and plain films can be unremarkable.[86] Disturbances of sweating, cyanosis, and edema have been reported in both intramedullary and extramedullary tumors and do not appear to be helpful in discriminating between them.[64]

Temporal Course

Intramedullary tumors cannot be differentiated from extramedullary benign growths such as meningiomas and nerve sheath tumors or from malignant epidural tumors on the basis of the time course of the symptoms and signs. While there are differences in the average period of time in which the clinical spinal syndrome evolves, frequent individual exceptions preclude definite conclusions. For example, while most malignant epidural tumors have a time course measured over days, to weeks or months, intramedullary growths as well as meningiomas and nerve sheath tumors may have a similar acute or subacute presentation or, occasionally, evolution over many years.

Spinal tumors of any location may present with a remitting/relapsing course often mistaken for multiple sclerosis. Schliack and Stille[144] cite a neurinoma in a young man that caused a progressive paraparesis with sphincter involvement over a few months and subsequently resolved to a complete remission lasting 4 years, at which time the symptoms recurred rapidly to a near-complete transection of the cord. The same authors cite several other cases of meningiomas and intramedullary tumors that presented with relapsing and remitting courses over several years. When a relapsing and remitting clinical syndrome involves one location of the nervous system, one should consider a structural etiology as responsible. Although the side of the clinical involvement may vary during subsequent attacks owing to the close anatomical relationship of the tracts, when the same segmental level is repeatedly involved, a mass lesion needs to be considered.

UNUSUAL CLINICAL FEATURES OF SPINAL TUMORS

Raised Intracranial Pressure and Dementia

Rarely, spinal tumors present with symptoms and signs of intracranial disease.[5, 48, 61, 78, 97, 98, 100, 108] For example, headache and papilledema secondary to raised intracranial pressure has rarely been reported as a presenting complaint. As of 1984, Michowiz and associates[107] found 53 cases of papilledema in association with spinal lesions. In each case, the papilledema resolved upon surgical removal of the spinal lesion.

The majority of reported spinal tumors causing increased intracranial pressure papilledema have been ependymomas-ependymoblastomas.[64,129] However, extramedullary tumors have also been found to cause papilledema.[64,108,142] Most spinal tumors causing increased intracranial pressure have been in the lower spinal canal, with half of the cases reviewed by Schliack and Stille[144] occurring in the lumbar area.

Among the patients with raised intracranial pressure secondary to spinal neoplasms, approximately 50 percent have associated ventriculomegaly.[48, 56, 69] Recently, Feldman and colleagues[48] reported a case of hydrocephalic dementia secondary to a benign lumbar schwannoma. Removal of the schwannoma resulted in a rapid resolution of the hydrocephalus and dementia. These authors reviewed five other cases[6, 114, 132] in which a caudal intradural tumor was associated with increased intracranial pressure, ventriculomegaly, and dementia. While over 50 percent of cases of papilledema due to spinal tumors are due to ependymomas-ependymoblastomas,[107] the spinal tumors in these six cases of dementia were two

cases of neurofibroma, three of schwannoma, and one of oligodendroglioma.

The pathophysiological mechanism of raised intracranial pressure secondary to spinal tumors has not been adequately explained. Although elevated CSF protein content has been suggested as a cause of impaired CSF resorption,[53] experimentally induced elevated CSF protein in monkeys did not cause papilledema.[72] Another explanation is that CSF normally absorbed in the lumbar subarachnoid region cannot be absorbed in such cases, resulting in increased intracranial pressure.[144] Intracranial basilar arachnoiditis may be the cause in some cases.[5]

Cranial Nerve Disturbances and Nystagmus

Surprisingly, lesions of the high cervical spine seldom give rise to lower cranial nerve symptoms and signs.[46] In one report of foramen magnum lesions,[161] disturbances of cranial nerves V (sensory loss), XI, and XII, and vertigo and nystagmus were only occasionally seen. After reviewing their own experience and that of others,[45] the authors commented on the relative rarity of these complaints in patients with foramen magnum tumors. They concluded that when cranial nerve symptoms did occur, they were overshadowed by the symptoms of spinal cord compression unless the lesion was located primarily in the posterior fossa.

Sensory disturbances involving the trigeminal distribution may occur in high cervical lesions, including both intramedullary and extramedullary tumors, since the descending trigeminal tract extends as far as the upper cervical spine.[26] Although high cervical intramedullary tumors may cause sensory loss in the distribution of the trigeminal nerve alone before long tract signs develop, extramedullary spinal growths produce long tract signs before trigeminal sensory loss is found.[144]

Nystagmus has been reported in several cases of both intramedullary and extramedullary cervical spine tumors.[46, 144, 161] The mechanism may be due to involvement of the medial longitudinal fasciculus in the cervical spine, extension of the tumor into the posterior fossa, distant vascular effects in the medulla, or other reasons.[144]

Cranial nerve symptoms and signs and raised intracranial pressure also may occur in patients with spinal tumors when the tumor has spread to the intracranial space. This may occur due to a second primary tumor intracranially, as is often seen in neurofibromatosis. Intracranial metastases may occur from primary spinal tumors or may develop independently in cases where the spinal tumor is itself a metastasis. Finally, cerebral and brainstem symptoms and signs may, of course, be due to an independent, unrelated disease.

Subarachnoid Hemorrhage

Spontaneous spinal subarachnoid hemorrhage is responsible for less than 1 percent of all cases of subarachnoid hemorrhage.[21] Unlike the intracranial causes, in which aneurysm is the most important etiology, spinal aneurysms are rare.[21] Spinal arteriovenous malformations are the most common cause of spinal subarachnoid hemorrhage. Rarely, spinal tumors may be responsible. According to one review,[64] the neoplasm is usually found in the lower spinal cord or cauda equina. The most common histological tumor type appears to be ependymoma. Other intramedullary tumors may also be responsible, and meningiomas and neurinomas have been reported to cause spinal subarachnoid hemorrhage. The same review[64] fails to cite any cases caused by epidural spinal tumors, and we are unaware of any such cases.

REFERENCES

1. Adams, RD and Victor, M: Diseases of the spinal cord. In Adams, RD and Victor, M (eds): Principles of Neurology. McGraw-Hill, New York, 1985, pp. 665–698.
2. Adams, RD and Victor, M: Principles of Neurology, ed 3. McGraw-Hill, New York, 1985.
3. Albert, ML, Greer, WER, and Kantrowitz, W: Paraplegia secondary to hypotension and cardiac arrest in a patient who has had previous thoracic surgery. Neurology 19:915–918, 1969.
4. Alter, M: Statistical aspects of spinal cord tumors. In Vinken, PJ and Bruyn, GW (eds): Handbook of Clinical Neurology, Vol 19. North-Holland Publishing, Amsterdam, 1975, pp 1–22.
5. Arseni, C and Maretsis, M: Tumors of the lower spinal cord associated with increased intracranial pressure and papilledema. J Neurosurg 27:105–110, 1967.
6. Bamford, CR and Labadie, EL: Reversal of dementia in normotensive hydrocephalus after removal of cauda equina tumor. J Neurosurg 45:104–107, 1976.
7. Barron, KD, Hirano, A, Araki, S, et al: Experiences with metastatic neoplasms involving the spinal cord. Neurology 9:91–106, 1959.
8. Benninger, TR and Patterson, VH: Lhermitte's sign as a presenting symptom of B_{12} deficiency. Ulster Med J 53:162–163, 1984.
9. Berger, L, Mitchell, RA, and Servinghaus, JW: Regulation of respiration (3 part series). N Engl J Med 297:92–97; 138–143; 194–201, 1977.
10. Bharucha, EP and Dastur, HM: Craniovertebral anomalies (a report on 40 cases). Brain 87:469–480, 1964.
11. Blackwood, W: Discussion on the vascular disease of the spinal cord. Proc R Soc Med 51:543–547, 1958.
12. Blight, AR: Axonal physiology of chronic spinal cord injury in the cat: Intracellular recordings in vitro. Neuroscience 10: 1471–1486, 1983.
13. Booth, RE and Rothman, RH: Cervical angina. Spine 1:28–32, 1976.
14. Bosley, TM, Cohen, DA, Schatz, NJ, Zimmerman, RA, Bilaniuk, LT, Savino, PJ, and Sergott, RS: Comparison of metrizamide computed tomography and magnetic resonance imaging in the evaluation of lesions at the cervicomedullary junction. Neurology 35:485–492, 1985.
15. Broager, B: Spinal neurinoma. Acta Psychiat Scand (Suppl)85:1–241, 1953.
16. Brodal, A: Neurological Anatomy: In Relation to Clinical Medicine, ed 3. Oxford University Press, New York, 1981.
17. Brodsky, A: Cervical angina: A correlative study with emphasis on the use of coronary arteriography. Spine 10:699–709, 1985.
18. Brooker, AE and Barter, AW: Cervical spondylosis. Clinical study with comparative radiology. Brain 88:925–936, 1965.
19. Brown-Séquard, CE: Physiology and Pathology of the Central Nervous System. Collins, Printer, Philadelphia, 1860.
20. Brown-Séquard, CE: Truth of Sir Charles Bell's theory as regards the existence of two distinct sets of nervous conductors: The sensitive and the motor. In Brown-Séquard, CE (ed): Physiology and Pathology of the Central Nervous System. Collins, Printer, Philadelphia, 1860, pp 1–12.
21. Buchan, AM and Barnett, JM: Vascular malfor-

mations and hemorrhage of the spinal cord. In Barnett, HJM, Mohr, JP, Stein, BM, and Yatsu, FM (eds): Stroke: Pathophysiology, Diagnosis and Management. Churchill Livingstone, New York, 1986, pp 721–730.

22. Bucy, PC, Keplinger, JE, and Siqueira, EB: Destruction of the pyramidal tract in man. J Neurosurg 21:385–398, 1964.

23. Bucy, PC, Ladpli, R, and Ehrlich, A: Destruction of the pyramidal tract in the monkey: The effects of bilateral destruction of the cerebral peduncles. J Neurosurg 25:1–20, 1966.

24. Burke, D: Spasticity as an adaptation to pyramidal tract injury. In Waxman, SG (ed): Functional Recovery in Neurological Disease. Raven Press, New York, 1988.

25. Cairns, H and Riddoch, G: Observations on the treatment of ependymal gliomas of the spinal cord. Brain 54:117–146, 1931.

26. Carpenter, MB: Human Neuroanatomy, ed 7. Williams & Wilkins, Baltimore, 1976, pp 213–384.

27. Cascino, TL, Kori, S, Krol, G, and Foley, KM: CT of the brachial plexus in patients with cancer. Neurology 33:1553–1557, 1983.

28. Chade, HO: Metastatic tumours of the spine and spinal cord. In Vinken, PJ and Bruyn, GW (eds): Handbook of Clinical Neurology, Vol 20. North-Holland Publishing, Amsterdam, 1976, pp 415–433.

29. Chambers, WW, Liu, CN, and McCouch, GP: Anatomical and physiological correlates of plasticity in the central nervous system. Brain Behav Evol 8:5–26, 1973.

30. Chan, RC and Steinboh, P: Delayed onset of Lhermitte's sign following head and/or neck injuries. J Neurosurg 60:609–612, 1984.

31. Coggeshall, RE, Applebaum, ML, Fazen, M, et al: Unmyelinated axons in human ventral roots, a possible explanation for the failure of dorsal root rhizotomy to relieve pain. Brain 98:157–166, 1975.

32. Csuka, M and McCarty, DJ: Simple method for measurement of lower extremity muscle strength. Am J Med 78:77–81, 1978.

33. Davis, RA and Washburn, PL: Spinal cord meningiomas. Brain 90:359–394, 1970.

34. DeJong, RN: Sensation. In Vinken, PJ and Bruyn, GW (eds): Handbook of Clinical Neurology, Vol 1. North-Holland Publishing, Amsterdam, 1969, pp 80–113.

35. DeJong, RN: The Neurologic Examination, ed 4. Harper & Row, Hagerstown, MD, 1979.

36. Denny-Brown, D, Kirk, EJ, and Yanigasawa, N: The tract of Lissauer in relation to sensory transmission in the dorsal horn of spinal cord in the macaque monkey. J Compar Neurol 151:175–200, 1973.

37. Deyo, RA, Diehl, AK, and Rosenthal, M: How many days of bed rest for acute low back pain? A randomized clinical trial. N Engl J Med 315:1064–1070, 1986.

38. Dimitriyevic, MR: Residual motor functions in spinal cord injury. In Waxman, SG (ed):

Functional Recovery in Neurological Disease. Raven Press, New York, 1987.

39. Djindjian, R: Angiography in angiomas of the spinal cord. In Pia, HW and Djindjian, R (eds): Spinal Angiomas: Advances in Diagnosis and Therapy. Springer-Verlag, New York, 1978, p 98.

40. Dodge, HW, Love, JG, and Gottlieb, CM: Benign tumors at the foramen magnum. J Neurosurg 13:603–617, 1956.

41. Dykes, RW and Terzis, JK: Spinal nerve distribution in the upper limb: The organization of the dermatome and afferent myotome. Philosophical Transactions of the Royal Society of London (Biol) 293:509–554, 1981.

42. Dynes, JB and Smedal, MI: Radiation myelitis. AJR 83:78–87, 1960.

43. Eaton, LM and Craig, WM: Tumor of the spinal cord: Sudden paralysis following lumbar puncture. Proceedings of the Staff Meetings of the Mayo Clinic 15:170–172, 1940.

44. Elkins, CW and Wegner, WR: Newer concepts in the treatment of the paralyzed patient due to wartime injuries of the spine. Neurosurgical complications. Ann Surg 123:516–522, 1946.

45. Elsberg, CA: Tumors of the Spinal Cord and Membranes. Paul B Hoeber, New York, 1925.

46. Elsberg, CA: Surgical Diseases of the Spinal Cord, Membranes and Nerve Root. Paul B Hoeber, New York, 1941.

47. Ely, LW: Subluxation of the atlas. Ann Surg 54:20–29, 1911.

48. Feldman, E, Bromfield, E, Navia, B, Pasternak, GW, and Posner, JB: Hydrocephalic dementia and spinal cord tumor: A report of a case and review of the literature. Arch Neurol 43:714–718, 1986.

49. Fitzgerald, M: The course and termination of primary afferent fibers. In Wall, PD and Melzack, R (eds): Textbook of Pain. Churchill Livingstone, Edinburgh, 1984, p 40.

50. Foerster, O: The dermatomes in man. Brain 56:1, 1933.

51. Frykholm, R, Norlen, G, and Skoglund, CR: On pain sensations produced by stimulation of ventral roots in man. Acta Physiol Scand 29:455–469, 1953.

52. Fulton, JE, Liddell, EGT, and Rioch, D McK: The influence of the vestibular nuclei upon posture and the knee jerk. Brain 53:327–343, 1930.

53. Gardner, WJ, Spitler, DK, and Whitten, C: Increased intracranial pressure caused by increased protein content in the cerebrospinal fluid: An explanation of papilledema in certain cases of small intracranial and intraspinal tumors and in Guillain-Barré syndrome. N Engl J Med 250:932–936, 1954.

54. Gautier-Smith, PC: Clinical aspects of spinal neurofibromas. Brain 90:359–394, 1970.

55. Gautier-Smith, PC: Lhermitte's sign in subacute degeneration of the cord. J Neurol Neurosurg Psychiatry 36:861–863, 1973.

56. Gibberd, FB, Ngan, H, and Swann, GF: Hydro-cephalus, subarachnoid hemorrhage and ependymomas of the cauda equina. Clin Radiol 23:422–426, 1972.

57. Gijn, J van: The Babinski response and the pyramidal syndrome. J Neurol Neurosurg Psychiatry 41:865–873, 1978.

58. Gilbert, RW, Kim, JH, and Posner, JB: Epidural spinal cord compression from metastatic tumor: Diagnosis and treatment. Ann Neurol 3:40–51, 1978.

59. Gilles, FH: Hypotensive brain stem necrosis. Arch Pathol 88:32, 1969.

60. Gilles, FH and Nag, D: Vulnerability of human spinal cord in transient cardiac arrest. Neurology 21:833, 1971.

61. Glasauer, FE: Thoracic and lumbar intraspinal tumors associated with increased intracranial pressure. J. Neurol Neurosurg Psychiatry 27:451–458, 1964.

62. Good, DC, Couch, JR, and Wacasar, L: "Numb, clumsy hands" and high cervical spondylosis. Surg Neurol 22:285–291, 1984.

63. Greenberg, AD: Atlanto-axial dislocations. Brain 91:655–684, 1968.

64. Guidetti, B and Fortuna, A: Differential diagnosis of intramedullary and extramedullary tumors. In Vinken, PJ and Bruyn, GE (eds): Handbook of Clinical Neurology, Vol 19. North-Holland Publishing, Amsterdam, 1975, pp 51–75.

65. Guidetti, B, Fortuna, A, Moscatelli, G, et al: I Tumori intramidollari: Relazione al XVI Congr Soc Ital di Neurochir Genova, Nov 1964. Lav Neuropsychiat 35:1–409, 1964.

66. Guttman, L: Rehabilitation after injury to the spinal cord and cauda equina. Br J Phys Med 9:130, 1946.

67. Guttman, L: Studies on reflex activity of the isolated spinal cord in spinal man. J Nerv Ment Dis 116:957–972, 1946.

68. Guttman, L: Clinical symptomatology of spinal cord lesions. In Vinken, PJ and Bruyn, GW (eds): Handbook of Clinical Neurology, Vol 2. North-Holland Publishing, Amsterdam, 1969, pp 178–216.

69. Harris, P: Chronic progressive communicating hydrocephalus due to protein transudates from brain and spinal tumors. Dev Med Child Neurol 4:270–278, 1962.

70. Hastings, DE, Macnab, I, and Lawson, V: Neoplasms of the atlas and axis. Can J Surg 11:290–296, 1968.

71. Haymaker, W: Bing's Local Diagnosis in Neurological Diseases, ed 15. CV Mosby, St Louis, 1969, pp 57–59.

72. Hayreh, SS: Pathogenesis of edema of the optic disc (papilledema). A preliminary report. Br J Ophthalmol 48:522–543, 1964.

73. Head, H: On disturbances of sensation with special reference to visceral disease. Brain 16:1–132, 1893.

74. Hensinger, RN and Mac Ewen, GD: Congenital anomalies of the spine. In Rothman, RH and Simeone, FA (eds): The Spine. WB Saunders, Philadelphia, 1982, pp 188–316.

75. Hogan, EL and Romanul, FCA: Spinal cord infarction occurring during insertion of aortic graft. Neurology 16:67–74, 1966.

76. Hollis, PH, Malis, LI, and Zappulla, RA: Neurological deterioration after lumbar puncture below complete spinal subarachnoid block. J Neurosurg 64:253–256, 1986.

77. Hughes, JT and MacIntyre, AG: Spinal cord infarction occurring during thoracolumbar sympathectomy. J Neurol Neurosurg Psychiatry 26:418–421, 1963.

78. Iob, I, Androli, GC, Rigobello, L, et al: An unusual onset of a spinal cord tumor: Subarachnoid bleeding and papilledema. Neurochirurgia 23:112–116, 1980.

79. Iraci, G, Peserico, L, and Salar, G: Intraspinal neurinomas and meningiomas. A clinical survey of 172 cases. International Journal of Surgery 56:289–303, 1971.

80. Jones, A: Transient radiation myelopathy (with reference to Lhermitte's sign of electrical paresthesia). Br J Radiol 37:727–744, 1964.

81. Karnofsky, DA and Burchenal, JH: The clinical evaluation of chemotherapeutic agents in cancer. In McCleod, CM (ed): Evaluation of Chemotherapeutic Agents. Columbia University Press, New York, pp 191–205.

82. Karp, SJ and Ho, RTK: Gait ataxia as a presenting symptom of malignant epidural spinal cord compression. Postgrad Med J 62:745–747, 1986.

83. Kato, A, Ushio, Y, Hayakawa, T, et al: Circulatory disturbance of the spinal cord with epidural neoplasm in rats. J Neurosurg 63:260–265, 1985.

84. Kellgren, JH: On the distribution of pain arising from deep somatic structures with charts of segmental pain areas. Clin Sci 4:35–46, 1939.

85. Khanchandani, R and Howe, JG: Lhermitte's sign in multiple sclerosis: A clinical survey and review of the literature. J Neurol Neurosurg Psychiatry 45:308–312, 1982.

86. Kori, SH, Foley, KM, and Posner, JB: Brachial plexus lesions in patients with cancer: 100 cases. Neurology 31:45–50, 1981.

87. Kuhn, RA: Functional capacity of the isolated human spinal cord. Brain 73:1–51, 1950.

88. Lance, JW: The control of muscle tone, reflexes, and movement: Robert Wartenberg Lecture. Neurology 30:1303–1313, 1980.

89. Landau, WM and Clare, MH: The plantar reflex in man, with special reference to some conditions where the extensor response is unexpectedly absent. Brain 82:321–355, 1959.

90. Lederman, RJ and Wilbourn, AJ: Brachial plexopathy: Recurrent cancer or radiation?. Neurology 34:1331–1335, 1984.

91. Levitt, P, Ransohoff, J, and Spielholz, N: The differential diagnosis of tumors of the conus medullaris and cauda equina. In Vinken, PJ and Bruyn, GW (eds): Handbook of Clinical Neurology, Vol 19. North-Holland Publishing, Amsterdam, 1975, pp 77–90.

92. Lhermitte, J, Bollak, NM and Nicolas, M: Les douleurs a type de décharge électrique consecutives a la flexion céphalique dans la sclérose en plaque. Rev Neurol (Paris) 42:56–62, 1924.

93. Lindenbaum, J, Healton, EB, Savage, DG, et al: Neuropsychiatric disorders caused by cobalamin deficiency in the absence of anemia or macrocytosis. N Engl J Med 318:1720–1728, 1988.

94. Lipson, S: Cervical myelopathy and posterior atlanto-axial subluxation in patients with rheumatoid arthritis. J Bone Joint Surg 67A:593–597, 1985.

95. Longeval, E, Holdebrand, J, and Vollont, GH: Early diagnosis of metastases in the epidural space. Acta Neurochir 31:177–184, 1975.

96. Love, JG, Thelen, EP, and Dodge, HW: Tumors of the foramen magnum. Journal of the International College of Surgeons 22:1–17, 1954.

97. Love, JG, Wagner, HP, and Woltman, HW: Tumors of the spinal cord associated with choking of the optic disks. Arch Neurol 66:171–177, 1951.

98. Luzecky, M, Siegel, BA, Coxe, WS, et al: Papilledema and communicating hydrocephalus: Association with a lumbar neurofibroma. Arch Neurol 30:487–489, 1974.

99. Matsumoto, S, Okuda, B, Imai, T, and Kameyama, M: A sensory level on the trunk in lower lateral brainstem lesions. Neurology 38:1515–1519, 1988.

100. Maurice-Williams, RS and Lucey, JJ: Raised intracranial pressure due to spinal tumors: Three rare cases with a probable common mechanism. Br J Surg 62:92–95, 1975.

101. Maynard, CW, Leonard, RB, Coulter, JD, et al: Central connections of ventral root afferents as demonstrated by the HRP method. J Comp Neurol 172:601–608, 1977.

102. McAfee, PC, Bohlman, HH, Han, JS, et al: Comparison of nuclear magnetic resonance imaging and computed tomography in the diagnosis of upper cervical spinal cord compression. Spine 11:295–304, 1986.

103. McAlhany, HJ and Netsky, MG: Compression of the spinal cord by extramedullary neoplasms: A clinical and pathological study. J Neuropath Exp Neurol 14:276–287, 1955.

104. McCall, IW, Park, WM, and O'Brien, JP: Induced pain referral from posterior lumbar elements in normal subjects. Spine 4:441–446, 1979.

105. McRae, DL: Bony abnormalities in the region of the foramen magnum: Correlation of the anatomic and neurologic findings. Acta Radiol 40:335–354, 1953.

106. McRae, DL: The significance of abnormalities of the cervical spine. AJR 84:3–25, 1960.

107. Michowiz, SD, Rappaport, HZ, Shaked, I, Yellin, A, and Sahar, A: Thoracic disc herniation associated with papilledema: Case report. J Neurosurg 61:1132–1134, 1984.

108. Mittal, MM, Gupta, NC, and Sharma, ML: Spinal epidural meningioma associated with increased intracranial pressure. Neurology 20:818–820, 1970.

109. MRC: Aids to the Investigation of Peripheral Nerve Injuries. Her Majesty's Royal Stationery Office, London, 1953.

110. Nachlas, I: Pseudo-angina pectoris originating in the cervical spine. JAMA 103:323, 1934.

111. Nassar, SI, Correll, JW, and Housepian, EM: Intramedullary cystic lesions of the conus medullaris. J Neurol Neurosurg Psychiatry 31:106–109, 1968.

112. Nathan, P and Smith, M: The centrifugal pathways for micturition within the spinal cord. J Neurol Neurosurg Psychiatry 21:177, 1958.

113. Nathan, PW and Smith, MC: The Babinski response: A review and new observations. Brain 18:250–259, 1955.

114. Neil-Dwyer, G: Tentorial block of cerebrospinal fluid associated with a lumbar neurofibroma. J Neurosurg 38:767–770, 1973.

115. Nicholas, JJ and Christy, WC: Spinal pain made worse by recumbency: A clue to spinal cord tumors. Arch Phys Med Rehabil 67:598–600, 1986.

116. Norstrom, CW, Kernohan, JW, and Love, JG: One hundred primary caudal tumors. JAMA 178:1071–1077, 1961.

117. O'Rourke, T. George, CB, Redmond, J, et al: Spinal computed tomography and computed tomographic metrizamide myelography in the early diagnosis of metastatic disease. J Clin Oncol 4:576–583, 1986.

118. Paillas, J-E, Alliez, B, and Pellet, W: Primary and secondary tumours of the spine. In Vinken, PJ and Bruyn, GE (eds): Handbook of Clinical Neurology, Vol 20. North-Holland Publishing, Amsterdam, 1976, pp 19–54.

119. Pallis, C, Jones, AM, and Spillane, JD: Cervical spondylosis. Brain 77:274–289, 1954.

120. Pancoast, HK: Superior pulmonary sulcus tumor: Tumor characterized by pain, Horner's syndrome, destruction of bone and atrophy of hand muscles. JAMA 99:1391–1396, 1932.

121. Patten, J: Neurological Differential Diagnosis. Springer-Verlag, New York, 1977, p 195.

122. Patten, J: Neurological Differential Diagnosis. Springer-Verlag, New York, 1977, p 211.

123. Phillips, J: The importance of examination of the spine in the presence of intrathoracic or abdominal pain. Proceedings of the International Postgraduate Medical Association of North America 3:70, 1927.

124. Plum, F: Neurological integration of behavioural and metabolic control of breathing. In Porter, R (ed): Breathing: Hering-Breuer Centenary Symposium. Churchill, London, 1970, pp 159–175.

125. Portenoy, R, Lipton, RB, and Foley, KM: Back pain in the cancer patient: An algorithm for the evaluation and management. Neurology 37:124–137, 1987.

126. Posner, JB: Back pain and epidural spinal cord

compression. Med Clin North Am 71:185–204, 1987.

127. Preobrajensky, PA: Syphilitic paraplegias with dissociated disturbances of sensibility. J Neuropat Psikhiat 4:594, 1904.

128. Rasmussen, TB, Kernohan, JW, and Adson, AW: Pathologic classification, with surgical consideration, of intraspinal tumors. Ann Surg 111:513–530, 1940.

129. Raynor, RB: Papilledema associated with tumors of the spinal cord. Neurology 19:700–704, 1969.

130. Rewcastle, NB and Berry, K: Neoplasms of the lower spinal canal. Neurology 14:608–615, 1964.

131. Riddoch, G: The reflex functions of the completely divided spinal cord in man, compared with those associated with the less severe lesions. Brain 40:264, 1917.

132. Ridsdale, L and Moseley, I: Thoracolumbar intraspinal tumors presenting features of raised intracranial pressure. J Neurol Neurosurg Psychiatry 41:737–745, 1978.

133. Rodichok, LD, Harper, GR, Ruckdeschel, JC, et al: Early diagnosis of spinal epidural metastases. Am J Med 70: 1181–1188, 1981.

134. Rodichok, LD, Ruckdeschel, JC, Harper, GR, et al: Early detection and treatment of spinal epidural metastases: The role of myelography. Ann Neurol 20:696–702, 1986.

135. Rodriguez, M and Dinapoli, RP: Spinal cord compression: With special reference to metastatic epidural tumors. Mayo Clin Proc 55:442–448, 1980.

136. Ropper, AH, Fisher, CM, and Kleinman, GM: Pyramidal infarction in the medulla: A cause of pure motor hemiplegia sparing the face. Neurology 29:91–95, 1979.

137. Ropper, AH and Poskanzer, DC: The prognosis of acute and subacute transverse myelopathy based on early signs and symptoms. Ann Neurol 4:51–59, 1978.

138. Rowe, ML: Low back pain in industry: A position paper. J Occup Med 11:161–169, 1969.

139. Russell, JSR, Batten, FE, and Collier, J: Subacute combined degeneration of the spinal cord. Brain 23: 39–110, 1900.

140. Sandyk, R and Brennan, MJW: Lhermitte's sign as a presenting symptom of subacute degeneration of the cord. Ann Neurol 13:215–216, 1983.

141. Savitsky, N and Madonick, MJ: Statistical control studies in neurology: Babinski sign. Archives of Neurology and Psychiatry 49:272–276, 1943.

142. Schijman, E, Zuccaro, G, and Monges, JA: Spinal tumors and hydrocephalus. Childs Brain 8:401–405, 1981.

143. Schliack, H: Segmental innervation and the clinical aspects of spinal nerve root syndromes. In Vinken, PJ and Bruyn, GW (eds): Handbook of Clinical Neurology, Vol 2. North-Holland Publishing, Amsterdam, 1969, pp 157–177.

144. Schliack, H and Stille, D: Clinical symptomatol-ogy of intraspinal tumors. In Vinken, PJ and Bruyn, GW (eds): Handbook of Clinical Neurology, Vol 19. North-Holland Publishing, Amsterdam, 1975, pp 23–49.

145. Schneider, RC, Cherry, G, and Pantek, H: The syndrome of acute central cervical spinal cord injury with special reference of mechanisms involved in hyperextension injuries of the cervical spine. J Neurosurg 11:546–577, 1954.

146. Schold, SC, Cho, E-S, Somasundaram, M, and Posner, JB: Subacute motor neuronopathy: A remote effect of lymphoma. Ann Neurol 5:271–287, 1979.

147. Shenkin, HA and Alpers, BJ: Clinical and pathological features of gliomas of the spinal cord. Archives of Neurology and Psychiatry 52:87–105, 1944.

148. Sherrington, CS: Experiments in the examination of the peripheral distribution of the fibers of the posterior roots of some spinal nerves. Part II. Philosophical Transactions B 190:45–186, 1898.

149. Sherrington, CS: The Integrative Action of the Nervous System. Yale University Press, New Haven, 1923.

150. Silver, JR and Buxton, PH: Spinal stroke. Brain 97:539–551, 1974.

151. Simmons, Z, Biller, J, Beck, DW, et al: Painless compressive cervical myelopathy with false localizing sensory findings. Spine 11:869–872, 1986.

152. Simons, DG and Travell, JG: Myofascial origins of low back pain. Postgrad Med 73:66–108, 1983.

153. Simons, DG and Travell, JG: Myofascial pain syndromes. In Wall, PD and Melzack, R (eds): Textbook of Pain. Churchill Livingstone, Edinburgh, 1984, pp 263–276.

154. Sinclair, DC, Feindel, WH, and Falconer, MA: The intervertebral ligaments as a source of segmental pain. J Bone Joint Surg 30B:515–521, 1948.

155. Sloof, JL, Kernohan, JW, and MacCarty, CS: Primary Intramedullary Tumors of the Spinal Cord and Filum Terminale. WB Saunders, Philadelphia, 1964.

156. Smith, KJ and McDonald, WI: Spontaneous and evoked electrical discharges from a central demyelinating lesion. J Neurol Sci 55:39–47, 1982.

157. Spillane, JD, Pallis, C, and Jones, AM: Developmental abnormalities in the region of the foramen magnum. Brain 80:11–48, 1957.

158. St. John, JR and Rand, CW: Stab wounds of the spinal cord. Bulletin of the Los Angeles Neurological Society 18:1–24, 1953.

159. Stark, RJ, Henson, RA, and Evans, SJW: Spinal metastases: A retrospective survey from a general hospital. Brain 105:189–213, 1982.

160. Stein, B, Leeds, NE, Taveras, J, and others: Meningiomas of the foramen magnum. J Neurosurg 20:740–751, 1963.

161. Symonds, C and Meadows, SP: Compression of

the spinal cord in the neighborhood of the foramen magnum. Brain 60:52–84, 1937.

162. Tilney, F and Elsberg, CA: Sensory disturbances in tumors of the cervical spinal cord: Arrangement of fibers in the sensory pathways. Archives of Neurology and Psychiatry 15:444–454, 1926.

163. Torma, T: Malignant tumors of the spine and the spinal extradural space. Acta Chir Scand (Suppl)225:1–176, 1957.

164. Tower, SS: Pyramidal lesion in the monkey. Brain 63:36–90, 1940.

165. Ushio, Y, Posner, R, Posner, JB, et al: Experimental spinal cord compression by epidural neoplasms. Neurology 27:422–429, 1977.

166. Vignos, PJ and Archibald, KC: Maintenance of ambulation in childhood muscular dystrophy. J Chronic Dis 12:273–290, 1960.

167. Walther, PJ, Rossitch, E, and Bullard, DE: The development of Lhermitte's sign during cisplatin chemotherapy: Possible drug-induced toxicity causing spinal cord demyelination. Cancer 60:2170–2172, 1987.

168. Walton, J: Clinical examination of the neuromuscular system. In Walton, J (ed): Disorders of Voluntary Muscle. Churchill Livingstone, Edinburgh, 1981, pp 448–480.

169. Warrington, WB: A case of tumor of the cauda equina removed by operation with remarks on the diagnosis and nature of lesions in that situation. Lancet 83(2):749–753, 1905.

170. Waxman, SG: Membrane, myelin and the pathophysiology of multiple sclerosis. N Engl J Med 306:1529–1533, 1982.

171. Willis, WD and Coggeshall, RE: Peripheral nerves, sensory receptors, and spinal roots. In Willis, WD and Coggeshall, RE (eds): Sensory Mechanisms of the Spinal Cord. Plenum Press, New York, 1978, pp 9–52.

172. Wolfe, BS, Kilnani, M, and Malis, L: The sagittal diameter of the bony cervical spinal canal and its significance in cervical spondylosis. J Mt Sinai Hosp (NY) 23:283–292, 1965.

173. Word, JA, Kalokhe, UP, Aron, BS, and Elson, HR: Transient radiation myelopathy (Lhermitte's sign) in patients with Hodgkin's disease treated by mantle radiation. In J Radiat Oncol Biol Phys 6:1731–1733, 1980.

174. Yakovlev, P and Farrell, MJ: Influence of locomotion on the plantar reflex in normal and in physically and mentally inferior persons: Theoretic and practical implications. Archives of Neurology and Psychiatry 46:322–330, 1941.

175. Yamamoto, T, Takahashi, K, Satomi, H, et al: Origins of primary afferent fibers in the spinal ventral roots in the cat as demonstrated by the horseradish peroxidase method. Brain Res 126:350–354, 1977.

Chapter 3

CLINICAL APPROACH TO PAIN ARISING FROM THE SPINE

Back pain, neck pain, and referred pain to the trunk and extremities are common and often represent diagnostically challenging problems for the physician. In the United States, low back pain is second only to colds as the most common reason for patients' visits to physicians[14] and is reported to occur at some time in the lives of approximately 65–80 percent of individuals.[10, 38, 66, 77] Back pain is reported to be the most expensive chronic illness among persons 30 to 60 years of age in our society.[66] The number of individuals disabled from low back pain grew at a rate 14 times that of the United States population growth between 1971 and 1981.[64]

Despite its major importance, in many cases the precise etiology and pathogenesis of this pain syndrome is uncertain.[55] While some authors report disc disease as a leading cause,[66] others cite musculoligamentous strain and degenerative osteoarthritis as the major culprits.[44, 60, 87] Fortunately, in the majority of such instances of regional back pain (i.e., those not caused by systemic illness), the pain is self-limited and the individual is able to return to normal activities in a few weeks with only rest and analgesics.[21, 38, 43]

Among the great number of individuals complaining of back and/or neck pain, with or without pain referral elsewhere, there are a few in whom it will be a manifestation of serious underlying disease. Metastatic cancer to the spine is an example of such a disease. For example, in a recent series of 1975 outpatients with a chief complaint of back pain, 13(0.66 percent) proved to have underlying cancer.[20]

Findings significantly associated with cancer were:[20]

1. Age $\geq$ 50 years
2. Duration of pain greater than one month
3. Prior history of cancer or other systemic signs of underlying disease (e.g., weight loss, hematuria)
4. Lack of improvement with conservative therapy
5. Anemia
6. An elevated erythrocyte sedimentation rate.

Among patients with a history of malignancy, back pain secondary to metastases frequently occurs at some time during the course of the disease. For example, vertebral metastases develop in nearly one third of patients dying from cancer.[41] In approximately 5 percent of dying cancer patients, vertebral metastases progress to cause epidural spinal cord compression.[4] In approximately 90 percent of this latter group, pain localized to the spine or referred elsewhere is the presenting manifestation of spinal cord compression.[75] It is important to detect spinal cord compression from malignancy when pain is the only symptom and the patient is ambulatory, because the prognosis for neurological function is far better than in patients who have signs of myelopathy at the time of diagnosis.

In addition to back pain arising from pathology of the spine, pain may be referred to the back from other organs. For example, back pain may be the first symptom of life-threatening intra-abdominal or intrathoracic disease such as dissecting aortic aneurysm, neoplasm, pleural disease, or infection.

Given the broad range of causes of back pain, radiological studies of the spine are often ordered in the expectation that they will identify the correct etiology. However, as discussed later in this chapter, radiological studies such as plain radiographs, CT scanning, or magnetic resonance imaging (MRI) performed in the evaluation of back pain may reveal clinically irrelevant information. A large number of asymptomatic individuals harbor radiological evidence of osteoarthritis and even herniated lumbar discs.[39, 48, 107] Therefore, in order to be considered clinically significant, *radiological findings must be correlated with the patient's clinical history and physical examination.* If this is not done properly, the correct diagnosis may be delayed or, worse, laminectomy and discectomy may be performed in a patient with an asymptomatic herniated disc who has serious disease elsewhere that is responsible for the pain.

Recognized in these terms, the diagnostic challenge of back pain, and its frequently associated referred pain, is daunting. This chapter summarizes the clinical features that are most helpful in achieving an accurate assessment of back, neck, referred, and radicular pain.

ANATOMICAL BASIS OF BACK AND NECK PAIN

Knowledge of the innervation of the vertebral column and its associated supporting structures is essential to understanding pain of spinal origin. Many of the pain-sensitive structures of the anterior segment of the spine are innervated by the sinuvertebral nerve,[7] whereas the facet joints of the posterior segment are innervated by the posterior ramus of the spinal nerve [74] (Fig. 3–1).

The sinuvertebral nerve, sometimes called the recurrent meningeal nerve, originates as a branch of the spinal nerve just distal to the dorsal root ganglion. This branch exits the root of the spinal nerve as it passes through the intervertebral foramen. As this recurrent branch reflects back towards the intervertebral foramen, it is joined by an autonomic branch from a nearby gray ramus communicans.[106] These two branches usually fuse to form the sinuvertebral nerve, which reenters the spinal canal through the superior part of the intervertebral foramen. Upon reentry into the spinal canal, the sinuvertebral nerve ramifies into multiple branches that innervate the periosteum of the vertebral body, posterior longitudinal ligament, posterior aspect of annulus fibrosus, anterior aspect of dura, and blood vessels.[7, 24, 86]

The segmental distribution of the sinuvertebral nerves is controversial. Early studies[79] suggested that the sinuvertebral nerve courses only caudally and innervates the posterior longitudinal ligament for one or two segments below the level of entry into the vertebral canal. More recent investigations have failed to confirm this[62], and report that the branches of the sinuvertebral nerve course in a cephalad direction for one segment and a caudal direction for two segments.[7, 25, 56] This results in considerable overlap of innervation between adjacent segments and could account for why sectioning of a single root does not result in loss of pain from a herniated disc.

The dura mater is innervated only on its anterior surface by the sinuvertebral nerve.[25] The posterior region of the dura is sparsely innervated, which may explain why puncture of the dura with a spinal needle is painless although the patient may feel a pop as the needle passes through the dura.

The nucleus pulposus and the inner layers of the annulus fibrosus are not innervated and are not, therefore, considered pain-sensitive. There has been debate over the extent of innervation of the peripheral region of the annulus fibrosus. Although early studies[79] did not identify nerve fibers, recent investigators[61], have suggested the existence of innervation. Many of these nerve fibers have free nerve endings, which may be considered to mediate pain sensibility, whereas others on the surface of the annulus have encapsulated endings that may conduct position sensibility.[61] Despite this network of innervation of the annulus fibrosus,[8, 112]

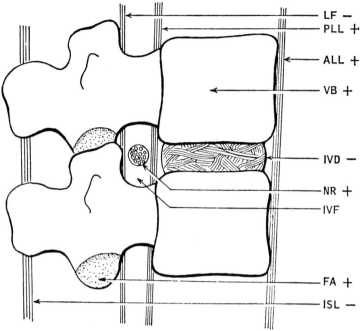

LF —
PLL +
ALL +
VB +
IVD —
NR +
IVF
FA +
ISL —

Figure 3–1. The pain-sensitive tissues of the functional unit of the spine. The tissues labeled + are pain-sensitive, containing sensory nerve endings capable of causing pain when irritated. Tissues labled − are devoid of sensory innervation. [LF, ligamentum flavum; PLL, posterior longitudinal ligament; ALL, anterior longitudinal ligament; VB, vertebral body; IVD, annulus fibrosus of intervertebral disc; IVF, intervertebral foramen containing nerve root (NR); FA, facet articular cartilage; ISL, interspinous ligament.] (From Cailliet, R, [13] p 26, with permission.)

there is controversy as to whether the annulus is pain-sensitive.[47, 68]

Experimental studies have demonstrated that if the intradiscal pressure is increased by injection of saline, normal subjects experience no pain. If the annulus fibrosus is degenerated (fragmented), however, then pain may be experienced.[46] These experiments have been extended by anesthetizing the posterior longitudinal ligament in subjects with a degenerated disc.[13] In this situation, the same procedure does not result in pain, leading to the conclusion that the posterior longitudinal ligament is the site responsible for mediating much of the pain arising from herniated discs. According to this hypothesis, pain results from the stimulation of free nerve endings when a herniated disc dissects the posterior longitudinal ligament away from the annulus and the vertebral body.

The anterior and lateral aspects of each annulus fibrosus and the anterior longitudinal ligaments are not innervated by the sinuvertebral nerve. These structures are innervated by branches of the anterior ramus of the spinal nerves and by autonomic branches of the gray rami communicans or of the sympathetic trunk.

The synovial, or facet, joints of the posterior segment of the spine are innervated by branches of the posterior ramus of the spinal nerve.[74] As in the anterior segments, there is considerable overlap in innervation by adjacent spinal roots. Each facet joint in the lumbar spine is innervated by three segmental levels.[84] Like synovial joints elsewhere, the facet joints may become inflamed, so that they become a source of pain. In addition to the unmyelinated fibers with free nerve endings, which probably mediate pain, there are myelinated fibers with complex encapsulated nerve endings that appear to mediate tension and position sensation within the facet joints.[47, 53] These terminations are probably important in controlling posture and movement.[74]

Innervation of the ligamentum flavum and the interspinous ligament has been reported by some authors[74] but denied by others.[93] The source of innervation of the ligamentum flavum is uncertain but is thought to be the posterior ramus.[7] In the cervical spine, the supraspinous ligament expands between the spinous processes of C2 and C7 to form the nuchal ligament. Recent investigations have shown that the nuchal ligament is innervated. Proprioceptive impulses might be conducted through some of these nerve endings,[30] which could be a mechanism of controlling head and neck position and movement.

In addition to spinal pain-sensitive structures, a common source of pain is spasm of the paravertebral muscles. This pain may be local and associated with physical findings of spasm, but it also may be referred, as in cases of myofascial pain syndromes.

CLASSIFICATION OF SPINAL PAIN

Several characteristic forms of pain arise from disease of the vertebral column and its associated supporting structures, as well as from diseases of the spinal cord and the nerve roots. Pain can be classified as local, referred, radicular, funicular, and secondary to muscle spasm (myofascial pain syndromes) (Table 3–1). Each of these forms of pain has a unique pathophysiology and clinical significance. Furthermore, distinguishing the form of pain is often very helpful in determining its etiology.

Local Pain

Local back or neck pain is usually characterized by a deep, boring, and aching quality. Often this pain results from degenerative joint disease and musculoskeletal strain, exacerbated by mechanical stresses on the weight-bearing spine. Therefore, activities that increase the load on the spine or are related to skeletal movement often exacerbate the pain, and bed rest usually alleviates it. When the pattern of pain deviates from this course, etiologies of pain other than the common-musculoskeletal causes should be considered. For example, back pain referred from visceral structures may share the qualities of deep, boring, aching pain and yet is less likely to be exacerbated by musculoskeletal movements. A gastrointestinal source of pain is likely to be temporally related to dietary and bowel habits rather than to musculoskeletal movements.

Table 3–1 CLASSIFICATION OF PAIN

1. Local
   - Characteristics: Deep, boring, and aching.
   - Tenderness may be present.
   - If exacerbated by lying down, strongly consider tumor.[67, 76]
2. Referred
   - Characteristics: Aching and diffuse.
   - Pain arising from irritation of lumbar spine referred to flank, pelvis, groin, and lower extremities but not generally below the knee.
   - The location of this pain is not truly segmental and does not, therefore, have localizing value.[54, 62, 91]
   - Areas of pain referral may be tender.
   - Referred pain is aggravated and relieved in tandem with local pain.
3. Radicular
   - Characteristics: Sharp, stabbing pain superimposed on chronic ache in the distribution of nerve root.
   - Commonly radiates to the distal portion of the extremity when due to cervical spondylosis at C5–7 or lumbar spondylosis at L4–S1; below knee if from L4–S1.
   - Has excellent localizing value.
   - Tenderness and sensory disturbance along the root distribution are common.
   - Exacerbated by stretching or further compression of root (e.g., straight leg raising, reversed straight leg raising, Valsalva maneuvers, hyperextension of spine, neck flexion).
4. Funicular
   - Characteristics: Diffuse, poorly localized, burning sensation or abrupt stabbing pain.
   - Not radicular in distribution but rather involves unilateral or bilateral limbs, trunk, or entire body.
   - Triggered by movements of spine or incidental cutaneous sensation.
5. Pain secondary to muscle spasm
   - Usually associated with local pain.
   - Physical findings of spasm present.
   - Myofascial pain syndromes (see text).

As previously discussed, local back or neck pain typically arises from irritation of the innervated portions of the vertebral column and its supporting structures. Since only innervated tissues are pain-sensitive, the cancellous region of the vertebral bodies may be invaded by tumor (as often shown by CT scan) in the absence of pain. When a neoplasm invades the innervated cortical region of bone and the periosteum, however, local pain is experienced. As reviewed in Chapter 5, most cases of malignant epidural spinal cord compression originate from metastases to the vertebrae. In order for neural compression to occur, the metastasis must first invade the cortex of bone and periosteum, causing local pain as the earliest symptom in the vast majority of cases. Similarly, patients with osteoporosis experience pain when the cortex of bone is fractured and the innervated bone and periosteum are irritated.

Since degenerative joint disease (e.g., cervical and lumbar spondylosis) and herniated discs are so frequent, one of the most common clinical problems in the patient with known cancer is that of distinguishing the local pain caused by such benign disorders from that caused by spine metastases. Some clinical features help to differentiate between these etiologies. As shown, pain due to disc disease is usually provoked by activity and alleviated by bed rest, but *when the cause of local back pain is spinal tumor, the pain may be exacerbated by the recumbent position rather than relieved by it.* This clinical phenomenon was recognized in an early study of intraspinal tumors: the pain "awakens the patient . . . after he has retired. It often becomes so severe as to compel him to walk the floor or to sleep in a sitting position."[76]

Patients with degenerative joint disease often give a history of chronic pain exacerbated and alleviated by familiar maneuvers. For example, most forms of spondylosis occur in the lower cervical and lower lumbar regions, resulting in local pain in these areas together with radicular pain radiating to distal regions of the extremities. In contrast, the thoracic spine is an infrequent location for spondylosis and disc disease but is a frequent region of spine metastases. Therefore, *one should be especially wary of attributing symptoms and signs to spondylosis or degenerative disc disease in the thoracic spine.*

Another important clinical clue is the chronicity and familiarity of the complaint. When patients with cancer develop a new and different form of pain, metastasis must be considered a likely cause. For example, among cancer patients, Foley[31] found that direct tumor invasion was responsible for 78 percent of pain problems in an inpatient population and 62 percent among an outpatient group. Although some complained of referred and radicular pain, many experienced local pain due to bone or viscus invasion. Thus, in the cancer patient, a new pain syndrome in the back, neck, or elsewhere is frequently due to direct tumor invasion and the work-up should be so directed.

Case Illustration

A 30-year-old former drug abuser with a history of colon cancer treated by abdominoperineal resection presented with progressive buttock and pelvic pain. The pain did not radiate elsewhere and Valsalva maneuver did not exacerbate it. Physical examination demonstrated no evidence for recurrent cancer and neurological examination was normal with no mechanical signs of spine disease. Laboratory studies were remarkable for a rising CEA, and CT scan of the abdomen and pelvis demonstrated irregularity of the posterior pelvic wall and probable postoperative scarring, but no definite tumor was visualized. As no definite cause for the pain could be established, no specific therapy was rendered.

The patient returned three weeks later with severe pain in the same location that had developed into burning pain exacerbated by sitting. Physical examination demonstrated an enlarged liver and tenderness of the sciatic notch on the left. A repeat CEA was higher than the earlier assays. A repeat CT scan of the abdomen and pelvis demonstrated metastatic cancer in the liver and an enlarging pelvic mass in the region earlier considered to be scar formation. The patient underwent radiation therapy and chemotherapy but the pain persisted unabated until he died of metastatic disease.

Comment. This case illustrates the importance of close and continued follow-up of patients with pain and known malignancy. Patients with malignancy who develop a new pain syndrome should be evaluated for recurrence of disease; if the work-up proves negative and the symptoms persist, the evaluation should be repeated.

Referred Pain

Pain that arises from the spine may be projected elsewhere in a radicular or nonradicular pattern. Although both are forms of referred pain, "referred pain" in this chapter is used to denote nonradicular projected pain arising from the spine or other tissue. Myofascial pain syndromes are another example of referred pain that may be difficult to differentiate from pain referred from the spine. As discussed in Chapter 2, these types of pain should be distinguished, because radicular pain has localizing value but referred pain usually does not. Interpreting referred pain as radicular may be misleading. Also, referred and radicular pain can coexist.[6] In one series of 1293 patients seen in a low back pain clinic over a 12-year period, referred pain was nearly twice as common as radicular pain; in some cases the two forms of pain coexisted.[6]

As reported in Chapter 2, when referred pain from the spine was studied experimentally by injecting hypertonic saline into facet joints of L1–2 and L4–5,[62] cramping, aching referred pain radiated into the flank, groin, buttocks, and thigh. Despite two noncontiguous levels of saline injection, the areas of pain referral overlapped significantly and the pain did not radiate below the knee in either case. Although there may be paresthesias and tenderness in the area of pain referral, no objective neurological abnormalities were found. Maneuvers that exacerbate and alleviate local pain generally have the same effect on the associated referred pain.

In a study designed to identify the characteristics of back and leg pain arising from facet disease, local anesthetic was injected into the most tender facet joint in a group of patients with acute low back pain with or without associated leg pain.[28] If pain was relieved by this injection, patients were termed responders and the pain was considered to be secondary to facet disease. Responders had pain that often was exacerbated by sitting, and by flexion and extension of the lumbar spine, and sometimes was relieved by walking. Pain in the back and lower leg rarely responded to facet injection, whereas back pain associated with thigh pain often did respond. This result confirms the report[62] that spinal referred pain infrequently radiates below the knee. Although straight leg raising often caused back pain in responders, it largely did not cause referred leg pain. Straight leg raising typically exacerbates radicular pain arising from the lower lumbar spine.

Somewhat different results have been obtained by others in a similar series of investigations. Mooney and Robertson[65] studied the effect of saline and anesthetic injections of the lower lumbar facet joints in two groups of subjects, one without a history of back pain and sciatica and another with such symptoms. They injected facet joints at the L3–4, L4–5, or L5–S1 levels with hypertonic saline and recorded the pattern of pain. The distribution of referred pain was similar for the L4–5 and L5–S1 levels and was located in the low back, greater trochanter, and posterior thigh and calf. The pain from the L3–4 facet injection usually produced pain in a more lateral distribution (Fig. 3–2). The pattern of pain referral was often that of sciatica. These authors then injected a local anesthetic into the facet joint and found that the referred pain resolved. Furthermore, in a group of patients suffering from the facet syndrome,

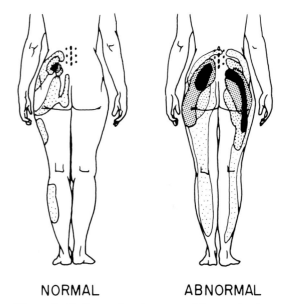

NORMAL   ABNORMAL

Figure 3–2. Pain referral patterns following lumbar facet injection in normal and symptomatic (abnormal) subjects. The investigators concluded that the pattern of pain referral from irritation of lumbar facet joints is similar to that seen in sciatica. (From Mooney, V and Robertson, J [65] p 152, with permission.)

this anesthetic injection normalized their previous positive straight-leg-raising test; in three patients, a depressed deep tendon reflex returned to normal. The authors speculated that the painful stimuli arising from the facet joint might inhibit the anterior horn cells innervating the reflex.

In summary, referred pain is usually poorly localized, deep, and ill-defined with respect to the distribution of a sclerotome. When arising from the low back, it can radiate into the buttock, thigh and, occasionally, the calf in the same distribution as an L5 or S1 radicular pain. Unlike radicular pain, however, the foot is usually not involved. Subjective motor weakness may occur but objective weakness or atrophy is rare. Sensory loss is atypical. Deep tendon reflex abnormalities have been rarely reported. Tension signs such as straight leg raising may cause an increase in low back pain or reveal tight hamstrings.[6] Referred pain into the lower extremity is often due to lumbar spondylosis; referred pain into the neck and upper extremity is frequently seen in cervical spondylosis. (See Chapter 4.)

Radicular Pain

DERMATOMAL PAIN

Radicular pain, which arises from irritation of the dorsal roots, is projected in the dermatomal distribution of the specific root involved (see Table 2–6). Unlike referred pain, it can have exquisite localizing value. Radicular pain is frequently sharp, stabbing, shooting, and superimposed on a chronic ache. The pain is generally aggravated by activities that increase compression of the nerve or further stretch the root, such as coughing, sneezing, straining, straight leg raising, external rotation and extension of the arm,[100] and hyperextension of the spine.

Since radicular pain usually radiates in the distribution of the injured nerve root, accurate localization of the site of pathology depends upon knowledge of the dermatomal map. (Exceptions to this radicular pain pattern may be due to ventral root injury, discussed below.) Unlike the case in referred pain, neurological abnormalities referable to the root involved also may be found, including reflex loss, sensory disturbance and/or motor abnormalities (discussed in Chapter 2). One of the most common causes of radicular pain is spondylosis and disc disease. Since cervical and lumbar spondylosis and disc disease typically involve nerve roots C6, C7 and L5, S1, respectively, radicular pain often is referred to the dermatomal distribution of roots in distal parts of the extremities.

MYOTOMAL PAIN

Another form of radicular pain is thought to arise from ventral spinal root irritation.[37] This pain has been described as deep, aching, diffuse, and dull in character and thus may be difficult to differentiate from visceral pain. It typically is referred to the myotome of the ventral root involved.

An example of this form of pain is anginoid pain arising from the cervical spine. Compression of the lower cervical spinal roots has been recognized as causing precordial pain that can simulate angina.[11, 12] In a large series reported from a cardiovascular referral center,[12] many patients had been carried with a diagnosis of cardiac ischemia for several years before the cervical spine was discovered as the source of pain and the condition was corrected by surgery. "Cervical angina" may be very difficult to differentiate from pain due to coronary artery insufficiency. Of course, at times, the two can coexist.

The pain in cervical angina may arise from compression of the ventral nerve roots of C6, C7, and C8, because these roots innervate chest wall muscles[11] (Fig. 3–3). This pain is, therefore, referred to the myotome rather than the dermatome of the involved nerve root. Pain of similar character may be projected to other sites (such as the leg) when ventral nerve roots at other levels are irritated. The fact that cervical spondylosis usually involves the dorsal roots and dorsal root ganglia more severely than the ventral roots[11] might explain the much greater frequency of dermatomal radicular pain to the upper extremity from the dorsal root, as com-

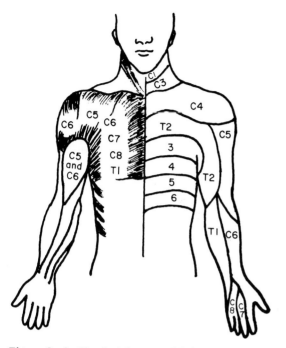

Figure 3–3. The distribution of (left) ventral (myotomal) and (right) dorsal (dermatomal) cervical root innervation. (From Booth, RE and Rothman, RH, [11] with permission.)

voked by incidental cutaneous stimulation or by movements of the spine such as neck flexion, straight leg raising, and Valsalva maneuver—movements that cause mechanical deformation of the involved ascending tracts.

When caused by neoplasms, funicular pain appears to result more often from intramedullary than extramedullary tumors. Funicular pain was found in more than 50 percent of a series of intramedullary tumors,[85] but less than 5 percent of cases of extramedullary tumors.[95]

Another form of funicular sensation is electric-like paresthesias that radiate down the back and into the legs on neck flexion, known as "Lhermitte's sign".[59] It probably reflects increased mechanosensitivity of damaged axons.[92] Similar sensations can be produced experimentally in man by stimulating the posterior funiculus.[42] Lhermitte's sign occurs in demyelinating disease, but may also be due to spinal cord compression from cervical spondylosis[16] or neoplasms of the cervical or thoracic spine, as well as other causes.[3, 82, 99, 101, 111]

pared to the myotomal pattern of radicular pain in cervical spondylosis.

Myotomal pain referral may, of course, be due to causes other than spondylosis, such as malignancy or infection. The character of the myotomal type of pain may also be similar to the referred pain from the spine. As in the case of dermatomal radicular pain, one often will find neurological signs of root dysfunction such as reflex, motor, or sensory disturbance[11] in the setting of ventral root pain.

Funicular Pain

In its complete form, funicular pain is characterized by a poorly localized, diffuse, burning pain syndrome with superimposed sharp, jabbing sensations.[42] It may be present in one or more extremities or the trunk in a unilateral or bilateral distribution. It appears to arise from irritation or compression of the spinothalamic tracts or posterior columns and has been induced experimentally.[2, 42] It is often pro-

Pain Due to Muscle Spasm

Muscle spasm is a common response to irritation of nerves and other tissues. As mentioned earlier, injured axons are sensitive to mechanical stimulation. Paravertebral muscle spasm, which is seen in spinal disorders and is reflexive in nature, guards against further mechanical irritation of the damaged tissues. When chronic, such spasm often results in a pain syndrome of its own.

The pain that arises from such spasm is of two types: The first is the well-recognized form of local pain that is cramping and aching in nature. Physical examination usually reveals evidence of muscle spasm. The second type of pain, termed a myofascial pain syndrome, is both local and referred in nature.[87–89] Myofascial pain syndromes may not be recognized as easily as pain from local spasm because the referred pain is usually the chief complaint and is often not associated with spasm or other abnormal findings at the site of referred pain.

Referred myofascial pain is caused by stimulation of trigger points, which have been described as "self-sustaining hyperirritable foci located in skeletal muscle or its associated fascia."[87] Although the location of the projected pain does not follow a root or peripheral nerve distribution, there are several distinctive myofascial pain syndromes that may be differentiated based upon the location of the trigger point or its associated pain.

Other physical findings in myofascial pain syndromes include a decreased range of motion and decreased apparent strength of the involved muscle group. Shortened tight bands of muscle fibers may give the muscle a ropey or nodular texture. Although the trigger point is typically not the site of reported pain, it is often the site of marked soft-tissue tenderness. Among conditions that may initiate and perpetuate myofascial pain syndromes are muscle strain and structural abnormalities such as unequal leg lengths.

Because myofascial pain syndromes cause referred pain and are associated with subjective weakness,[6, 87] they fall within the differential diagnosis of diseases of the spine or peripheral nervous system. As there are no specific laboratory tests to confirm it, the diagnosis is a clinical one. Extreme care and close follow-up should be exercised, however, because the early pain of many cases of spinal cord neoplasm or other serious pathology is often initially attributed to muscle strain.

The quadratus lumborum is the most common muscle to cause low back myofascial pain.[87] When the trigger points of this muscle are stimulated, pain is referred downward towards the iliac crest, buttocks, and greater trochanter, and occasionally to the lower abdomen and groin. As in other cases of referred pain, the region of referred pain may be tender, resulting in the incorrect clinical impression that the pain is due to local pathology at the site of pain referral.

The gluteal muscles may also be the source of pain in the buttock and posterolateral thigh and calf, and this may be difficult to differentiate from nerve root compression or sciatica. The distinction may be made by identifying the tender spot or trigger point on the muscle and reproducing the patient's chief complaint by pressure on that spot.

PIRIFORM SYNDROME

Sciatica may also be secondary to the piriform syndrome.[70] The pain may be poorly localized but often involves the hip, buttock, and groin and radiates down the posterolateral leg in a sciatic distribution.[71] In one large series, women were more frequently affected than men by a ratio of 6 to 1, and they often complained of dyspareunia.[71]

Since a portion of the sciatic nerve often passes through or is extremely close to the piriform muscle,[33] the nerve may become compressed and irritated when the muscle is in spasm. The result is referred pain in a truly sciatic distribution. The etiology of the piriform syndrome is uncertain in most cases.[13, 71]

The physical examination reveals normal mobility of the lumbar spine.[13] Straight leg raising may be restricted, especially when the leg is simultaneously internally rotated, as this places the piriform muscle under tension.[13] Because the piriform muscle is an abductor and external rotator of the thigh, pain and weakness may be elicited when forced abduction and external rotation of the thigh are tested in a seated position.[34, 71] The rectal examination, along with a pelvic examination in the woman, is very important in the diagnosis. Tenderness of the lateral pelvic wall is often found, and this reproduces the patient's pain.[71] The sciatic notch may also be tender.[78]

There are no diagnostic laboratory tests. The differential diagnosis includes other causes of low back, pelvic, hip, and leg pain. Unlike cases of spondylosis and radiculopathy, no neurological deficit is found in the piriform syndrome despite the fact that the sciatic nerve may be irritated. Tenderness of the lateral pelvic wall, pain and weakness of resisted hip abduction and external rotation, and pain on internal rotation of the hip are clinical clues suggestive of the piriform syndrome.[71]

Neurogenic Claudication

One cause of local back and projected pain that does not have the typical features of a monoradiculopathy has been termed neurogenic claudication. This specific clinical syndrome is usually secondary to a narrowed lumbar spinal canal, often due to lumbar spondylosis, with or without associated congenital spinal stenosis.[96, 97] The major clinical features are pain, weakness, and numbness.[45] The clinical manifestations and laboratory studies found in spinal stenosis and neurogenic claudication are reviewed in the next chapter.

CLINICAL ASSESSMENT OF THE PATIENT

This section focuses on the more frequent clinical features of neck, back, and referred pain identified during the history and physical examination that may help distinguish among the various etiologies (Table 3–2). These are general clinical features; aspects of the history and physical examination may be misleading in the assessment of any individual patient. The clinical features should only be considered a guide in the assessment of patients, for often, laboratory studies must be used to confirm the clinical impression or reveal an unexpected diagnosis.

History

The medical history is often the most important component of the evaluation of back or neck pain. The most important historical features are the location, character, onset, duration, and aggravating and palliating features of pain, because they help establish its source and mechanism. The circumstances at or prior to the onset of pain may be helpful in establishing the cause. The patient should be asked about trauma and the occurrence of similar pain in the past. A list of medications used for pain or other conditions should be obtained.

Patients should be asked to describe the pain first in their own words. If the de-

Table 3–2 SOME FREQUENT CAUSES OF SPINAL PAIN*

Traumatic or Mechanical

Musculoligamentous strain
Myofascial pain syndrome
Herniated intervertebral disc
Spondylosis (osteoarthritis; usually lower cervical or lumbar)
Spinal stenosis
Vertebral fracture
Postoperative

Metabolic

Osteopenia with vertebral collapse
Gout, Paget's disease, diabetic neuropathy

Congenital

Spondylolysis/spondylolisthesis

Neoplasms (primary and metastatic, malignant and benign)

Epidural
Extramedullary-intradural
Intramedullary
Leptomeningeal metastases

Inflammatory Diseases

Ankylosing spondylitis, rheumatoid arthritis
Arachnoiditis

Infections

Discitis, osteomyelitis, paraspinal and spinal abscess, zoster, meningitis

Referred pain

Visceral (e.g., neoplastic and inflammatory) and vascular lesions of chest, abdomen, and pelvis
Retroperitoneal lesions

Pregnancy[29]

Nonorganic Causes

Psychiatric causes
Malingering
Substance abuse

*Adapted from Howell, DS,[50] p. 1955.

scription offered by the patient is inadequate to help discriminate among the myriad etiologies, then the physician should specifically ask about these clinical manifestations. Dull, aching pain has an entirely different significance from shooting or burning pain. Aching or boring pain usually arises from locally irritated tissues, but burning pain is most suggestive of neural injury. Sharp, stabbing pains are often seen in radiculopathies. Dysesthesias and pain on tactile stimulation of the skin also point towards a neural cause.

The correct localization of pain is critical to the evaluation of patients. Many patients identify the location of pain referral and consider it to be the site of pathology. For example, patients may believe they have a hip or knee problem and become surprised or annoyed when the physician seems more concerned with their lumbar spine. Rather than use anatomical terms that may prejudice the evaluation, it is preferable to ask the patient to point to the location and extent of pain. A pain diagram drawn by the patient may be helpful.

Most mechanical causes of pain are never elucidated but are attributed to muscle strain or unusual activity despite the fact that there may be no identifiable precipitating event. As mentioned earlier, pain due to muscle strain is usually dull and aching. It is typically exacerbated by activity and self-limited with rest and mild analgesics. Individuals often awaken the morning after strenuous activity with stiffness of the neck or back accompanied by pain. When the pain has been recurrent over many years and is familiar to patients, they usually will not seek medical attention. They do frequently present when the pain is more severe than usual or when it is not identical to their previous complaint. In such cases, it is important to determine whether the other characteristics of their pain (location, type, and provocative and palliating features) are similar to those of the pain they have had in the past. As mentioned above, when the pain is exacerbated by bed rest, one should consider neoplasm or other more serious causes.

When the pain projects from the spine to other regions, associated symptoms and physical findings may help discriminate between referred and radicular pain. The patient should be queried as to associated sensory loss, weakness, or sphincter disturbances. When pain is associated with these abnormalities, a radicular component should be considered. When the pa-

tient reports that the pain is exacerbated by coughing, sneezing, and the Valsalva maneuver, it often signifies structural disease of the spine, because the epidural venous plexus, a collateral site of blood flow from intrathoracic and intra-abdominal locations, becomes engorged under these circumstances and further compromises the spinal canal.[5]

Pain secondary to cervical and lumbar spondylosis and intervertebral disc disease is common. In the cervical region, the lower cervical spine is most commonly affected. In such cases, the patient usually complains of a stiff neck and pain radiating into the shoulder and arm. The C5−6 and/or C6−7 levels are most commonly involved and posterolateral disc herniation causes compression of the nerve root at their respective levels (Fig. 3−4). In one series, the C7 root was compressed in 69 percent of cases and the C6 root in 19 percent.[113] When the C6 root is involved, pain and sensory loss typically radiate along the radial border of the forearm and hand, into the thumb. When the C7 nerve root is compressed, the sensory disturbance is more medial and tends to involve the middle finger (See dermatomal map, Fig. 2−2).

In the case of lumbar spondylosis and disc disease, the levels most commonly involved are L4−5 and L5−S1. In one study of single prolapsed lumbar intervertebral discs, the L4−5 and L5−S1 levels were involved in 97 percent of cases.[36] Among all lumbar levels, L4−5 and L5−S1 were the levels of symptomatic spondylosis causing single-level radiculopathy in 98 percent of cases.[36] Thinning of the posterior longitudinal ligament laterally along the posterior surface of the vertebral bodies and the intervertebral discs makes posterolateral herniation of the nucleus pulposus most common. In contrast to cervical roots, each lumbar nerve root exits above the corresponding intervertebral disc, so herniation of the disc most frequently compresses the exiting root just caudal to the level of disc herniation (Fig. 3−5). Consequently in lumbar disc disease, a unilateral L5 or S1 radiculopathy most commonly arises from a disc herniation at L4−5 or L5−S1, respectively.

Patients with disc disease usually com-

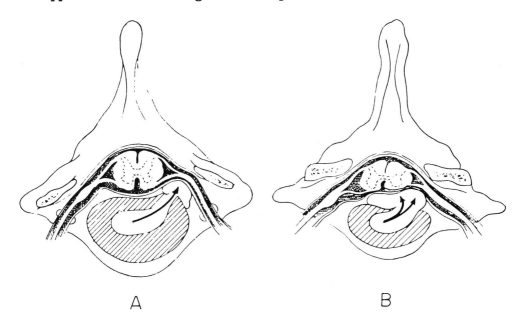

Figure 3–4. (A) Lateral cervical disc herniation causing nerve root compression. (B) Central cervical disc herniation causing spinal cord and nerve root compression. (From Adams, RD and Victor, M, [1] with permission and adapted from Kristoff, FV and Odom, GL. [57])

plain of pain in the low back and pain radiating in a sciatic distribution. When the L5 nerve root is compressed, the radicular pain radiates down the posterolateral thigh and calf to the medial aspect of the foot. When the S1 nerve root is compressed, pain radiates down the posterolateral thigh and calf to the lateral aspect of

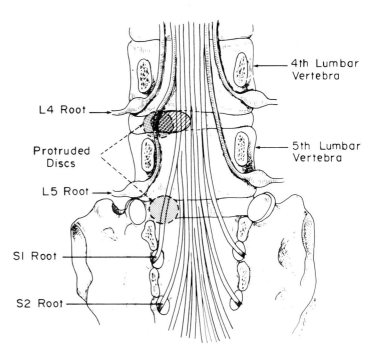

Figure 3–5. The mechanism of lateral disc herniation at L4–5 and L5–S1 causing L5 and S1 nerve root compression, respectively. A more medially placed disc protrusion may cause cauda equina compression. (From Adams, RD and Victor, M, [1] with permission.)

4th Lumbar Vertebra

L4 Root

Protruded Discs

5th Lumbar Vertebra

L5 Root

S1 Root

S2 Root

the foot. As would be expected, such radicular pain is often provoked by coughing, sneezing, and Valsalva maneuvers.

Spondylolisthesis, subluxation of one vertebral body on another, in the lower lumbar region may be asymptomatic but may also clinically present with low back pain and pain radiating into the lower extremities. In some cases, spondylolisthesis is secondary to spondylolysis, a bony defect in the pars interarticularis, but it may also be classified as degenerative, traumatic, or pathologic. With anterior subluxation of one vertebral body on another, palpation of the spinous processes may reveal a "step." Since spondylolisthesis most commonly occurs at the L5-Sl level (less commonly at L4-L5), pain in the sciatic distribution and neurologic impairments referable to the compressed nerve roots is commonly seen and must be differentiated from sciatica secondary to herniated disc disease, spondylosis and other causes. Sponylolisthesis may also cause spinal stenosis (See Chapter 4).

In obtaining the history of pain, it is imperative to review the patient's past medical history. A history of malignancy immediately suggests the possibility of metastasis even if the cancer has been considered cured for many years. A history of fever, chills, or recent infection would raise concern for a discitis and/or epidural abscess. Diabetics and patients with AIDS seem especially prone to such infections. In the young adult, insidious onset and progression of stiffness and pain that are exacerbated by rest suggest a spondyloarthropathy such as ankylosing spondylitis. A family history of back pain early in life may also suggest the possibility of one of the spondyloarthropathies. Pain in the back, buttocks, and legs that is exacerbated by walking and relieved by lying down, sitting, or bending forward might indicate lumbar spinal stenosis.

Finally, it is important in the diagnosis of back pain to consider visceral disease, which may project pain to the spine. The patient should be queried regarding a change in bowel habits, hematuria, pyuria, fever and, in women, vaginal bleeding or discharge, because pathology in any one of these organ systems may result in pain referred to the back. A recent study, for example, demonstrated that back pain and tenderness in the costovertebral angle were important findings in nearly one third of women with urinary tract infections.[108] In addition, low back pain is present in 56 percent of women during pregnancy;[29] in 45 percent of such cases, the pain radiated into the lower extremities. Finally, intrathoracic pathology may also result in upper back pain through compression of paravertebral structures or through referred pain from visceral disease (Table 2−3).

Physical Examination

To search for an undiagnosed systemic illness, the patient should undergo a thorough general physical examination. The abdominal examination may reveal evidence of an abdominal aortic aneurysm or other mass that may be the cause of back pain. A rectal exam, including stool guaiac test, should be performed to screen for cases of gastrointestinal cancer, ulcer disease, or other sources of bleeding that may relate to the back pain. In women complaining of low back pain, a thorough pelvic examination is important because pathology of pelvic viscera is such a common cause. The vascular examination should include palpation of peripheral pulses.

The examination is then directed to the musculoskeletal system, including posture and mobility. During this portion of the examination, the physician may be able to elucidate the mechanism provoking the pain. The posture and spontaneous movements of the patient are often best assessed prior to the initiation of the formal physical examination. At this time one can often identify limitation of neck or back movement due to pain and muscle spasm (or normal mobility) when the patient is unaware that he or she is being examined. If these findings are at variance with those found during the formal physical examination, they need to be reconciled.

The formal physical examination of the musculoskeletal system begins by examining the patient in the standing position. In the presence of a herniated lower lumbar disc causing sciatica, the patient may maintain the affected leg in a flexed position at the hip, knee, and ankle, preventing the heel from reaching the ground. Such a leg posture releases the traction on the sciatic nerve roots that occurs when the leg is extended, as is demonstrated with the straight-leg-raising test. The spine tends to list to the side that places the least traction on the nerve root, resulting in a functional scoliosis. When the disc is lateral to the nerve root, the list is usually away from the side of herniation, and when the disc is medial to the nerve root, the list is toward the side of herniation.[105] Although these findings are commonly seen in lumbar disc disease, they are not specific for this etiology, for they may also be found in patients with metastatic disease to the spine or other structural abnormalities of the spine.

Palpation of the entire spine and paravertebral structures is performed. Pain that can be elicited by palpation or percussion of the spine suggests structural disease at that site and in the cancer patient strongly suggests the possibility of metastasis. However, the absence of spine tenderness does not rule out the existence of spine metastasis. In one study, only 13 of 20 (65 percent) patients with epidural metastases had percussion tenderness at the time of diagnosis.[69]

The examination is then directed to identifying those positions or movements that provoke pain, as this will help elucidate the mechanism and often the source of pain. As already mentioned, movement of inflamed or irritated tissues generally causes pain and even passive movements are prevented by muscle spasm and splinting. In patients complaining of neck or back pain, a gentle attempt to flex, extend, and rotate the neck should be performed to determine if the pain arises from these structures. Passive extension of the cervical spine is especially helpful in evaluating patients with neck pain; because cervical extension narrows the intervertebral foramina, patients with cervical radiculopathy due to foraminal compromise will commonly complain of pain with cervical spine extension. If slow and gentle movement of the spine is associated with severe pain in the neck, then one should consider the possibility of major structural pathology of the spine such as fracture or dislocation.

The shoulder-abduction test has been cited as a reliable means to identify cervical monoradiculopathies secondary to extradural compressive disease such as cervical spondylosis, disc disease, and possibly neoplasm in the lower cervical spine.[15] When shoulder abduction (with the elbow in flexion) results in pain relief, the patient is considered to have a positive test and a high probability of extradural compression of a cervical nerve root.[15] Alternatively, if the abducted arm is extended at the elbow and laterally rotated (Fig. 3–6), pain is usually increased in cases of cervical root and brachial plexus disorders.[100] This latter maneuver is similar to the hyperabduction test, or Allen test, used in the diagnosis of thoracic outlet syndrome, or scalenus anticus syndrome.[17] In the case of thoracic outlet syndrome, the patient will experience an increase in symptoms with this maneuver.

If neck flexion causes pain in the thoracic or lumbar region, especially if the pain is radicular, then spinal cord compression should seriously be considered and excluded with alacrity. The following illustration demonstrates a case where the history initially suggested cranial disease, but maneuvers on physical examination led to the correct diagnosis of metastasis to the spinal column.

Case Illustration

A 42-year-old woman with known metastatic colon cancer was referred for evaluation of headaches. She was reported to have a normal neurological examination and negative head CT scan prior to neurological referral. Her headaches, primarily occipital in location, were worsened by sitting up or standing and relieved by lying down. Her neurological examination, including funduscopic examination, was normal. She had severe limitation of neck movement and paravertebral cervical muscle spasm with exacerbation of her pain with these maneuvers. Gentle downward compression of the head when she was sitting resulted in severe occipital pain.

Given the marked limitation of neck movement, a presumptive diagnosis of cervical spine metastasis was made. She was referred for cervical spine films, which demonstrated destruction of C2 vertebral body by neoplasm. A

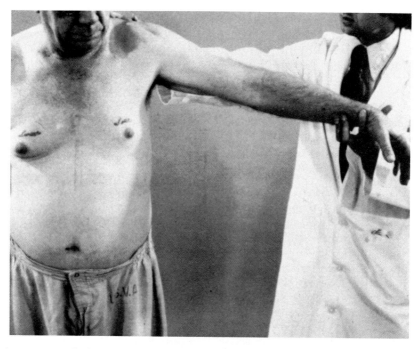

Figure 3—6. A maneuver which may produce radicular pain in a patient with cervical radiculopathy. The arm is abducted, laterally rotated and the elbow is in extension. (From Waxman, SG [100] with permission.)

CT scan with intravenous contrast through the area confirmed the diagnosis and demonstrated epidural extension of the metastasis without spinal cord compression. The patient was placed in a collar and underwent radiation therapy to the region with improvement of her pain. Although she died several months later due to widespread metastatic disease, she never developed clinical signs of spinal cord compression.

The examination of the low back includes testing mobility by forward flexion, lateral bending, rotation, and hyperextension. In cases of herniation of a lumbar disc causing compression of a nerve root, the lumbar spine often assumes a protective posture to prevent further compression or stretch of the nerve root. As described above, the direction of the list is that which places the least traction on the nerve root.[105] Under these circumstances, lateral bending to the side away from the list is usually limited.

Most causes of low back pain limit forward flexion due to the associated muscle spasm. Herniated lumbar discs and other causes of mass within the lumbar canal

(e.g., metastatic cancer or spinal sepsis) may be associated with increased pain during maneuvers that increase the lumbar lordosis, such as hyperextension of the lumbar spine.

STRAIGHT-LEG-RAISING TEST

Several clinical tests have developed over the last century to evaluate the patient with low back pain with or without radiation into the leg. The most well known is the straight-leg-raising test. Often referred to as the Lasègue sign, the test actually was described by Lasègue's student, Forst, in 1881.[23] The sciatic nerve is stretched over the ischial tuberosity as the extended leg is flexed at the hip, so that pain is elicited or exacerbated in cases where the sciatic nerve or root is already compressed.[23] Forst proposed the test as a means of differentiating hip disease from sciatica but, as noted below, the maneuver does not confidently do this.

The straight-leg-raising test is performed on the supine patient by flexing the thigh at the hip with the knee extended

(Fig. 3–7). If pain radiating down the leg in a sciatic distribution is provoked, then the test results are considered positive. If the foot is also dorsiflexed during the straight leg raising, the pain will often be intensified.

Positive results on the straight-leg-raising test are often considered evidence for L5 or S1 nerve root compression as often occurs with herniated discs at L4–5 and L5–S1, respectively. It was shown by Falconer at surgical operation that the L5 nerve root moves 2–6 mm caudally during the act of straight leg raising,[27, 28a] supporting this concept. Positive results on the straight-leg-raising test may also be seen in diseases of the hip, thigh, and pelvis, however, and are not, therefore, specific for lumbar spine disease and radiculopathy. This impression was confirmed in a recent neurosurgical series[51] (intended to study patients with herniated discs and, therefore, excluding patients with spinal tumors) in which patients with low back pain, leg pain, or both were tested for straight leg raising. Of 351 patients with positive results, only 64 percent proved to have a disc herniation. This study underscores the lack of specificity of this sign. Moreover, positive results are not invariably present in cases of prolapsed lower lumbar intervertebral discs. One study found that only 80 percent of individuals with surgically proven herniated lower lumbar discs had positive results on straight-leg-raising tests.[26]

Occasional patients report sciatica and appear to have positive results but actually have a nonorganic component to their pain. In order to distinguish between organic and nonorganic pain, the flip test has been recommended.[90, 98] This maneuver is a modification of the straight-leg-raising test and is performed on the seated patient by extending the knee. When it is performed as described by Waddell and colleagues[98] to identify a nonorganic component to pain, the patient is distracted during the maneuver. One method of performing the test involves extending the leg at the knee with the patient in a seated position in order to test the plantar reflex. The patient with a nonorganic component to sciatic-type pain may report pain with straight leg raising but no pain with the flip test.[98] Waddell and colleagues[98] have presented several nonorganic physical signs in low back pain that they recommend as part of the evaluation of these patients. Even so, the presence of such a nonorganic sign does not rule out the possibility of coexisting organic diesase.

CROSSED-STRAIGHT-LEG-RAISING TEST

Another helpful clinical test is the crossed-straight-leg-raising test. This test is performed in a manner similar to the straight-leg-raising test, but in this case, positive results are defined as pain projected to the affected leg when the unaffected leg is raised. Positive results are explained by the observation that straight leg raising causes the contralateral as well as the ipsilateral L5 and S1 roots to be pulled caudally.

Woodhall and Hayes[110] found that of 95 patients with positive results, 90 had a herniated disc at laminectomy. All but two of the herniated discs were at the L4–5 or L5–S1 level. In another study, 54 of 56 (97 percent) patients who had positive results were found to have a herniated disc.[51] These findings suggest that the test is highly specific for localizing disease to the spine. Although herniated discs were found in these two studies, spinal tumors

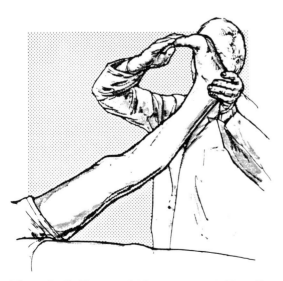

Figure 3–7. The straight-leg-raising test. (From De-Jong, RN, [17] with permission.)

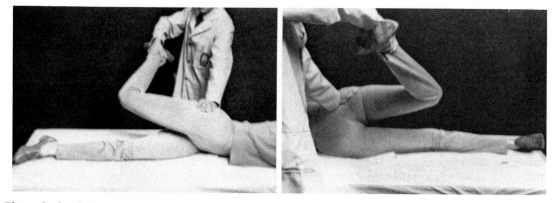

Figure 3—8. The "reversed-straight-leg-raising test." Left, anterior view. Right, posterior view. (From Jabre, JF and Bryan, RW, [52] with permission.)

in the same location also may give rise to positive results on this test. Thus, positive results on this test more accurately indicate a compressive lesion in the lower lumbar spinal canal than do positive results on the straight-leg-raising test. When the subjective response has been accurately reported and interpreted, this sign is exceedingly reliable in localizing disease to the spine. In our experience, cases in which the localization has been misleading have been those rare patients with severe metastatic disease to the pelvis. In that instance, any movement of one leg may cause pain in the contralateral leg as well.

REVERSED-STRAIGHT-LEG-RAISING TEST

A useful clinical test to evaluate patients with suspected upper lumbar spine disease and radiculopathies is termed the femoral-nerve-traction test[22, 27, 52] or the reversed-straight-leg-raising test. The test is not specific for spinal disease or a radiculopathy, as positive results are often seen with femoral neuropathy due to ischemia in diabetes mellitus or with retroperitoneal masses such as psoas hematoma or abscess.

The test may be performed with the patient lying on the painless side and with the neck flexed to increase tension on the cauda equina. The painful leg is then pulled back by the examiner to hyperextend it at the hip and then the knee is flexed, further stretching the upper lum-

bar roots (Fig. 3—8). In an alternative technique, the test may be performed by flexing the knee of the patient, who is in a prone position. In cases of L3 radiculopathy, pain will often radiate to the anterior thigh. In cases of L4 radiculopathy, the pain is more apt to radiate below the knee. The results of this test are negative in cases of L5 and S1 radiculopathies[52] but positive in cases of upper lumbar radiculopathy.

PATRICK'S MANEUVER

Buttock, hip, and knee pain may arise from hip disease such as metastasis, osteoarthritis, or infection. The location and pattern of pain referral is often similar to that of radicular pain arising from the lumbar spine. When positive, the Patrick sign is often helpful in localizing the source of pain to the hip.[17, 49]

This test is performed by placing the heel of the lower extremity being tested on the contralateral knee; downward and outward pressure is then exerted on the ipsilateral knee. The resultant movement is flexion, abduction, and external rotation of the involved hip. Flexion of the knee helps to relieve tension on the nerve roots. If the patient's pain complaint is reproduced in the hip or ipsilateral thigh, the hip may be the source of pain. Since stretch is not placed on the sciatic nerve with this test, Patrick's maneuver helps in distinguishing between sciatica and referred pain from the hip. Other lesions of the pelvis and lower extremity such as metastases, of course, may also give rise to a positive Patrick sign.

Neurological Examination

When abnormalities are found on the neurological examination, they may not only localize the level of the lesion but may also suggest the etiology. For example, as already mentioned, cervical disc disease most frequently occurs at the C5−6 and C6−7 levels and lumbar disc disease most frequently involves the L4−5 and L5−S1 levels. Although metastases, infection, or other diseases may be responsible, when radicular signs place the lesion at these levels, spondylosis and disc disease are prominent considerations. When the neurological signs localize the lesion to levels other than these, while spondylosis may be the cause, there is a greater likelihood of other causes. One of the most common sources of delay in diagnosis of metastatic cancer to the spine occurs when the physician attributes neurological abnormalities to spondylosis and disc disease in the upper lumbar region or thoracic area; these are levels that are rarely involved clinically in these disorders.

Deep tendon reflexes should be tested carefully to detect asymmetry. In the upper extremity, depressed or asymmetric reflexes at the biceps (C5, C6), brachioradialis (C5, C6), or triceps (C7) are often seen in association with cervical spondylosis at these levels. Asymmetrical Hoffmann's reflex suggests pathology at the C7−T1 level or the lower brachial plexus levels, which is not common for spondylosis but is frequently found in patients with superior sulcus tumors.[73] In the lower extremity, an absent ankle jerk (S1) is a common finding in lumbar spondylosis and disc disease. However, an absent knee reflex is an unusual sign of spondylosis because over 90 percent of herniated lumbar discs occur at the L4−5 or L5−S1 levels.[36]

Muscle strength, bulk, and tone are usually not severely affected in cases of monoradiculopathy. Some abnormalities may be found, however, in cases of radiculopathy upon testing muscles that receive a preponderance of innervation from the affected nerve root. These segment-pointer muscles[83] are presented in Chapter 2. However, muscle spasm and guarding may be responsible for abnormalities. If the abnormalities are thought to be related to pain, the examination should be repeated after the pain has been controlled with analgesics.

In suspected spine disease, the sensory examination is performed to distinguish between a sensory level and a dermatomal sensory loss. When sensory testing is performed in patients suffering from peripheral neuropathy, decreased sensation distally in the lower extremities is often found. This distal type of sensory loss is not necessarily confined to the limbs. In many peripheral neuropathies, there is a relative invariance over the entire body surface of the distance from the spinal or cranial root of origin to the border of normal sensation.[81] If the neuropathy is advanced, sensory loss over the distal part of the intercostal distribution in the midanterior trunk, may be seen in the context of sensory loss in the distal limbs.[9] This anterior distribution of truncal sensory loss widens with progression of the neuropathy (Fig. 3−9A and B). Anterior truncal sensory loss due to peripheral neuropathy can be mistakenly attributed to a spinal cord lesion. Confusion can be avoided if the sensory examination includes the back and buttocks, because the thoracic, lumbar, and sacral dermatomes are represented posteriorly as well as anteriorly. The distinction between sensory loss due to peripheral neuropathy and that due to spinal cord pathology often needs to be made in patients with cancer receiving vinca alkaloids who complain of numbness of their legs, because these drugs commonly cause a peripheral neuropathy. Such patients may also have painful dysesthesias of the distal legs secondary to the peripheral neuropathy. If they complain of back, neck, or radicular pain, or if they have a sensory level on the trunk, their symptoms should not be attributed to peripheral neuropathy; they should be considered candidates for a diagnosis of spinal disease.

Superficial reflexes are often abnormal in patients suffering from spinal cord or cauda equina disease. The pathophysiol-

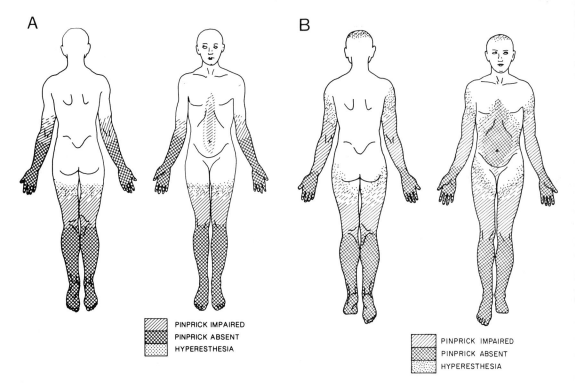

Figure 3–9. (A) Sensory map in patient with moderately advanced diabetic neuropathy. Note distal sensory loss in arms and legs, and in the most distal part of the territory served by truncal nerves. (B) Sensory map in severe diabetic neuropathy. Sensory loss has progressed to include anterior thorax, in addition to the arms and legs which show an advanced "glove-and-stocking" pattern. Note that unless the posterior thorax is examined, the pattern of sensory loss over the trunk can be confused with a sensory level due to spinal cord compression. (From Waxman, SG and Sabin, TD, [102] with permission.)

ogy and methods of obtaining the superficial abdominal, cremasteric, anal, and Babinski reflexes were reviewed in Chapter 2. It should be emphasized that in spinal cord disease involving descending pathways, there may be an increase in deep tendon reflexes in conjunction with a diminution of superficial abdominal, anal, and cremasteric reflexes. This dissociation of reflexes should alert the physician to pathology of the pyramidal tracts.

Laboratory and Diagnostic Imaging Studies

In most cases of acute low back or neck pain where the history and physical examination do not lead to a suspicion of serious underlying disease, no laboratory investigations are required, as the pain is often due to musculoligamentous strain and is self-limited. However, these patients require close clinical observation before one can confidently exclude more serious underlying pathology.

In persistent or atypical cases, or if the history and physical examination lead to the suspicion of underlying systemic disease, a more thorough evaluation should be undertaken. Any relevant leads already uncovered should be pursued. In addition, a CBC, sedimentation rate, urinalysis, and serum chemistry profile may yield clues to the existence and identity of more serious disease. For example, acid phosphatase or prostatic specific antigen may be elevated in men with carcinoma of the prostate. If multiple myeloma is in the differential diagnosis, a serum and urine protein electrophoresis may be helpful. When inflammatory disease is suspected, a tuberculin test, antinuclear antibody, rheumatoid factor, HLA B-27, and other screening studies for autoimmune and infectious causes may be helpful.

In 1977, back pain was the most common symptom associated with roentgenogram use in ambulatory settings in the U.S.[18] In most cases, the purpose of ordering such plain films is to detect serious underlying diseases such as cancer, fractures, infections, and spondyloarthropathies. Although compression fractures may be seen in 3 percent of cases, cancer is found in approximately 6 per 1,000 cases and vertebral osteomyelitis is seen in 1 in 100,000 patients with acute low back pain in primary care settings.[18, 19, 32] In an attempt to establish selective criteria for ordering radiological studies in the patient with acute low back pain, Deyo and Diehl[19] suggested in 1986 that spinal radiographs are indicated when the patient meets any of the following criteria:

1. When the patient is over 50 years of age.
2. When there has been significant trauma.
3. When the history or physical examination suggests ankylosing spondylitis or demonstrates a neuromotor deficit.
4. When there is a history of drug or alcohol abuse, a history of treatment with corticosteroids, or temperature over 37.8°C.
5. When there is a history of cancer, pain at rest, or unexplained weight loss.
6. When there has been a recent visit for the same problem, which has not improved.
7. When the patient is seeking compensation.

In a more recent study, however, Frazier and colleagues[32] concluded that adoption of these criteria would increase the use of roentgenographic studies. The difficulty in establishing strict criteria for the use of roentgenographic studies for this problem remains.[18]

In cases of subacute or chronic back pain, spine films are often performed. Since radiological studies often reveal cervical and/or lumbar spondylosis in asymptomatic individuals,[39, 44, 66, 109] however, the physician must be wary of attributing a patient's symptom or sign to a finding that may be incidental and asymptomatic. This section reviews some of the more common abnormal radiological findings in the asymptomatic general population.

In a recent epidemiological study of the frequency of abnormal spine radiographs, plain anteroposterior and lateral films of the lumbar spine were taken in a randomly selected group of men between the ages of 18 and 55.[39] One group had a history of no low back pain, the second group had a history of moderate low back pain, and the third had severe low back pain. The authors found no difference among these groups in the incidence of transitional vertebrae, Schmorl's nodes, narrowing of the disc spaces between the third and fourth lumbar vertebrae and between the fifth lumbar and first sacral vertebrae, or of other abnormalities. Only the presence of traction spurs and/or disc space narrowing between the fourth and fifth lumbar vertebrae correlated with the symptoms of severe low back pain and numbness, weakness, and pain in the lower extremities. As in other studies,[39, 40] these authors found a high degree of interobserver variation in the interpretation of conventional roentgenograms, which might have contributed to the lack of correlation between the patients' histories and the radiological studies. As noted below, similar findings have been reported with other imaging modalities.

In a study using CT scanning of the lumbar spine in a group of asymptomatic adults, 35 percent were abnormal.[107] Over 50 percent of individuals over 40 years of age had abnormal scans. The most common abnormality in the entire group of asymptomatic subjects was a herniated nucleus pulposus, found in 20 percent of individuals.

Similarly, radiological evidence of cervical spondylosis has been reported in a large proportion of individuals without specific complaints.[35] Such evidence was found on the plain films of 50 percent of individuals over the age of 50 and 75 percent of those over the age of 65;[72] many of these individuals were asymptomatic.

The abnormalities found on plain x-ray and CT scanning have been corroborated by the findings on total spine myelography in asymptomatic patients. In a study of

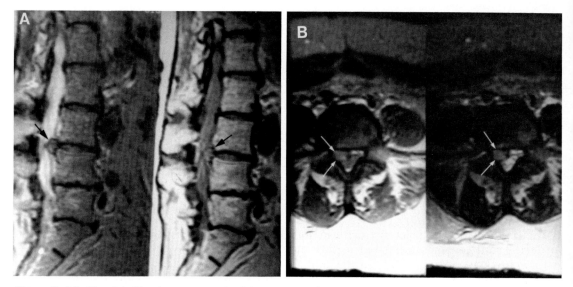

Figure 3–10. Herniated lumbar intervertebral disc (arrows) demonstrated on MRI. (A) Sagittal image. (B) Axial image. (Courtesy of Dr. Helmuth Gehbauer)

total myelograms incidentally performed in the evaluation of possible acoustic neuromas, 37 percent of 300 otherwise asymptomatic individuals with no history of neck, back, or radicular pain had spinal abnormalities on their myelograms.[48] The abnormalities ranged from deformed nerve root sleeves and ruptured discs to nearly complete obstruction. The defects were solitary in 19 percent and multiple in 18 percent. Lumbar abnormalities were present in 24 percent and cervical abnormalities in 21 percent of these asymptomatic individuals.

In a smaller study of asymptomatic intervertebral disc protrusions, McCrae[63] performed postmortem myelograms and dissections of 18 complete spines in individuals over 30 years of age. He concluded that "nearly everybody, 40 years of age or older, has at least one posterior cervical and one posterior lumbar disc protrusion."[63]

These reports underscore the importance of making a correct clinical diagnosis and not relying exclusively on the radiological studies in the absence of clinical data. Radiographic studies in many cases demonstrate structural abnormalities that are not related to the patient's complaint. With its exquisite sensitivity,

MRI is expected to increase the frequency of identifying asymptomatic abnormalities[58, 94, 103] (Fig. 3–10).

Management

In the vast majority of cases, acute low back and neck pain are self-limited disorders in which no specific pathoanatomic diagnosis can be made and no specific therapy is required. In such cases, the term musculoligamentous strain is often used. In some of these cases, however, the pain is sufficient to require a brief period of bed rest, anti-inflammatory agents, analgesics, and local heat. In the case of neck pain, a collar and cervical traction may be used with benefit. A recent study of the duration of bed rest for acute mechanical low back pain without significant neurological deficit showed that 2 days of bed rest were as effective as 7 days.[21] Because non-narcotic analgesics are usually effective, the use of narcotics should be strictly limited. After the acute bout of pain, exercise programs may be used to reduce the risk of recurrence.[38]

The management of cases of low back pain with or without radicular pain due to a herniated lumbar disc is similar to that of mechanical low back pain just discussed, except that the necessary period of bed rest is often longer. It is important to reassure the patient that in the majority of cases of low back pain (with or without sciatica) due to a herniated lumbar disc, the pain will resolve with nonsurgical therapy.[80] The use of bed rest, analgesics, anti-inflammatory agents, and muscle relaxants, along with avoidance of activities that provoke leg pain, is usually sufficient. In most cases of severe pain, bed rest should be complete except for bathroom privileges until there is significant improvement of pain. Gradual increase in activity is allowed as the pain permits; activities that exacerbate the radicular pain should be avoided. Usually pain from a herniated disc improves with such conservative treatment and the patient will benefit from instruction in an exercise program to prevent recurrence of pain.

Some physicians recommend that in suspected herniated lumbar disc disease, if after one week of conservative therapy there are no signs of improvement of pain and amount of tolerated straight leg raising, radiological studies and other laboratory studies be undertaken to exclude other serious pathology, and consideration be given, when appropriate, to referral to a surgeon or other specialist.[80] Indications for surgery of lumbar disc disease are discussed in Chapter 4, as is the management of herniated cervical discs.

The management of chronic low back pain and sciatica, as in the case of other chronic illnesses, requires definition of the pathophysiological mechanism. Therefore, in addition to the history and physical examination, laboratory and radiological examinations should be undertaken to identify serious underlying disease. In the majority of cases, however, lumbar spondylosis and/or herniated disc disease is found and the management options again include nonsurgical and surgical intervention discussed above. According to Frymoyer,[38] less than 10 percent of patients with unrelenting sciatica require an operation; thus the management of most patients includes the nonsurgical approaches discussed earlier, supplemented, when necessary, with a multidisciplinary chronic pain management program.[38]

REFERENCES

1. Adams, RD and Victor, M: Diseases of the spinal cord. In Adams, RD and Victor, M (eds): Principles of Neurology, ed 3. McGraw-Hill, New York, 1985, pp 665–698.
2. Austin, GM: The significance and nature of pain in tumors of the spinal cord. Surgical Forum 10:782–785, 1959.
3. Baldwin, RN and Chadwick, D: Lhermitte's "sign" due to thoracic cord compression (letter to the editor). J Neurol Neurosurg Psychiatry 49:840–841, 1986.
4. Barron, KD, Hirano, A, Araki, S, et al: Experiences with metastatic neoplasms involving the spinal cord. Neurology 9:91–106, 1959.
5. Batson, OV: The function of the vertebral veins and their role in the spread of metastases. Ann Surg 112:138–148, 1940.
6. Bernard, TN and Kirkaldy-Willis, WH: Recognizing specific characteristics of nonspecific low back pain. Spine 217:266–280, 1987.
7. Bogduk, N: The innervation of the lumbar spine. Spine 8:286–293, 1983.
8. Bogduk, N, Tynan, W, and Wilson, AS: The nerve supply to the human lumbar intervertebral discs. J Anat 132:29–56, 1981.
9. Bolton, B: Blood supply of the human spinal cord. J Neurol Neurosurg Psychiatry 2:137–148, 1939.
10. Bonica, JJ: Historical, socioeconomic and diagnostic aspects of the problem. In Carron, H and McLaughlin, RE (eds): Management of Low Back Pain. The Stonebridge Press, Bristol, 1982, pp 1–15.
11. Booth, RE and Rothman, RH: Cervical angina. Spine 1:28–32, 1976.
12. Brodsky, A: Cervical angina: A correlative study with emphasis on the use of coronary arteriography. Spine 10:699–709, 1985.
13. Cailliet, R: Low Back Pain Syndrome, ed 3. FA Davis, Philadelphia, 1981.
14. Cypress, BK: Characteristics of physician visits for back symptoms: A national perspective. Am J Public Health 73:389–395, 1983.
15. Davidson, RI, Dunn, EJ, and Metzmaker, JN: The shoulder abduction test in the diagnosis of radicular pain in cervical extradural compressive monoradiculopathies. Spine 6:441–446, 1981.
16. DeJong, RN: Sensation. In Vinken, PJ and Bruyn, GW (eds): Handbook of Clinical Neurology, Vol 1. North-Holland Publishing, Amsterdam, 1969, pp 80–113.
17. DeJong, RN: The Neurologic Examination, ed 4. Harper & Row, Hagerstown, Md, 1979.
18. Deyo, RA: Plain roentgenography for low-back pain: Finding needles in a haystack (editorial). Arch Intern Med 149:27–29, 1989.

19. Deyo, RA and Diehl, AK: Lumbar spine films in primary care: Current use and effects of selective ordering criteria. J Gen Intern Med 1:20–25, 1986.
20. Deyo, RA and Diehl, AK: Cancer as a cause of back pain: Frequency, clinical presentation and diagnostic strategies. J Gen Intern Med 3:230–238, 1988.
21. Deyo, RA, Diehl, AK, and Rosenthal, M: How many days of bed rest for acute low back pain? A randomized clinical trial. N Engl J Med 315:1064–1070, 1986.
22. Dyck, P: The femoral nerve traction test with lumbar disc protrusion. Surg Neurol 6:163–166, 1976.
23. Dyck, P: Lumbar nerve root: The enigmatic eponyms. Spine 9:3–6, 1984.
24. Edgar, MA and Ghadially, JA: Innervation of the lumbar spine. Clin Orthop 115:35–41, 1976.
25. Edgar, MA and Nundy, S: Innervation of the spinal dura mater. J Neurol Neurosurg Psychiatry 29:530–534, 1966.
26. Edgar, MA and Park, WM: Induced pain patterns on passive straight-leg raising in lower lumbar disc protrusion. J Bone Joint Surg 56B:658–667, 1974.
27. Estridge, MN, Rouhe, SA, and Johnson, NG: The femoral stretching test: A valuable sign in diagnosing upper lumbar disc herniations. J Neurosurg 57:813–817, 1982.
28. Fairbank, JCT, Park, WM, McCall, IA, et al: Apophyseal injection of local anesthetic as a diagnostic aid in primary low-back pain syndromes. Spine 6:598–605, 1981.
28a. Falconer, MA, McGeorge, M and Begg, AC: Observations on the cause and mechanism of symptom-production in sciatica and low-back pain. J Neurol Neurosurg Psychiatry 11:13–26, 1948.
29. Fast, A, Shapiro, D, Ducommun, EJ, et al: Low-back pain in pregnancy. Spine 12:368–371, 1987.
30. Fielding, JW, Burstein, AH, and Frankel, VH: The nuchal ligament. Spine 1:3–14, 1976.
31. Foley, KM: Pain syndromes in patients with cancer. Med Clin North Am 71:169–184, 1987.
32. Frazier, LM, Carey, TS, Lyles, MF, et al: Selective criteria may increase lumbosacral spine roentgenogram use in acute low–back pain. Arch Intern Med 149:47–50, 1989.
33. Frieberg, AH: Sciatic pain and its relief by operations on muscle and fascia. Arch Surg 34:337–350, 1937.
34. Freiburg, AH and Vinke, TH: Sciatica and the sacro-iliac joint. J Bone J Surg 16:126–136, 1934.
35. Freidenberg, ZB and Miller, WT: Degenerative disc disease of the cervical spine: A comparative study of asymptomatic and symptomatic patients. J Bone Joint Surg 45A:1171–1178, 1963.
36. Friis, ML, Gulliksen, GC, and Rasmussen, P: Distribution of pain with nerve root compression. Acta Neurosurgica 39:241, 1977.
37. Frykholm, R, Norlen, G, and Skoglund, CR: On pain sensations produced by stimulation of ventral roots in man. Acta Physiol Scand 29:455–469, 1953.
38. Frymoyer, JW: Back pain and sciatica. N Engl J Med 318:291–300, 1988.
39. Frymoyer, JW, Newberg, A, Pope, MH, Wilder, DG, Clements, J, and MacPherson, B: Spine radiographs in patients with low-back pain. J Bone Joint Surg 66A:1048–1055, 1984.
40. Frymoyer, JW, Phillips, RB, Newberg, AH, et al: A comparative analysis of the interpretations of lumbar spinal radiographs by chiropractors and medical doctors. Spine 11:1020–1023, 1986.
41. Galasko, CSB: The anatomy and pathways of skeletal metastases. In Weiss, L and Gilbert, HA (eds): Bone Metastasis. GK Hall, Boston, 1981, pp 49–63.
42. Guidetti, B and Fortuna, A: Differential diagnosis of intramedullary and extramedullary tumors. In Vinken, PJ and Bruyn, GW (eds): Handbook of Clinical Neurology, Vol 19. North-Holland Publishing, Amsterdam, 1975, pp 51–75.
43. Hadler, N: Regional back pain (editorial). N Engl J Med 315:1090–1092, 1986.
44. Hall, FM: Overutilization of radiological examinations. Radiology 120:443–448, 1976.
45. Hall, SH, Bartleson, JD, Onofrio, BM, et al: Lumbar spinal stenosis: Clinical features, diagnostic procedures, and results of surgical treatment in 68 patients. Ann Intern Med 103:271–275, 1985.
46. Hirsch, C: An attempt to diagnose the level of a disc lesion clinically by disc puncture. Acta Orthop Scand 18:132–140, 1948.
47. Hirsch, C, Ingelmark, B-E, and Miller, M: The anatomical basis for low back pain: Studies on the presence of nerve endings in ligamentous capsular and intervertebral disc structures in the human lumbar spine. Acta Orthop Scand 33:1–17, 1963.
48. Hitselberger, WE and Witten, RM: Abnormal myelograms in asymptomatic patients. J Neurosurg 28:204–206, 1968.
49. Hoppenfeld, S: Physical Examination of Spine and Extremities. Appleton-Century-Crofts, New York, 1976.
50. Howell, DS: The painful back. In Wyngaarden, JB and Smith, LH (eds): Cecil Textbook of Medicine, ed 17. WB Saunders, Philadelphia, 1985, p 1955.
51. Hudgins, WR: The crossed straight leg raising test: A diagnostic sign of herniated disc. J Occup Med 21:407–408, 1979.
52. Jabre, JF and Bryan, RW: Bent-knee pulling in the diagnosis of upper lumbar root lesions. Arch Neurol 39:669–670, 1982.
53. Jackson, HC, Winkelman, RK, and Bickel, WH: Nerve endings in the human lumbar spinal column and related structures. J Bone Joint Surg 48A:1272–1281, 1966.
54. Kellgren, JH: On the distribution of pain arising from deep somatic structures with charts of

segmental pain areas. Clin Sci 4:35–46, 1939.

55. Kelsey, JL and White, AA: Epidemiology and impact of low-back pain. Spine 5:133–142, 1980.

56. Kimmel, D: Innervation of spinal dura mater and dura mater of the posterior cranial fossa. Neurology 10:800–809, 1961.

57. Kristoff, FV and Odom, GL: Ruptured intervertebral disc in the cervical region. Arch Surg 54:287–304, 1947.

58. Lee, SH, Coleman, PE, and Hahn, FJ: Magnetic resonance imaging of degenerative disk disease of the spine. Radiol Clin North Am 26:949–964, 1988.

59. Lhermitte, J and Bollak, NM: Les douleurs a type de decharge electrique consecutives a la flexion cephalique dans la sclerose en plaque. Rev Neurol (Paris) 31:36–52, 1924.

60. Lippitt, AB: The facet joint and its role in spine pain: Management with facet joint injections. Spine 9:746–750, 1984.

61. Malinsky, J: The ontogenetic development of nerve terminations in the intervertebral discs of man. Acta Anat 38:96–113, 1959.

62. McCall, IW, Park, WM, and O'Brien, JP: Induced pain referral from posterior lumbar elements in normal subjects. Spine 4:441–446, 1979.

63. McCrae, DL: Asymptomatic intervertebral disc protrusions. Acta Radiol 46:9–27, 1956.

64. Mooney, V: Where is the pain coming from? Spine 12:754–759, 1987.

65. Mooney, V and Robertson, J: The facet syndrome. Clin Orthop 115:149–156, 1976.

66. Nachemson, AL: The lumbar spine: An orthopaedic challenge. Spine 1:59–71, 1976.

67. Nicholas, JJ and Christy, WC: Spinal pain made worse by recumbency: A clue to spinal cord tumors. Arch Phys Med Rehabil 67:598–600, 1986.

68. O'Brien, JP: Mechanisms of spinal pain. In Wall, PD and Melzak, R (eds): Textbook of Pain. Churchill Livingstone, Edinburgh, 1984.

69. O'Rourke, T, George, CB, Redmond, J, et al: Spinal computed tomography and computed tomographic metrizamide myelography in the early diagnosis of metastatic disease. J Clin Oncol 4:576–583, 1986.

70. Pace, JB and Naghle, D: Piriform syndrome. West J Med 124:435–439, 1976.

71. Pace, JB: Commonly overlooked pain syndromes. Postgrad Med 58:107–113, 1975.

72. Pallis, C, Jones, AM, and Spillane, JD: Cervical spondylosis. Brain 77:274–289, 1954.

73. Pancoast, HK: Superior pulmonary sulcus tumor: Tumor characterized by pain, Horner's syndrome, destruction of bone and atrophy of hand muscles. JAMA 99:1391–1396, 1932.

74. Parke, WW: Applied anatomy of the spine. In Rothman, RH and Simeone, FA (eds): The Spine. WB Saunders, Philadelphia, 1982, pp 18–51.

75. Posner, JB: Back pain and epidural spinal cord compression. Med Clin North Am 71:185–204, 1987.

76. Rasmussen, TB, Kernohan, JW, and Adson, AW: Pathologic classification, with surgical consideration, of intraspinal tumors. Ann Surg 111:513–530, 1940.

77. Reisbord, LS and Greenland, S: Factors associated with self-reported back pain prevalence: A population-based study. J Chronic Dis 38:691–702, 1985.

78. Robinson, DR: Piriformis syndrome in relation to sciatic pain. Am J Surg 73:355–358, 1947.

79. Roofe, PG: Innervation of annulus fibrosus and posterior longitudinal ligament. Archives of Neurology and Psychiatry 44:100–103, 1940.

80. Rybock, JD: Acute back pain and disc herniation. In Johnson, RT (ed): Current Therapy in Neurological Disease—2. BC Decker, Toronto, 1987, pp 48–50.

81. Sabin, TD, Geschwind, N, and Waxman, SG: Patterns of clinical deficit in peripheral nerve disease. In Waxman, SG (ed): Physiology and Pathobiology of Axons. Raven Press, New York, 1978, pp 431–439.

82. Sandyk, R and Brennan, MJW: Lhermitte's sign as a presenting symptom of subacute degeneration of the cord. Ann Neurol 13:215–216, 1983.

83. Schliack, H: Segmental innervation and the clinical aspects of spinal nerve root syndromes. In Vinken, PJ and Bruyn, GW (eds): Handbook of Clinical Neurology, Vol 2. North-Holland Publishing, Amsterdam, 1969, pp 157–177.

84. Selby, DK and Paris, SV: Anatomy of facet joints and its clinical correlation with low back pain. Contemporary Orthopaedics 3:20–23, 1981.

85. Shenkin, HA and Alpers, BJ: Clinical and pathological features of gliomas of the spinal cord. Arch Neurol Psychiatry 52:87–105, 1944.

86. Sherman, MS: The nerves of bone. J Bone Joint Surg 45A:522–528, 1963.

87. Simons, DG and Travell, JG: Myofascial origins of low back pain. Postgrad Med 73:66–108, 1983.

88. Simons, DG and Travell, JG: Myofascial Pain and Dysfunction: The Trigger Point Manual. Williams & Wilkins, Baltimore, 1983.

89. Simons, DG and Travell, JG: Myofascial Pain Syndromes. In Wall, PD and Melzack, R (eds): Textbook of Pain. Churchill Livingstone, Edinburgh, 1984, pp 263–276.

90. Simpson, JF: Meningeal Signs. In Vinken, PJ and Bruyn, GW (eds): Handbook of Clinical Neurology, Vol 1. North-Holland Publishing, Amsterdam, 1969, p 546.

91. Sinclair, DC, Feindel, WH, and Falconer, MA: The intervertebral ligaments as a source of segmental pain. J Bone Joint Surg 30B:515–521, 1948.

92. Smith, KJ and McDonald, WI: Spontaneous and mechanically evoked activity due to central

demyelinating lesions. Nature 286:154–155, 1980.

93. Stillwell, DL: The nerve supply of the vertebral column and its associated structures in the monkey. Anat Rec 125:132–140, 1948.

94. Sze, G: Gadolinium-DTPA in spinal disease. Radiol Clin North Am 26:1009–1024, 1988.

95. Torma, T: Malignant tumors of the spine and the spinal extradural space. Acta Chir Scand (Suppl)225:1–176, 1957.

96. Verbiest, H: Further experiences on the pathologic influence of a developmental narrowness of the bony lumbar vertebral canal. J Bone Joint Surg 37:576–583, 1955.

97. Verbiest, H: The significance and principles of computerized axial tomography in idiopathic developmental stenosis of the lumbar vertebral canal. Spine 4:369–378, 1979.

98. Waddell, G, McCulloch, JA, Kummel, E, et al: Nonorganic physical signs in low-back pain. Spine 5:117–125, 1980.

99. Walther, PJ, Rossitch, E, and Bullard, DE: The development of Lhermitte's sign during cisplatin chemotherapy: Possible drug-induced toxicity causing spinal cord demyelination. Cancer 60:2170–2172, 1987.

100. Waxman, SG: The flexion-adduction sign in neuralgic amyotrophy. Neurology 29:1301–1304, 1979.

101. Waxman, SG: Clinicopathological correlations in multiple sclerosis and related diseases. In Waxman, SG and Ritchie, JM (eds): Demyelinating Diseases: Basic and Clinical Electrophysiology. Raven Press, New York, 1981, pp 169–182.

102. Waxman, SG and Sabin, TD: Diabetic truncal polyneuropathy. Arch Neurol 38:46–47, 1981.

103. Weisz, GM and Kitchener, PN: The use of MR in diagnosing postoperative lumbar conditions. Med J Aust 146:99–101, 1987.

104. Weisz, GM, Lamond, TS, and Kitchener, PN: Spinal imaging: Will MRI replace myelography? Spine 13:65–68, 1988.

105. Weitz, EM: The lateral bending sign. Spine 6:388–397, 1981.

106. Wiberg, G: Back pain in relation to the nerve supply of the intervertebral disc. Acta Orthopaedica 19:211–221, 1947.

107. Wiesel, SW, Tsourmas, N, Feffer, HL, et al: A study of computer-assisted tomography. 1. The incidence of positive CAT scans in an asymptomatic group of patients. Spine 9:549–551, 1984.

108. Wigton, RS, Hoellerich, VL, Ornato, JP, Leu, V, Mazzotta, LA, and Cheng, I-H: Use of clinical findings in the diagnosis of urinary tract infection in women. Arch Intern Med 145:2222–2227, 1985.

109. Witt, I, Vestergaard, A, and Rosenklint, A: A comparative analysis of X-ray findings of the lumbar spine in patients with and without lumbar pain. Spine 9:298–300, 1984.

110. Woodhall, B and Hayes, GJ: The well-leg-raising test of Fajerstajn in the diagnosis of ruptured lumbar intervertebral disc. J Bone Joint Surg 32A:786–792, 1950.

111. Word, JA, Kalokhe, UP, Aron, BS, and Elson, HR: Transient radiation myelopathy (Lhermitte's sign) in patients with Hodgkin's disease treated by mantle radiation. Int J Radiat Oncol Biol Phys 6:1731–1733, 1980.

112. Yoshizawa, H, O'Brien, JP, Smith, WT, et al: The neuropathology of intervertebral discs removed for low back pain. J Pathol 132:95–104, 1980.

113. Yoss, RE, Corbin, KB, MacCarty, CS, and Love, JG: Significance of symptoms and signs in localization of involved root in cervical disc protrusion. Neurology 7:673–683, 1957.

Chapter 4

NON-NEOPLASTIC CAUSES OF SPINAL CORD COMPRESSION

SPONDYLOSIS

Spondylosis, a common cause of pain and disability in middle and later years, frequently occurs in the cervical and lumbar regions. In the cervical spine, it is a common cause of radiculopathy and/or myelopathy, and, in the lumbar region, it commonly causes low back pain, radiculopathy, a cauda equina syndrome and/or neurogenic claudication.

Stenosis of the spinal canal and intervertebral foramina is the mechanism whereby spondylosis causes symptoms and signs.[210] The primary event in the development of spondylosis appears to be degeneration of the intervertebral disc, which results in disc space narrowing and allows the disc to bulge centrifugally. In response to this narrowing of the disc space, the adjacent vertebral bodies produce osteophytes, which consist of new bone formation. The osteophytes, along with cartilaginous and fibrous tissue overgrowth, may combine to bulge posteriorly into the spinal canal and intervertebral foramina, resulting in compression of the adjacent spinal cord and nerve root(s). Unlike acute prolapse of an intervertebral disc, which often occurs after trauma, there is usually no herniation of the nucleus pulposus in spondylosis; rather, an expansion of the circumference of the disc in association with osteophyte, cartilaginous, and fibrous growth is found.[180]

Although neurologic symptoms and signs do not occur in many cases of spondylosis, the degenerative changes that cause progressive narrowing of the spinal canal and intervertebral foramina frequently give rise to myelopathy and radiculopathy in cases of cervical spondylosis, and radiculopathy in lumbar spondylosis. The clinical importance of cervical spondylosis is underscored by its frequency; according to Adams and Victor,[7] it is the most common cause of myelopathy found in patients in the general hospital population. In addition, many cases of low back pain and sciatica may be attributed to lumbar spondylosis. The clinical manifestations of lumbar spondylosis are presented in Chapter 3 and in the section in this chapter entitled Spinal Stenosis and Neurogenic Claudication.

Cervical Spondylotic Myelopathy (CSM)

In 1911, Bailey and Casamajor[25] reported a series of patients with cervical spondylosis and speculated on the pathogenesis of the disorder; thinning of the intervertebral disc was considered the primary pathological event that led to trauma of the adjacent vertebral bodies and, secondarily, bony overgrowth. This mechanism of production of spondylosis is still favored today. They further suggested that posteriorly placed osteophytes could cause spinal cord compression. Some years later, Stookey[339, 340] classified extradural cervical chondromas into three clinical groups: (1) those midline anterior lesions compressing both sides of the spinal cord; (2) those just lateral to the midline that compress only one half of the cord, producing a

Brown-Séquard syndrome; and (3) those laterally placed lesions that compress only the cervical nerve root. Thus the protean clinical manifestations of cervical spondylosis were recognized in the first decades of this century. It was not until 1934, though, that the chondromata which had previously been considered neoplastic in origin were recognized as protrusions of intervertebral discs.[255, 256, 282] Interested readers may wish to read more about the history of cervical spondylotic myelopathy.[62, 143]

A study reported in 1954[274] found that among individuals without neurologic complaints, there was radiological evidence of cervical spondylosis in 50 percent of individuals over the age of 50 years and in 75 percent of those over 65. Limitation of neck movement was found in 40 percent of those over 50. Furthermore, 60 percent had some neurologic abnormality referable to their cervical spondylosis.

PATHOGENESIS OF CERVICAL SPONDYLOSIS AND SPONDYLOTIC MYELOPATHY

Although no portion of the cervical spine is immune to the development of spondylosis, the lower cervical spine is most vulnerable. The reason is uncertain but has been considered to be due to its extensive mobility.[2, 7] During flexion and extension, the vertebral bodies roll on one another with the nucleus pulposus of each intervertebral disc acting as a ball bearing.[192] As discussed earlier, the water content of the intervertebral disc declines with age and the nucleus pulposus becomes replaced with fibrocartilage, resulting in narrowing of the disc space. Degeneration of the annulus fibrosus results in tears that allow bulging or frank herniation of disc material into the spinal canal.

With this change in architecture, the ball-bearing movement at the intervertebral joint is lost and is replaced by a sliding motion that places stress on the anterior and posterior longitudinal ligaments and vertebrae, resulting in osteophyte formation.[2] Most commonly, disc degeneration occurs at multiple levels with aging and thus spondylosis is typically seen at more than a single level. However, when a single intervertebral disc herniates, spondy-

losis may form at that level without involvement elsewhere, through a similar mechanism.[269]

Although there has been controversy surrounding the pathogenesis of cervical spondylotic myelopathy, the most important factors appear to be spinal canal size, impairment of blood supply to the spinal cord, and mechanical factors.[44, 267] The observation that the anteroposterior diameter of the spinal canal of patients with CSM is, on average, smaller than that of patients without myelopathy suggests that simple compression would explain the myelopathy.[270, 280, 353] In an anatomicopathological study of the cervical spines of patients with myelopathy secondary to cervical spondylosis, Payne and Spillane[280] found that the average anteroposterior diameter of the spinal canal at the C4–C7 levels was smaller than in those without myelopathy. Although spondylosis reduced the diameter of the vertebral canal of all patients, those patients with spondylotic myelopathy had original spinal canal diameters that were smaller than those with spondylosis but without myelopathy. As the degenerating cervical disc narrowed, the resulting apposition of the vertebral bodies caused deformity of the uncovertebral joints, narrowing of the intervertebral foramen, and formation of an osteophytic bar along the anterior spinal canal wall.

However, although in population studies there is a correlation between a narrow sagittal diameter of the spinal canal and CSM, there is a considerable degree of overlap between the frequency histograms for the minimum anteroposterior diameter of the asymptomatic population and those with CSM.[267] Interference with the blood supply to the cord was suggested by Brain[49] as a probable cause of spondylotic myelopathy. Pathological studies[225, 345] supported this hypothesis. Moreover, Allen's observation of blanching of the spinal cord with neck flexion during laminectomy further corroborated the ischemic explanation.[11] However, it has been noted that the temporal profile of CSM is unlike that of other ischemic disorders.[2] In addition, anterior spinal artery thrombosis has only rarely been verified pathologically.[181]

An alternative hypothesis that has found considerable support is that during the natural movements of the neck, the spinal cord is intermittently compressed and injured.[2, 7, 44, 371, 372] When the neck is flexed and extended, the spinal cord moves up and down the spinal canal.[3-5] During hyperextension, the ligamenta flava bulge, thereby compressing the cord posteriorly.[344] Given the triangular anatomical configuration of the cervical spinal canal, a hypertrophied and bulging ligamenta flava would compress the posterior and lateral columns and the dorsal root entry zone.[338] In addition, during extension, the cross-sectional area of the cervical spinal cord has been found to enlarge.[3, 361] These findings may explain the occasional exacerbation of symptoms and myelographic and manometric block that is encountered with hyperextension of the cervical spine and the clinical improvement often seen with immobilization of the neck with a collar.[2, 4] Symptoms and signs may also be exacerbated with neck flexion. In this case, the spinal cord would be injured as it is stretched over an anterior osteophytic bar during flexion.[2-4, 269]

The pathogenesis of radiculopathy secondary to cervical spondylosis is usually considered to be due to compression of the nerve root arising secondary to adjacent osteophytes.[274] However, patients may have narrowed intervertebral foramina without associated radiculopathy, or radiculopathy without radiographic signs of narrowing of the intervertebral foramen.[59] It has been found, however, that radiological studies of the intervertebral foramina with the spine in a neutral position may not reveal narrowing that may develop with the neck in extension.[153, 361] Such narrowing may contribute to nerve root compression with extension and thus also explain the improvement seen, at times, with immobilization with a collar or surgical foraminotomy. Furthermore, radiculopathy might be aggravated during flexion of the neck secondary to stretching of the nerve root.[4]

PATHOLOGY

Although cervical spondylosis has been said to be the most common cause of spinal cord compression in general hospitals,[7] there are relatively few reports describing the pathological features of the disease.[2, 180] The tissues involved in cervical spondylosis are the joints and supporting structures surrounding the cervical spine, including the intervertebral disc joint, the Luschka and facet joints, ligaments, tendons, hyaline cartilage, subchondral bone, and other supporting extra-articular structures.

While any level may be involved, cervical spondylosis occurs most frequently at interspaces C3–4 to C6–7.[289] The C5–6 level is the level most commonly affected by cervical spondylosis.[2] The most easily recognized finding consists of osteophytes at the level of the affected intervertebral disc spaces. Such osteophytes form transverse bars that may extend the entire width of the spinal canal or involve only a portion of it (Fig. 4–1). Laterally placed bulging soft tissue and osteophytes may narrow the adjacent intervertebral foramina. The dura may be thickened and adherent to the adjacent bone.[180]

The spinal cord is often indented at the level of the offending osteophytes and may show a broad range of pathology, from minor changes to severe destruction (Fig. 4–1). The spinal cord is usually flattened in an anteroposterior direction. Hughes[180] has classified the changes into four groups: (1) posterior long-tract degeneration that is more prominent at the C1 level than the T1 level; (2) lateral tract degeneration that is more prominent at the T1 level than the C1 level; (3) white matter destruction, for example, myelin pallor or necrosis; and (4) gray matter destruction, for example, ischemic changes or neuronal loss.

The pathological findings in cervical spondylotic radiculopathy appear to be even more sparse than those of CSM.[2] The uncovertebral osteophyte is often responsible for the foraminal narrowing.[180] Because on pathological examination, spondylotic radiculopathy and myelopathy are often seen together, the findings secondary to radiculopathy alone are obscured. Nevertheless, because spondylotic radiculopathy typically involves part of the root proximal to the dorsal root ganglion, Wallerian degeneration may be seen in the posterior columns cephalad to the root compression.

CLINICAL FEATURES

We present the clinical features of cervical spondylotic radiculopathy and CSM

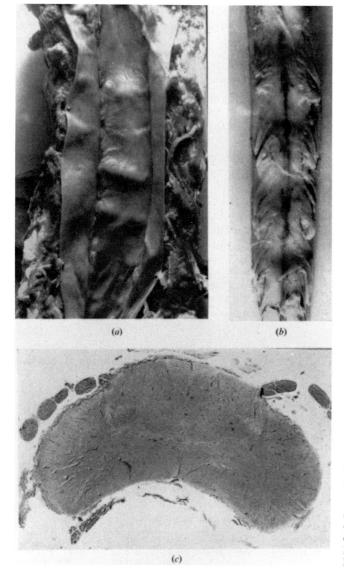

(a)   (b)

(c)

Figure 4–1. (a) The spinal canal is shown following a laminectomy in a case of cervical spondylosis. The spinal cord has been removed and spondylotic bars are seen bulging into the spinal canal. (b) The anterior aspect of the spinal cord is seen to contain indentations which have occurred secondary to the spondylotic bars. (c) A transverse section through the C6 level of the spinal cord is shown. The anterior aspect of the spinal cord has been indented. Leptomeningeal fibrosis and vascular proliferation within the cord is seen. Hematoxylin and Van Gieson X 8. (From Hughes, JT, [180] with permission.)

together because they are often found in the same patient. Symptoms may begin in either the upper or lower extremities. As in other forms of spinal cord compression, the symptoms and signs may include pain, and motor, sensory, or sphincter disturbances.

Symptoms most frequently begin between 50 and 70 years of age but may occur earlier or in advanced years; men are affected more frequently than women.[289] The clinical history typically is 1–2 years, but may extend over only weeks or date back over more than a decade. The symptoms may develop progressively or in a step-wise fashion, with remissions between periods of deterioration. Symptoms and signs may develop for the first time or be aggravated following injuries such as a fall, motor vehicle accident, or hyperextension of the neck.

Pain in the neck, shoulder, and/or arm is a common presenting complaint. Pain may radiate in a radicular distribution, usually dermatomal but occasionally in the distribution of the affected myotome. Muscle spasm usually occurs, resulting in a tilted and rotated posture and pain arising from the spasm. Paresthesias, fasciculations, and muscle weakness in the distribution of the affected nerve roots are often encountered. Reduction in the biceps (C5, C6), brachioradialis (C5, C6), or triceps (C7) reflexes may be seen. These depressed deep tendon reflexes may be associated with hyperactive reflexes caudal to the level of spondylosis when radiculopathy and myelopathy simultaneously occur. Thus when a depressed brachioradialis reflex is associated with hyperactivity of the finger flexors, the resulting reflex on stimulation of the brachioradialis is termed inverted finger flexors and may be a valuable localizing finding. Radicular symptoms and signs may be seen at levels of myelomalacia a few segments above and below the level of the spondylotic osteophyte; these areas, which may be secondary to ischemic changes, may create a perplexing clinical picture by causing lower motor neuron signs at multiple levels above and below the level of spondylosis.[140]

The symptoms and signs of myelopathy include spasticity, weakness, sensory findings, and bowel and bladder complaints. Often the earliest findings of CSM are reduced distal vibratory sensation with exaggeration of deep tendon reflexes and, occasionally, Babinski signs.[289] Although the patient may complain only of unilateral lower extremity symptoms, the neurologic examination usually reveals signs of bilateral disturbance of long tract function. Spasticity is an especially prominent sign and jumping legs may be reported. Sensory complaints in the lower extremities often are not prominent. When sensory abnormalities are found in the lower extremities, vibratory sensation usually is more impaired than position sense; pain and temperature are typically unimpaired unless spinal damage is advanced.[289] Lhermitte's sign also is often reported. Disturbances of sphincter function are late phenomena and generally do not occur in the absence of advanced cord dysfunction, which manifests itself earlier by dysfunction of other modalities.

LABORATORY AND DIAGNOSTIC IMAGING STUDIES

General laboratory studies are usually unremarkable in cervical spondylosis. Cerebrospinal fluid examination is typically normal or shows a nonspecific elevation in protein concentration.[76] Manometric testing may show a block, especially when the neck is extended.

In cervical spondylosis, plain radiographs of the cervical spine most frequently show narrowing of the intervertebral disc space(s), with adjacent osteophytes narrowing the spinal canal and/or the intervertebral foramina, and sclerosis of the vertebral end-plates. Osteophytes may develop on the facet joints and uncovertebral joints as well.[29] The range of normal dimensions of the sagittal diameter of the cervical spinal canal have been reported elsewhere.[29, 47, 280] Although there is not a good correlation between the specific findings on plain films and the clinical manifestations,[289] it has been suggested that if the anteroposterior dimension is greater than 13 mm, then cord compression from spondylotic changes alone is unlikely.[51] Alternatively, as noted previously, a frequent clinical pitfall lies in erroneously attributing neurologic symptoms to spondylosis in cases where these common radiological findings are incidental and asymptomatic.

In the setting of cervical spondylosis, myelography may show any of the following, alone or in combination: (1) extradural defects from osteophytes, disc material, ligamenta flava and other associated spondylotic changes protruding into the spinal canal; (2) non-filling of nerve root sleeves; (3) flattening and widening of the spinal cord (which may simulate an intramedullary mass lesion, especially when viewed in the anteroposterior projection alone); and (4) obstruction to the flow of contrast, which may be exacerbated by extension of the neck.[29]

Computerized tomography (CT) may show the dimensions of the spinal canal and may reveal the location of osteophytes in relation to the intervertebral foramina and spinal cord. In patients with a cervical radiculopathy due to spondylosis, CT scanning may confirm the presence of the offending osteophyte.[22, 78] A recent review[199] recommends initial study with myelography or MRI for patients with myelopathy suspected to be secondary to cervical spondylosis and/or a herniated cervical disc, because of the long extent of spinal canal that must be screened. Following such localization, CT scanning with intrathecal contrast agents may be able to differentiate soft disc herniation from spondylosis and define the relationship of the abnormality to the spinal cord[29, 89, 199, 321] (see Fig. 4–5).

In cases of CSM, CT has shown hypodense intramedullary cavitations of the spinal cord that extend above and below the levels of spondylotic cord compression.[221] Following the intrathecal administration of contrast material, many patients have delayed enhancement in the gray matter at and near the level of the spondylotic bar.[183, 186] These lesions have been described as snake-eyes or fried eggs in appearance when seen in the axial projection. These abnormalities correlate with the pathologists' findings of necrosis in the central gray matter in cases of CSM.[9] Extending several levels from the spondylotic bar, pencil-shaped softenings reported to occur in cases of spinal cord compression and ischemia[161] have been visualized with CT scanning.[186] More recently, snake-eyes and pencil-shaped zones have been seen on MRI of the spinal cords of CSM patients.[9] These findings may explain the neurologic changes seen distant from the level of spondylosis, such as atrophy and fasciculations of the hand muscles with spondylosis at middle cervical levels.[50, 140]

MRI is rapidly becoming a major diagnostic imaging technique for cervical spondylosis, and it may permit the differentiation of osteophytes from herniated discs. MRI is also an evolving imaging modality for the visualization of a narrowed spinal canal associated with thecal compression due to cervical spondylosis and degenerative disc disease.[206]

DIFFERENTIAL DIAGNOSIS

In its complete form, CSM is usually readily recognized as consisting of neck pain and brachialgia, with radicular motor-sensory-reflex signs in the upper extremities in association with myelopathy. However, other causes of spinal cord compression such as neoplasms and syringomyelia may cause symptoms and signs that are difficult to differentiate from cervical spondylosis on the basis of the clini-

cal history and physical examination alone. This problem is compounded by the fact that an erroneous clinical diagnosis of CSM might be supported by the presence of coincidental and asymptomatic spondylosis seen on imaging studies. It is wise to remember that cervical spondylosis most commonly involves the lower cervical spine. Clinical manifestations that point to other cervical levels or, certainly, to thoracic levels are atypical of spondylosis.

Extradural spinal neoplasms (Chapter 5) are usually associated with a more rapid temporal clinical evolution than spondylosis. In addition, there is often (although not invariably) a history of prior malignancy, and the radiographic studies generally show signs of neoplasm. Similar to spondylosis, intradural-extramedullary neoplasms (Chapter 6) may have a very long clinical history; imaging studies may show widening of the spinal canal, however, rather than narrowing. Intramedullary neoplasms and syringomyelia most frequently occur in younger age groups than is typical for cervical spondylosis. Furthermore, these intramedullary processes often give rise to dissociated sensory disturbances (loss of pain and temperature function with preservation of vibration and position sensation) in a cape-like distribution. Cervical spine plain films usually show widening of the spinal canal rather than narrowing. MRI has been useful in identifying intramedullary mass lesions.

Noncompressive forms of myelopathy such as multiple sclerosis (MS), subacute combined degeneration, and amyotrophic lateral sclerosis (ALS) may rarely present clinical syndromes similar to CSM (see Chapter 8). In multiple sclerosis, there is often a history or findings on examination of disease above the foramen magnum, such as optic neuritis, nystagmus, or internuclear ophthalmoplegia. Although progressive spinal forms occur (especially in middle-aged individuals), MS is usually a disease with remission and exacerbations that occurs most frequently in younger individuals.[208, 291] Early impairment of sphincter function also is often seen, whereas it is atypical for CSM. Localized root signs in the upper extremities are very unusual in MS. The CSF, evoked potentials, and MRI will usually differentiate demyelinating disease from CSM.

Motor neuron disease or ALS produces motor disturbances without sensory findings. Unlike spondylosis, pain is not typical and eventually signs of lower motor neuron disease are seen in muscles above the foramen magnum. The CSF and spine imaging studies are not revealing in ALS. Subacute combined degeneration secondary to vitamin B_{12} deficiency has protean clinical manifestations as discussed in Chapter 8. Unlike spondylosis, however, neck pain is not characteristic, and signs of peripheral neuropathy are often present. Loss of position sense in the lower extremities is more often seen in this kind of combined systems disease than in cervical spondylosis. Laboratory studies for vitamin B_{12} deficiency are usually diagnostic.

NATURAL HISTORY AND THERAPY

In general, the pain of cervical spondylosis can be successfully managed with rest, local heat, collar, anti-inflammatory agents, and analgesics. In cases with radiculopathy, these measures are often supplemented by cervical traction. Surgery is considered for patients with progressive, major neurologic impairment due to spondylotic radiculopathy unresponsive to optimal conservative management.

There are few studies of the natural history of CSM. Lees and Turner[207] reported their findings on the long-term follow-up in 44 patients who had CSM at the time they first attended the neurology department of St. Bartholomew's Hospital. (Only eight patients underwent surgical intervention). The clinical course of CSM in these patients is shown in Figure 4–2.

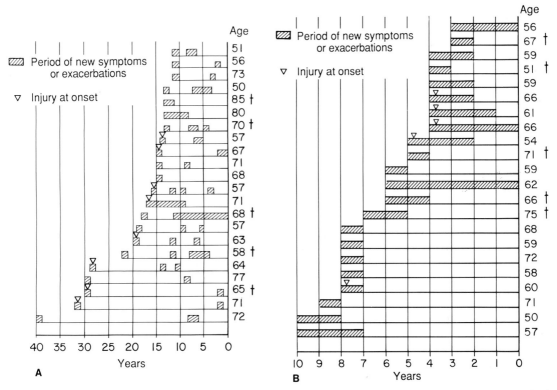

Figure 4–2. Clinical course of cervical spondylotic myelopathy. (A) Pattern of disease in 22 patients who had symptoms for more than 10 years. (B) Pattern of disease in 22 patients who had symptoms for 10 years or less. Each "block" represents the initial symptom or an exacerbation of symptoms. Between blocks, the horizontal lines represent periods in which no new symptoms or signs of myelopathy developed; patients were stable or improving. The vertical line on the right represents the last follow-up or death (indicated by cross at far right). (From Lees, F and Turner, JWA, [207] with permission.)

The maximal disability and disability at follow-up among the same patients is shown in Table 4–1. The authors concluded that in most patients, CSM is a chronic disorder characterized by long periods of nonprogressive disability interrupted by shorter periods of exacerbation of myelopathy. Disability may improve with conservative management alone (Table 4–1). In a minority of patients, these authors found that the course of CSM is characterized by progressive deterioration.

In another study of the long-term prognosis of CSM, Epstein and associates[118] found that among 114 nonsurgical patients culled from the literature, 36 percent improved, 38 percent remained stable, and 26 percent deteriorated. They found that when progressive myelopathy does occur, it may show a pattern of step-wise worsening interrupted by long periods of stability, improvement, or slow deterioration; the intervals of stability or improvement may last for many years. Alternatively, deterioration may be slow and steady without remissions or stabilization. In a recent review. LaRocca[204] concluded that it is not possible to predict the clinical course precisely in an individual patient. Unfortunately, this variability in prognosis jeopardizes the assessment of therapy and leads to controversy in the management of CSM.

Management of patients with CSM includes both nonsurgical and surgical means. In patients without major deficits or signs of progression, a conservative approach including rest, cervical traction, and stabilization of the neck with a collar, followed by physical therapy, is often successful. Alternatively, if the patient is moderately or severely disabled from progressive CSM, then surgery should be considered. Surgery should also be considered if the patient develops signs of progressive myelopathy despite conservative management.[204] Surgical approaches include discectomy and stabilization via an anterior approach,[368] or laminectomy by posterior approach.[117]

INTERVERTEBRAL DISC HERNIATION

Intervertebral disc herniation refers to a condition in which a portion of an intervertebral disc herniates beyond the confines of the surrounding annulus fibrosus.[180, 206] Although herniation into the adjacent vertebral body is very common (Schmorl's node), it has no clinical significance. On the other hand, herniation of disc material posteriorly into the spinal canal or intervertebral foramen may cause spinal cord or nerve root compression.

Using CT criteria, degenerative disc disease has been classified as: (1) annular protrusion or bulge; (2) herniation; or (3)

Table 4–1 DISABILITY AND EMPLOYMENT OF PATIENTS WITH CERVICAL SPONDYLOTIC MYELOPATHY*

Duration of Symptoms	Maximuum Disability			Disability at Follow-up				Unemployed
	Mild	Mod.	Sev.	Nil	Mild	Mod.	Sev.	
More than 10 years	1				1			0
		6				6		0
			15	1		5	9	3
10 years or less	3			1	2			0
		9				8	1	0
			10			2	8	3
Totals	4	15	25	2	3	21	18	6

*From Lees, F and Turner, JWA, [207] p 1608, with permission.

sequestration or free fragment.[206] Protrusion or bulging of the annulus is frequently seen in association with spondylosis. In this condition, the nucleus pulposus does not extend beyond the confines of the intact annulus fibrosus. Such a bulging disc usually suggests no focal nerve root compression.[206] A herniated disc refers to a focal extension of the nucleus pulposus beyond the outer margin of the annulus fibrosus. When herniation occurs into the spinal canal or intervertebral foramen, neural compression may ensue. A sequestered disc or free fragment refers to a herniated nucleus pulposus that has lost continuity with the original nucleus pulposus. When the free fragment is within the spinal canal, it may migrate rostrally or caudally under the posterior longitudinal ligament (PLL), lateral to the PLL, or rupture through the PLL. In the present context, the term herniated disc includes all forms of symptomatic extension of the nucleus pulposus beyond its normal boundaries.

In 1934, Mixter and Barr[256] surgically removed herniated cervical and lumbar disc material from a series of patients, establishing the relationship between disc herniation and neural compression. Kristoff and Odom[200] found a much higher frequency of root compression than cord compression and suggested that cervical disc protrusion should be divided into three stages: (1) root compression; (2) unilateral cord compression; and (3) bilateral cord compression. It is now recognized that spinal cord compression due to herniated intervertebral discs may occur without radicular symptoms or signs.[6] Although intervertebral disc protrusion may coexist with spondylosis, whenever possible, disc protrusion without spondylosis should be distinguished from that with spondylosis, since the etiologies, pathogeneses, and results of diagnostic studies usually differ.

Pathology

Herniation of an intervertebral disc is defined in pathological terms as an extension of the fluid nucleus pulposus through a tear in the annulus fibrosus.[180] This protrusion usually occurs through the posterior region of the annulus fibrosus, which is thinnest in this region.

Although the herniated nucleus pulposus may return to its normal position, it usually remains extruded, and often becomes calcified. However, there is no osteophyte formation unless secondary spondylosis develops.[268, 371] In some cases, the annulus fibrosus does not tear but rather bulges into the spinal canal or adjacent intervertebral foramina.[180] Such cases may be difficult to differentiate from those that occur in spondylosis.

Clinical Features

Although severe trauma may cause symptomatic protrusion of an intervertebral disc, more commonly, minor repeated trauma from activities of daily living will be found in the clinical history.[262] Occasionally, cervical discs and, rarely, thoracic discs may protrude to compress the spinal cord to cause myelopathy. In the lumbar region, intervertebral discs occasionally herniate posteriorly to cause cauda equina dysfunction. This section outlines the clinical features of herniated intervertebral discs in each region.

CERVICAL DISC HERNIATION

Although herniation of cervical intervertebral discs typically causes symptoms and signs of radiculopathy, it may occasionally cause a painless myelopathy that may mimic a degenerative disease of the spinal cord.[6] In such cases, the disc is often centrally herniated and does not cause a radiculopathy. The most common levels for herniated discs in the cervical spine are at the C5−6 and C6−7 levels.[6, 262, 385]

Cervical disc protrusion occurs much more commonly in men than in women.[385] Most patients are in middle age; in a series of 100 patients, their age at the time of operation ranged from 30 to 65 years, with a median of 46.[385] Symptoms and signs of myelopathy, including motor, sensory, and sphincter disturbances, are similar to other extrinsic lesions compressing the spinal cord. However, as in cases of cervical spondylosis, patients with herniated cervical discs may demonstrate evidence of both radicular and myelopathic signs in the arms and myelopathic signs in the lower extremities.

Diagnostic Imaging Studies. The diagnosis of a herniated cervical disc causing myelopathy is confirmed by myelography, CT scan, and/or MRI. Because the cervical spine lacks the large amount of epidural fat seen in the lumbar spine, cervical CT scanning has some limitations.[163] For CT evaluation of cervical disc disease and spondylosis, some investigators advocate the use of intravenous contrast material (Fig. 4–3) or intrathecal contrast material while others prefer conventional CT scans.[22, 89, 199] CT scanning with intrathecal contrast material is often able to differentiate a soft herniated disc from a spondylosis.[199] In the presence of myelopathy, myelography, MRI, or both have been recommended over CT because they have the advantage of being able to examine large areas of the spinal axis.[199] Lee and associates[206] have recently recommended MRI as the initial diagnostic imaging study of choice in suspected herniated cervical intervertebral disc disease.

THORACIC DISC HERNIATION

Herniation of thoracic discs is an unusual clinical problem and thus may not be readily recognized. Surgery for thoracic disc herniations represents only 3–5 cases per 1,000 disc operations.[105] In a surgical series at the Mayo Clinic,[220] 69 percent of cases of thoracic disc herniation were located at the last four interspaces, with the T11 space most commonly involved. Other studies have shown a similar predilection for the lower thoracic spine.[17] Herniation is more likely to occur in the midline than laterally; thus the spinal cord is jeopardized, especially given the narrow diameter of the spinal canal in this region.[105]

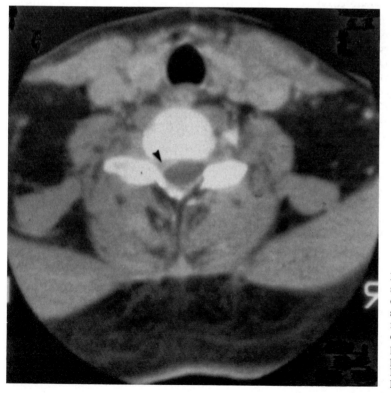

Figure 4–3. Cervical spine CT scan following intravenous contrast enhancement demonstrating intervertebral disc herniation on the left. Note the enhancing epidural venous plexus on the left (arrow) displaced posteriorly by the disc herniation. (Courtesy of Dr. Helmuth Gehbauer)

Thoracic disc herniations most commonly occur at ages 30 to 55; both sexes appear to be affected equally. Pain in the back, the root distribution, or both is the most common presenting manifestation. Occasionally spinal cord symptoms and signs without pain herald the onset of thoracic disc herniation.[20, 220] In one review,[105] pain or dysesthesias were the presenting complaints in 80 percent of cases and paresis in 15 percent. Sphincter disturbances were seen in 22 of the 61 cases reported from the Mayo Clinic.[220] This high frequency of sphincter disturbance may be due to the proximity of many cases to the conus medullaris. Thoracic discs also may cause compression of the artery of Adamkiewicz, causing ischemia of the caudal spinal cord.[69]

Diagnostic Imaging Studies. Conventional radiographs of the thoracic spine are frequently normal but calcification within the spinal canal at the level of intervertebral disc space narrowing may be seen in approximately 55 percent of cases.[238] CT scanning may be very helpful in demonstrating herniation of a calcified thoracic disc.[177, 320, 351] However, the relative paucity of epidural fat in the thoracic spine and the difficulty in defining the segmental level of involvement limit the value of CT in the diagnosis of this disorder.[199] CT myelography may be useful in defining small disc herniations.[17, 38] Lee and associates[206] recommend MRI as the initial diagnostic imaging procedure of choice for thoracic disc pathology.

LUMBAR DISC HERNIATION

Herniation of a lumbar disc usually causes low back pain and symptoms and signs of radiculopathy. Much less frequently, such herniation may result in a cauda equina syndrome. In this situation, paralysis of both legs and sphincters and sensory loss may develop acutely or subacutely. The sensory level and the distribution of weakness are usually determined by the level of disc herniation.

Lumbar disc disease more commonly affects males than females,[159] and most frequently affects young and middle-aged adults. According to Gathier,[135] 70 percent of individuals are between 20 and 40 years of age. Some authors, however, have found a greater frequency in those 40 to 49. Most emphasize the rarity of the disorder among individuals less than 20 years old[135] (Table 4−2).

The most frequent levels of involvement are L4−5 and L5−S1. Although there are differences among various series, these two levels appear to account for 90−98 percent of surgically treated lumbar disc herniations.[135] Furthermore, according to surgical series, the L4−5 and L5−S1 levels are approximately equally involved.[101, 159] The levels of involvement as found on CT scanning are shown in Table 4−3.[199] The clinical manifestations of pain, sensory complaints, reflex changes, and weakness generally follow the patterns predicted by the segmental level involved. Nonradicular referred pain, such as myofascial pain syndromes and the facet syndrome, must also be considered.[37] In general, sensory, motor, and reflex dysfunction are rarely prominent in such cases, and radicular pain is more sharp and localized than nonradicular referred pain.[37] Furthermore, signs of nerve root compression on physical examination (such as a positive straight-leg-raising test) are much more prominent in radicular pain syndromes.

Diagnostic Imaging Studies. Imaging modalities for evaluating lumbar disc disease are rapidly evolving. Many abnormalities seen in patients with back pain are similarly found among those without symptoms and thus do not necessarily confirm the diagnosis of symptomatic lumbar disc disease.[131] Studies using myelography[175, 245] and CT scans[370] have shown a high incidence of protruding or herni-

Table 4−2 FREQUENCY OF AGE (YEARS) AT OPERATION FOR LUMBAR DISC DISEASE*

< 20	1%
20−29	16%
30−39	39%
40−49	31%
50−59	11%
> 60	3%

*From Harkelius, A and Hindmarch, J,[159] p 234, with permission.

Table 4−3 FREQUENCY OF LUMBAR DISC HERNIATION BY DISC LEVEL AS DEMONSTRATED ON CT*

L5−S1	35−40%
L4−L5	50−60%
L3−L4	5−10%
L1−L2, L2−L3	< 1%

*From Kricun, R and Kricun, ME, [199] p 391, with permission.

ated discs among the asymptomatic population. Nevertheless, imaging of lumbar disc disease with both these modalities has been exceptionally helpful (Fig. 4−4). CT has been sensitive in diagnosing the axial location of lumbar disc herniations, found to occur with the following frequency: posterolaterally, 60−85 percent; centrally, 5−35 percent; and laterally, 5 percent.[199] CT has been reported more accurate than myelography in detecting: (1) a herniated disc at the L5−S1 level and (2) lateral disc herniation.[137, 199, 326] CT also may be valuable in recognizing a herniated nucleus pulposus that ex-

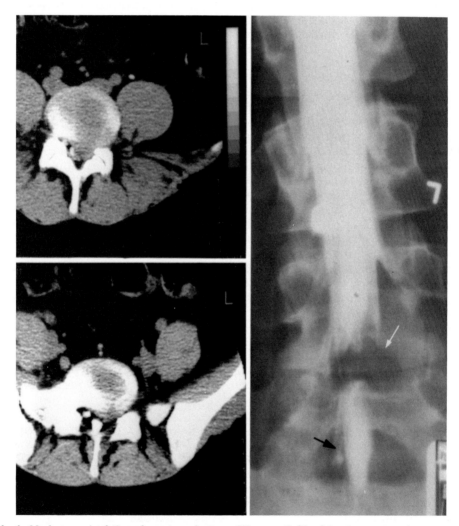

Figure 4−4. Myelogram (right) and post-myelogram CT scan (left) of lumbar spine demonstrating disc herniations at L4−5 and L5−S1. At L4−5, there is a large disc herniation effacing the intrathecal contrast material seen on the myelogram (white arrow) and CT scan (upper left panel). On the myelogram, the normal right S1 nerve root is shown (black arrow); alternatively, the left S1 nerve root sleeve is compressed by the L5−S1 disc and, therefore, not visualized on the myelogram and CT scan (lower left panel). (Courtesy of Dr. Helmuth Gehbauer)

tends through the posterior longitudinal ligament,[373] and the rarely found condition in which it has traversed the dura.[75, 100] It may be a useful in differentiating between a soft disc herniation and a hard disc, which may be a calcified herniated disc or an osteophyte secondary to spondylosis. The use of intravenous contrast enhancement with CT also helps to distinguish recurrent disc herniation from postoperative scar formation.[54] Preliminary studies of MRI in the evaluation of lumbar disc disease are encouraging but its full potential is yet to be established.[72, 258]

Therapy

The treatment of herniated discs, also discussed in Chapter 3, is controversial. As in spondylosis, most patients will respond to bed rest, anti-inflammatory agents, and muscle relaxants. In the case of cervical disc disease, in addition to these measures, a cervical collar and traction are often helpful. Following the acute phase of pain, a course of physical therapy and an exercise program are often useful in preventing recurrence.[130] If during recuperation or later, the patient experiences pain (especially radicular pain) reminiscent of that associated with the herniated disc, he or she should be advised that this is a warning and that activities should be modified to reduce the risk of further injury.[313]

Occasional patients with herniated disc disease require surgical intervention. When a sufficient trial of conservative management (many physicians require several weeks) fails to relieve incapacitating pain, surgery is often beneficial. Alternatively, urgent surgical consultation is recommended in the following: (1) acute cervical or thoracic disc herniation that causes significant myelopathy; (2) lumbar disc herniation causing cauda equina dysfunction (such as impaired bowel or bladder control due to cauda equina compression); and (3) major neurological deficit (for example, foot drop) that is severe or progresses despite conservative management.[313]

SPINAL STENOSIS AND NEUROGENIC CLAUDICATION

Intermittent claudication, first described in many humans by Charcot in 1858,[355] refers to the clinical syndrome of the onset of discomfort and weakness of the lower extremities while walking; these symptoms progressively worsen to a point at which walking becomes impossible, then disappear when the patient stops walking. Although intermittent claudication is commonly recognized as occurring secondary to ischemia of the muscles of the lower extremities and is considered a cardinal symptom of peripheral vascular disease, intermittent neurogenic claudication refers to a similar functional disturbance of the lower extremities that occurs secondary to disturbances of function of the spinal cord or cauda equina.[355] Distinguishing claudication due to peripheral vascular disease from that of neurogenic etiology is a common clinical problem.

Although ischemia of the spinal cord and cauda equina were originally considered the cause of neurogenic claudication, some authors[6, 155, 185] consider compression of these neural structures due to spinal stenosis to be primarily responsible. Recently, these two hypotheses have been reconciled by a proposed pathophysiological mechanism that includes both compressive and ischemic elements.[224] The following discussion reviews the classification of spinal stenosis and presents the pathogenesis, symptoms, and signs of neurogenic claudication symptoms and signs.

Spinal Stenosis

In anatomical or radiographic terms, spinal stenosis refers to a reduction in the cross-sectional area of the spinal canal and may be classified as congenital, acquired, or due to a combination of both[18] (Table 4−4 lists examples of causes of spinal stenosis).

CONGENITAL SPINAL STENOSIS

The congenital or developmental forms are usually idiopathic, associated with Klippel-Feil syndrome[113, 120, 294] or with

Table 4–4 CLASSIFICATION OF SPINAL STENOSIS*

Congenital-Developmental

Idiopathic
Achondroplastic
Morquio's disease
Klippel-Feil

Acquired

Degenerative
Spondylolisthetic
Postsurgical
Post-traumatic
Paget's disease[236, 365]
Acromegaly[109, 277]
Steroid-induced lipomatosis[19, 188]
Fluorosis
Ossification of posterior longitudinal
 ligament[160, 176, 285, 350]
Ossification of the ligamenta flava[199, 338]

Combined (acquired superimposed on congenital)

*Adapted from Kricun, R and Kricun, ME, [199] p 398.

achondroplasia.[114, 194] At the craniocervical junction, stenosis may be secondary to developmental anomalies of the foramen magnum, atlas, and axis.[115] Patients with developmental stenosis may be asymptomatic until superimposed acquired lesions such as spondylosis, trauma, or disc disease occur. Spinal stenosis may be familial.[292] Spondylolysis and spondylolisthesis may cause lumbar stenosis with root compression.

In developmental stenosis, the spinal canal tends to be uniformly stenotic along a region that can extend several levels along the spinal axis.[198] In addition, the pedicles are usually short, which decreases the anteroposterior diameter of the canal. Acquired stenosis, on the other hand, usually is segmental, with areas of normal canal dimensions apart from stenotic regions.

In achondroplasia, early fusion of the neurocentral synchondroses occurs, resulting in spinal stenosis.[10, 261] The thoracolumbar spine is the region that most commonly becomes symptomatic. The stenosis usually becomes symptomatic after degenerative changes develop that further compromise the spinal canal.[10, 199, 261] Other bony abnormalities such as scoliosis or gibbus deformity are common in achondroplasia and may aggravate symptoms.

Cervical spinal stenosis and deformities at the craniocervical junction are also common.[261, 264]

ACQUIRED SPINAL STENOSIS

As noted, the canal narrowing in acquired spinal stenosis is not uniform at several levels throughout the spinal axis but rather is narrowed segmentally. Although spondylosis is the most common cause, it may be post-traumatic due to spondylolisthesis or secondary to a number of other conditions (see Table 4–4).

When spondylosis is the cause, narrowing is typically found at the disc and facet levels[116] and the anteroposterior diameter of the canal often is normal between the discrete levels of narrowing. The stenosis arises secondary to a combination of factors that include disc hypertrophy of the face joints, vertebral osteophytes, hypertrophy of the ligamenta flava, and bulging annulus fibrosus.[115, 128, 199] (Figs. 4–5 and 4–6).

In the cervical spine, spondylotic stenosis usually occurs between the C4 and C6 levels.[115] In the thoracic spine, stenosis is usually secondary to generalized metabolic, rheumatologic, or orthopedic disorder, or is post-traumatic.[31, 276] It rarely occurs in the absence of these; when it does, it most commonly is due to hypertrophy of the ligamenta flava and articular processes in the lower thoracic spine.[31, 383] The more frequent involvement of the lower thoracic spine rather than higher levels may be related to the greater mobility of the lower segments.[367]

Lumbar stenosis secondary to spondylosis involves the lower lumbar spine more commonly than the more rostral lumbar levels.[114, 199] Among patients with cervical or lumbar stenosis, 5 percent have been reported to have symptoms secondary to stenosis at both levels.[119] This clinical constellation has been termed tandem lumbar and cervical stenosis.[86]

Pathogenesis of Intermittent Neurogenic Claudication

The pathogenesis of neurogenic claudication has been debated as secondary to

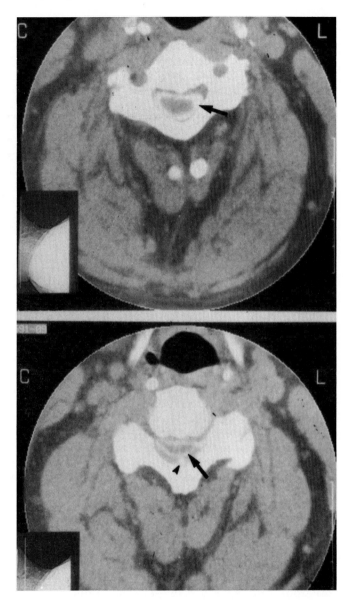

Figure 4–5. CT scan demonstrating acquired cervical spinal stenosis due to cervical spondylosis. The upper panel shows intrathecal contrast material (arrow) without spinal cord compression (normal). The lower panel demonstrates uncovertebral spondylosis, partial calcification of the ligamentum flavum (arrowhead), and secondary thecal and spinal cord compression (arrow). (Courtesy of Dr. Helmuth Gehbauer)

either ischemia or mechanical compression.[185] In some cases, arteriosclerotic vascular disease or vascular malformations have been found to be the cause.[224, 355, 382] More commonly, however, neurogenic claudication is secondary to compression of the spinal cord or cauda equina due to spinal stenosis.

Blau and Logue[42] have suggested that the increase in metabolic demand of neural tissue that occurs with exercise cannot be met by an increase in blood flow due to compression of blood vessels. Oth-

ers[185, 355] have shown that in many patients with claudication due to cauda equina dysfunction, symptoms correlate with posture and do not require exercise. In such patients, the lumbar lordosis alone is sufficient to provoke symptoms that are alleviated by flexing the lumbar spine. These findings suggest that mechanical compression of the cauda equina is more important than ischemic factors in the pathogenesis of clinical manifestations. A clinical study of lumbar stenosis[155] also suggests that mechanical factors are more

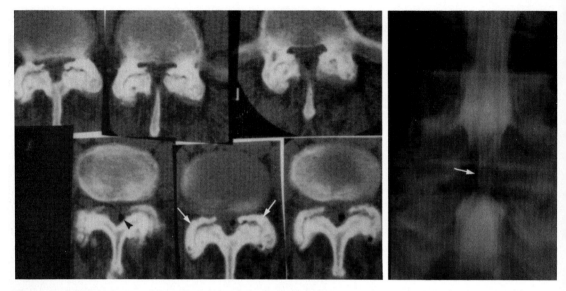

Figure 4–6. Myelogram and CT scan demonstrating acquired lumbar stenosis due to lumbar spondylosis. Note the air (black arrowhead) in the degenerated facet joint (white arrows) shown on the CT scan. The myelogram demonstrates a stenosis in the form of an hourglass deformity (white arrow) secondary to severe spondylosis. (Courtesy of Dr. Helmuth Gehbauer)

important than primary vascular causes in the pathogenesis of the disorder.

Recently Madsen and Heros[224] have postulated a pathogenesis of neurogenic claudication that may reconcile the vascular and mechanical-compressive hypotheses. These investigators have considered the potential role of venous hypertension in the development of neurogenic claudication (Fig. 4–7). Although arteriovenous malformations that may cause a rise in venous pressure were present in their two cases, they suggest that degenerative changes such as osteophytes, annular bulging, and hypertrophy of ligaments may compress both neural elements and the draining veins that exit the canal with the spinal roots. Lordotic postures such as that assumed with ambulation would further narrow the spinal canal and intervertebral foramina and would, therefore, further compress both nerves and veins. The resulting increased venous pressure could cause ischemia of the spinal cord or cauda equina, and neurogenic claudication. According to this hypothesis, a positive feedback loop would be created in which increases in venous pressure would cause greater mass effect, which in turn would further increase venous pressure. Progres-

sive neurogenic claudication would be the outcome, relieved only by maneuvers that break this cycle. Although their hypothesis arose from observations related to both spinal arteriovenous malformations and spinal stenosis, spinal stenosis alone could potentially cause neurogenic claudication through a similar mechanism.

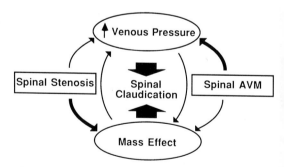

Figure 4–7. Proposed pathophysiological mechanism for the development of neurogenic claudication in patients with either spinal stenosis or a spinal arteriovenous malformation (AVM). Either lesion alone may contribute to mass effect or increase venous pressure, which in turn complicate one another, leading to neurogenic claudication. When spinal stenosis and spinal AVM coexist, they may further exacerbate one another. (From Madsen, JR and Heros, RC, [224] with permission.)

Intermittent Neurogenic Claudication of Spinal Cord Origin

CLINICAL FEATURES

Originally described by Dejerine,[95] claudication due to spinal cord dysfunction is characterized by progressive weakness of the lower extremities that occurs during walking and is relieved by rest. The weakness may initially be unilateral but usually progresses to bilateral. Sensory complaints may consist of paresthesias or dysesthesias. Unlike claudication due to cauda equina dysfunction, spinal claudication rarely causes severe pain, although cramps may occur.[355] With progression of the clinical syndrome, the amount of walking required to cause symptoms decreases.

The clinical hallmark of neurogenic claudication is the change in the neurologic examination following exercise. After a period of rest, the patient's neurologic examination may be entirely normal, but after a period of exercise, there may be spasticity and hyperreflexia of the lower extremities in association with Babinski signs described as afternoon Babinskis.[355] As with the symptoms of spinal claudication, these abnormal signs often resolve with rest.

As noted above, the lower cervical spine is the most common site of compression. Patients may therefore have symptoms and signs of associated radiculopathy at these levels in addition to intermittent spinal claudication. When the thoracic spine is the site of stenosis, most often the lower thoracic spine is involved.[31, 383] These patients may present with symptoms and signs suggestive either of spinal claudication or cauda equina claudication, since both upper and lower motor neurons are located at this level.[31, 206, 383]

DIAGNOSTIC IMAGING STUDIES

Radiographic studies of patients with spinal claudication often show signs of spinal stenosis. In cases of developmental stenosis, the spine imaging studies may reveal uniform stenosis. In patients with acquired stenosis, abnormalities suggestive of the diseases shown in Table 4–4 may be seen. The anteroposterior diameter of the stenotic cervical spinal canal is usually equal to or less than 10 mm.[86, 119, 160] Myelography and CT-myelography typically show evidence of partial or complete block of contrast material at several levels. Compression of the spinal cord is usually seen on these imaging studies and MRI.[86, 119]

Intermittent Neurogenic Claudication Due to Cauda Equina Dysfunction

CLINICAL FEATURES

The clinical syndrome of intermittent neurogenic claudication due to cauda equina dysfunction is typically characterized by back and leg pain, weakness, and numbness precipitated by walking (or standing) and alleviated by rest.[18, 185] Because it shares many of the features of claudication due to vascular insufficiency of the lower extremities, it has been termed pseudoclaudication or intermittent claudication of neurogenic origin.[185]

Claudication due to cauda equina dysfunction may be secondary to vascular malformations[224] and other vascular diseases of the cauda equina. However, it appears most commonly to be secondary to lumbar spinal stenosis,[185, 355] which may be developmental (congenital) in origin,[116, 194, 357] due to acquired disease such as spondylosis,[42, 114, 155] or due to acquired stenosis superimposed on a developmentally narrow canal.[356]

Originally described by Van Gelderen in 1948,[352] the clinical syndrome and pathophysiology of intermittent claudication secondary to lumbar stenosis has been studied extensively by Verbiest[354, 356, 357] and others.[42, 57, 273, 377] The principal clinical features are listed in Table 4–5.

Pseudoclaudication, considered to be any discomfort in the buttock(s), thigh(s), or leg(s) that develops with walking or standing and is relieved by rest, is the most common symptom. The discomfort could be described as pain, numbness, or weakness, and a combination of these complaints was frequent (Table 4–5). The sensory symptoms may ascend from the distal lower extremities to the buttocks or,

Table 4—5 SYMPTOMS AND SIGNS OF LUMBAR SPINAL STENOSIS IN 68 PATIENTS*

Symptom or Sign	Prevalence (%)
Pseudoclaudication	94
Standing discomfort	94
Description of discomfort	
Pain	93
Numbness	63
Weakness	43
Bilateral symptoms	69
Site	
Whole limb	78
Above knee alone	15
Below knee alone	7
Radicular pain only	6
Ankle reflex decreased or absent	43
Knee reflex decreased or absent	18
Objective weakness	37
Positive straight-leg-raising sign	10

*From Hall, SH et al, [155] p 272, with permission.

alternatively, descend the lower extremities. Such a 'sensory march' is considered common in cauda equina claudication but unusual for claudication due to peripheral vascular disease.[185, 377] Low back pain is a frequent complaint, being present in 65 percent of the patients in the Mayo Clinic series shown in Table 4—5. Although the symptoms are generally bilateral, they may not be symmetrical. The entire limb or part thereof may be affected. Radicular pain alone is unusual, in contrast to the pain of a herniated disc.

Intermittent dysfunction of autonomic fibers has also been found. For example, Ram and colleagues[297] reported on a 70-year-old man who developed priapism and urinary incontinence along with sensory disturbances and leg weakness while walking. Following decompressive lumbar surgery, the patient's exercise tolerance returned to normal and penile erection and urinary incontinence related to walking also resolved.

The symptoms of neurogenic claudication due to cauda equina dysfunction are typically relieved by lying with legs flexed, sitting, flexing the waist, or squatting. Thus patients may not be symptomatic if they lean forward to push a cart, or climb a hill, or if they ride a bicycle. However, descending a hill may exacerbate symptoms because this activity usually in-

creases the lumbar lordosis. Such a response to change in posture is atypical for claudication due to peripheral vascular disease.[185]

Although abnormal neurologic signs may be present in neurogenic claudication (Table 4—5), the neurologic examination may be entirely normal, particularly after a period of rest. A paucity of neurologic findings despite a history of severe disability is typical of spinal stenosis.[185] Characteristic in lumbar stenosis, however, is the development of neurologic signs when the patient is symptomatic after a period of walking.[185] In such cases, deep tendon reflexes may be lost and weakness and sensory loss may develop. Positive results on the straight-leg-raising test are rare.

Recently, a series of seven patients with thoracic spinal stenosis was reported with symptoms of pseudoclaudication resembling the syndrome of lumbar stenosis except that it was not accompanied by pain radiating down the legs.[383] The stenosis was in the low thoracic spine and was caused by thickening of the laminar arch and facet joints. The authors noted that a compressive lesion between T10 and T12 would cause a mixture of upper and lower motor neuron symptoms and signs in the lower extremities. It should be recalled, however, that thoracic spinal stenosis may also present with intermittent neurogenic claudication in which the spinal cord, not the cauda equina, is the primary site of involvement.

In summary, in differentiating claudication due to cauda equina dysfunction from claudication secondary to peripheral vascular disease, the following features may be considered more suggestive of cauda equina claudication:[185]

1. Worsening neurologic symptoms and signs following ambulation or with an increase of the lordotic posture of the lumbar spine.

2. A "march" of symptoms through the lower extremities.

3. Relief of symptoms with a change in posture alone while exercise continues (e.g., flexion of the lumbar spine while walking).

4. Symptoms not relieved after a few minutes of rest.[185]

LABORATORY AND DIAGNOSTIC IMAGING STUDIES

Laboratory findings including neurophysiologic and imaging investigations are very helpful in the diagnosis of lumbar spinal stenosis.[187] In the Mayo Clinic study cited above, the electromyogram (EMG) was abnormal in 34 of the 37 patients in whom it was performed; this test was considered to be more sensitive than the neurologic examination.[155] The EMG abnormalities consisted of denervation in muscles innervated by lumbosacral nerve roots. The findings are often bilateral and are located in the paraspinal areas. The cerebrospinal fluid usually shows a normal cell count but often demonstrates elevation of protein concentration.[185]

Although plain radiographs of the lumbar spine may be normal, they usually show evidence of degenerative disc disease, osteoarthritis of the facet joints, or other abnormalities.[155] Lumbar spinal stenosis most frequently involves the lower lumbar spine, especially the L4 level.[114, 198] The laminae may be hypertrophied. Although controversial (see below), a midsagittal diameter of the lumbar canal less than 15 mm radiographically identifies patients who are at risk for the development of symptoms, whereas those with a diameter greater than 20 mm have much lower risk of development of symptoms.[108] Other abnormalities often associated with lumbar spinal stenosis include Paget's disease, spondylolisthesis, acromegaly, ankylosing spondylosis, trauma, and congenital-developmental abnormalities.[155, 185, 198] Myelography has been considered extremely valuable in confirming the diagnosis of lumbar stenosis. It may show compression of the dural sac during extension that improves with flexion (Fig. 4–8). These anatomical findings correlate with the clinical presentation.

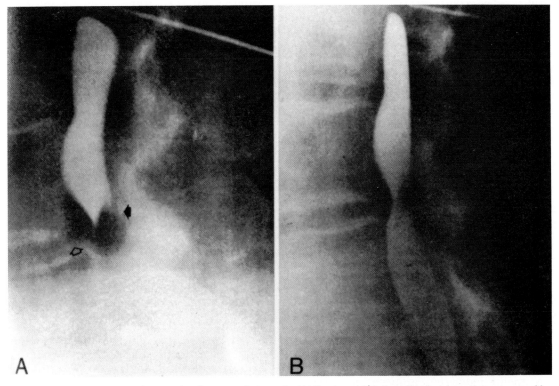

Figure 4–8. Myelograms showing lumbar spinal stenosis. (A) During extension, the dural sac is compressed by ligamentum flavum with obstruction (solid arrow). Note the spondylolisthesis of L4 on L5 (open arrow) with an intact neural arch. (B) With mild flexion, the stenosis at L4 due to a bulging annulus anteriorly and thickened ligamentum flavum posteriorly is decreased. (From Hall, SH et al,[155] with permission.)

CT scanning may demonstrate the short, thickened pedicles and decreased interpedicular distance often seen in developmental lumbar stenosis. In developmental stenosis, an anteroposterior diameter of less than 10 mm has been considered evidence of spinal stenosis, according to one study.[357] Alternatively, in degenerative cases, the anteroposterior dimensions have been found to be abnormal in only a minority of patients. In one study,[45] only 20 percent of patients had an anteroposterior posterior diameter less than 13 mm. For this reason, in cases of degenerative lumbar stenosis, some investigators have suggested that the cross-sectional area of the thecal sac should be considered a more accurate indicator of spinal stenosis. A normal cross-sectional area of the lumbar thecal sac has been reported to be 180 $mm^2 \pm 50$ mm^2; an area of less than 100 mm^2 was considered evidence of stenosis. Other authors[199] have suggested that the dimensions of the spinal canal are not necessary to make a CT diagnosis. Rather, the characteristic CT features, including segmental stenosis at disc and facet levels, hypertrophy of the ligamenta flava and articular processes, bulging of an annulus fibrosus, and obliteration of epidural fat may be sufficient to confirm the presence of lumbar spinal stenosis.[199] Recently, MRI has been reported to be valuable in assessing spinal stenosis, although osteophytes and facet hypertrophy generally may be better seen with CT.[206] In patients with combined spinal stenosis secondary to developmental disturbances and superimposed degenerative disease, the CT findings show features of both conditions.

Therapy

The therapy of spinal cord compression due to cervical spinal stenosis consists of conservative and surgical approaches as discussed in the section on CSM.[117] For neurogenic claudication due to lumbar stenosis, the results of surgery can be gratifying. For example, in a recent study, the mean distance of ambulation at which claudication developed increased from 180 m preoperatively to 2.4 km postoperatively.[155] After a period of follow-up (mean 4 years), 62 percent of patients reported

that laminectomy (often multilevel) gave good to excellent results.

PAGET'S DISEASE (OSTEITIS DEFORMANS)

The bony abnormalities of Paget's disease (osteitis deformans) occur as a result of a disturbance in bone modeling and remodeling.[330] Although Paget's disease of bone has been reported to occur in 3 percent of the population over the age of 40 in areas of prevalence,[330] neurologic complications are relatively unusual.[112] When they occur, they are often due to vertebral involvement. The clinical syndromes of spinal stenosis or spinal cord/cauda equina compression may develop.[319, 324] Back pain is a common complaint.[13, 388] Neural compression is usually due to flattening of the vertebral bodies, thickening of the vertebral arches, and projection of osteoid into the vertebral canal.[319] Neural compression may, however, also be secondary to vertebral compression fractures or subluxation, or to sarcomatous changes.[324] Although involvement of a single vertebra with Paget's disease may lead to neurologic complications, it is more common for multiple levels to be involved. The thoracic spine is most often involved, followed by the lumbar spine. The cervical spine is less frequently the site of Paget's disease.[319]

When spinal cord or cauda equina compression occurs, the symptoms and signs may evolve over several months or even years.[319] The clinical manifestations of progressive neurologic dysfunction resemble those due to other causes of spinal cord compression and depend upon the level involved. When spinal stenosis is present, intermittent neurogenic claudication may be the prominent presenting manifestation. Alternatively, in the setting of a vertebral compression fracture, acute severe pain and neurologic dysfunction may be the presenting clinical manifestation. Finally, syringomyelia has been attributed to cranial settling and basilar invagination secondary to Paget's disease.[112]

In some cases, progressive neurologic dysfunction in the absence of spinal cord compression may occur. In such cases, ischemia of the spinal cord and/or cauda equina has been suggested as the etiology.[104, 170]

The laboratory studies are usually characteristic of Paget's disease, with an elevated serum alkaline phosphatase and typical radiographic changes. However, with the high frequency of asymptomatic Paget's disease of bone in the general population, one must consider the possibility that the presence of Paget's disease is an incidental finding.[13] In most cases of spinal cord or cauda equina compression, imaging studies will reveal evidence of spinal canal narrowing. CT scanning and myelography have been helpful in demonstrating epidural compression.[388] CT scanning may reveal central spinal stenosis and/or a lateral recess syndrome.[388] In the latter case, radiculopathy may occur. The role of MRI in the evaluation of these patients is expected to increase as further experience is gained.

Treatment of Paget's disease includes both medical and surgical approaches. While some patients only require analgesics, the advent of calcitonin therapy has provided an effective treatment for many. Surgical decompression may be necessary in patients with neural compression.[330]

OSTEOPOROSIS

Osteoporosis, the most common metabolic bone disorder to involve the spine, is a condition in which there is less bone present than expected.[198] It may be associated with a variety of metabolic diseases but is most commonly found in the elderly, especially postmenopausal women. As osteoporosis progresses, vertebral collapse may occur, causing back and/or flank pain.

Although vertebral collapse due to osteoporosis is a common cause of complaints in the elderly, spinal cord compression appears to be a rarely reported complication. A recent report[342] of two cases of spinal cord compression due to osteoporosis (confirmed at necropsy) noted the clinical and radiographic findings. In both cases, back pain, leg weakness, sensory loss, and sphincter disturbance evolved over several days. Myelography demonstrated a complete block due to extradural mass at the level of a collapsed vertebral body that was considered secondary to metastatic disease on the basis of the radiographic findings. In both cases, however, necropsy revealed only osteoporotic compression fracture with secondary spinal cord compression. This report emphasized the rarity of this complication and the need to consider osteoporosis in the differential diagnosis of spinal cord compression.

SYRINGOMYELIA

Pathologically, syringomyelia is characterized by cavitation of the spinal cord. Although it has protean manifestations, traditionally it has been considered to be a chronically progressive disorder clinically manifested by brachial amyotrophy, dissociated anesthesia, neurogenic arthropathies, and long tract signs.[32] Its pathogenesis is controversial. Barnett, Foster, and Hudgson[32] have suggested that syringomyelia be classified into communicating and noncommunicating forms (Table 4–6). The communicating types are usually associated with obstructive lesions of the foramen magnum, leading some authors[134] to propose a hydrodynamic theory for its development. The noncommunicating type is usually associated with other diseases of the spinal cord, discussed below.

Pathology

The most common level of syringomyelia is in the cervicothoracic region. The cavity

Table 4–6 A CLASSIFICATION OF SYRINGOMYELIA*

1. Communicating (syringo-hydromyelia).
   a. Associated with developmental abnormalities of the cranial-cervical junction and posterior fossa (e.g., Chiari malformation).
   b. Associated with acquired obstructive lesions of the foramen magnum (e.g., basilar meningitis).
2. Secondary to traumatic myelopathy.
3. Secondary to spinal arachnoiditis.
4. Secondary to spinal cord tumors.
5. Idiopathic (unrelated to the above causes).

*Adapted from Barnett, HJM, Hudgson, P, and Foster, JB,[32] p 312.

often extends at least one half of the rostro-caudal extent of the spinal cord; the largest portion of the cavity is often in the cervical region but it is usually absent at the first cervical segment.[179, 180] The syrinx commonly extends into the lower end of the thoracic spinal cord. The lumbosacral cord is rarely involved, though occasionally the cavity may extend the entire length of the cord and even into the brainstem or cerebrum.[335]

At the level of the syrinx, the spinal cord may be of normal transverse size, wider than usual, or occasionally thinner than normal.[124] The cavity is usually located within the gray matter of the cord, posterior to the central canal[179] (Fig. 4—9), and is usually filled with clear fluid that has the composition of cerebrospinal fluid.[180] Occasionally, the fluid may be xanthochromic or may reveal signs of hemorrhage.[286] As the cavity enlarges, it may involve the lateral and posterior funiculi, and may extend to the pial surface. Although a communication with the central canal may be present, this is not found in all cases.

The wall of the cavity varies in histological appearance. It may be irregular and may contain degenerated neuroglial elements, strands of collagen, and blood vessels. When the cavity communicates with

the central canal, it frequently is lined by ependymal cells.[179] In noncommunicating cases associated with neoplasms, trauma, and arachnoiditis, for example, these pathological conditions will be present. In both communicating and noncommunicating syringomyelia, other associated pathological processes such as scoliosis and developmental disturbances may be present and should be sought.

Pathogenesis

Syringomyelia is associated with a diverse group of disorders, thwarting attempts to develop a unified understanding of the pathogenesis of the disorder and leading to intense debate.[32, 60, 134, 281]

Communicating syringomyelia may be part of a dysraphic state (for example, myelomeningocele, basilar invagination, Chiari malformation, or Klippel-Feil anomaly). Gardner[134] has proposed that communicating syringomyelia arises secondary to the obstruction of normal CSF flow through the outlets of the fourth ventricle. He suggests a water-hammer effect, in which CSF pulsations are transmitted to the central canal due to this obstruction (Fig. 4—10A and B). He postulated that the

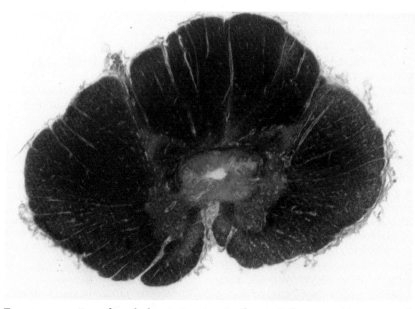

Figure 4—9. Transverse section of cord showing syrinx in the central gray matter surrounded by gliosis. (Courtesy of Dr. Lysia Forno)

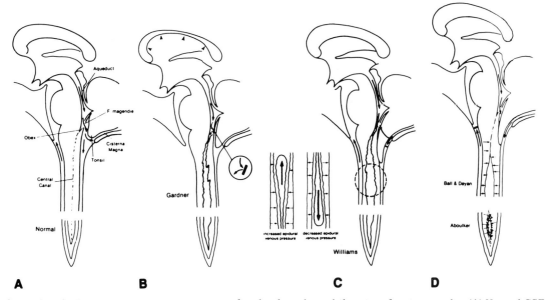

Figure 4–10. Diagrammatic representations of pathophysiological theories of syringomyelia. (A) Normal CSF flow. Note incomplete central canal of spinal cord. (B) Gardner's theory emphasizing imperforate foramen of Magendie (blocked arrow, insert). (C) Williams' theory emphasizing "ball-valve" effect of foramen magnum obstruction. Movement of intracranial CSF into the spinal canal is impeded and redirected into the central canal. The CSF movements in the syrinx are depicted (inset). (D) Theory of Ball and Dayan and Albouker. CSF movement from the spinal canal into cranial space is impeded (blocked arrow). CSF passes into the cord. From Sherman et al [328], with permission.

central canal thus dilates and, with rupture of the ependymal lining, a cystic cavity is formed within the spinal cord. This theory may apply in cases of syringomyelia associated with craniocervical anomalies.

Williams[375] has suggested that differences in intracranial, intraspinal, and venous and CSF pressures are important in the pathogenesis of syringomyelia. Coughing and other Valsalva maneuvers result in engorgement of the epidural venous plexus (Fig. 4–10C), causing displacement of spinal CSF intracranially. If there is any obstruction of CSF outflow from the fourth ventricle, then CSF enters the central spinal canal. When the epidural plexus fills, the fluid within the central canal and syrinx is displaced to the area of least resistance and lowest pressure. These fluid shifts result in extension of the cavity to other areas of the spinal cord. Ball and Dayan[28] propose that the CSF under increased pressure tracks along Virchow-Robin spaces to form cystic cavitations within the spinal cord (Fig. 4–10D). This theory explains the passage of intrathecal

contrast material into noncommunicating syrinxes.

Cases of noncommunicating syringomyelia may be associated with intramedullary tumors, post-traumatic states, spinal arachnoiditis, infarction, acute transverse myelopathy, and, rarely, extramedullary cord compression.[16, 71] Extensions of the cavities seen after spinal cord trauma may be due to transmission of venous backpressure, precipitated by Valsalva maneuvers, to the spinal cord.[32] Experimental studies have suggested that ischemia of the spinal cord caused by spinal arachnoiditis and tethering of the cord may be important in cases of syringomyelia associated with post-traumatic states and spinal arachnoiditis.[32]

The cystic cavitations associated with intramedullary spinal cord tumors are similar to the cysts formed in association with cerebral neoplasms. Poser[290] found that of 245 cases of syringomyelia, 40 patients (16 percent) had intramedullary spinal cord tumors; while among 209 patients with a diagnosis of spinal tumor, 65 cases

(31 percent) were associated with syringomyelia. The most common spinal tumors associated with syringomyelia are those in von Hippel-Lindau disease and von Recklinghausen's disease.[32] Approximately 20 percent of patients with von Recklinghausen's neurofibromatosis harboring multiple intraspinal and intracranial nerve sheath tumors or meningiomas also had spinal cord cavitation.[307] A high incidence of syringomyelia is found when spinal hemangioblastoma is a manifestation of von Hippel-Lindau disease.[247]

In addition to being a sensitive modality for the diagnosis of syringomyelia, MRI may be valuable in elucidating its pathogenesis.[71] Using MRI, 58 cases of syringomyelia were classified as: communicating (those associated with Chiari malformation), 40 percent; traumatic, 29 percent; neoplastic, 15 percent; and idiopathic, 15 percent. The average length of the syrinx was approximately seven spinal segments.[328]

Clinical Features

The clinical presentation of syringomyelia is dependent upon the location of the syrinx and the associated pathological changes noted above. Thus in some cases, an associated pathological condition such as Arnold-Chiari malformation (present in more than 60 percent of cases in some series) or hydrocephalus may overshadow the spinal findings.[66, 376] As noted, although syringomyelia may occur at any level, its most common location is in the cervicothoracic region, and the most typical syndrome includes brachial amyotrophy, dissociated segmental sensory loss, trophic disturbances, and long tract findings.

It may present at any age, but most commonly occurs between the ages of 25 and 40. Men are somewhat more frequently affected than are women.[241] Although familial occurrence has been reported infrequently, syringomyelia is considered a sporadic disease in most instances.[318]

The symptoms and signs of syringomyelia are shown in Table 4−7. Sensory ab

Table 4−7 FIRST SIGNS AND SYMPTOMS OF SYRINGOMYELIA NOTED BY PATIENTS*

Symptom/Sign	No. of patients (n = 172)	
Muscular weakness	52	(30%)
Sensory disturbances	32	(19%)
Paresthesias	32	(19%)
Pain	25	(14%)
Neurogenic arthropathy and scoliosis	11	(6%)
Muscular wasting	9	(5%)
Spastic gait	5	(3%)
Brain-stem signs	3	(2%)
Trophic skin disorders	3	(2%)

*From Schliep, G,[318] p 260, with permission.

normalities are the most common presenting complaint, with 52 percent of patients reporting sensory disturbances, pain, or paresthesias. The sensory loss is typically in a cape distribution, a pattern that is secondary to involvement of the decussating pain and temperature pathways with preservation of posterior column function. Occasionally, such sensory involvement will result in painless burns of one or both upper extremities as a presenting manifestation. When advanced, the sensory disturbances may result in painless ulcers and dystrophic changes (Morvan's syndrome). Infrequently, the posterior columns may also be involved and complete anesthesia may be seen.

Pain may be another presenting manifestation of syringomyelia.[336] It was reported in one third to one half of patients with idiopathic syringomyelia or with obstruction of the foramen magnum.[7] The pain is usually of a burning or aching nature and is often seen at the borders of sensory impairment. If it is exacerbated by a Valsalva maneuver, there is often an associated compressive lesion such as Arnold-Chiari malformation.

Muscle weakness, the second most common presenting complaint (see Table 4−7), is present in 30 percent of cases. It often is associated with wasting and diminution of the deep tendon reflexes. Kyphoscoliosis and neurogenic arthropathies account for approximately 6 percent of the presenting manifestations.[318] Kyphoscoliosis may reflect involvement of the tracts to axial musculature. Neurogenic arthropathies in the areas of anesthesia may be seen in approximately 25 percent of cases throughout the course of the disease.[252]

Autonomic involvement is frequently encountered in the form of trophic disturbances of the skin, Horner's syndrome, and sphincter disturbance. A Horner's syndrome may occur secondary to involvement of descending sympathetic pathways or involvement of the intermediolateral cells at C8, T1, and T2. Trophic changes in the upper extremities are also reported. Involvement of descending autonomic fibers may cause a neurogenic bladder, but this is usually a late phenomenon.

When syringomyelia is of the communicating variety, the brainstem and cerebellar signs (for example, ataxia, nystagmus, hoarseness, dysphagia, and hydrocephalus) may be present and dominate the clinical presentation. When a spinal cord tumor is the cause, the motor and sensory disturbances often extend over several segments.

TEMPORAL COURSE

Although the clinical onset is usually insidious and the temporal course is most commonly progressive, the course may vary. Among 79 patients followed for up to 20 years, Schliep[318] defined four different temporal profiles of syringomyelia: (1) chronic progression, 50 percent; (2) no progression during period of follow-up, 22 percent; (3) stationary and progressive stages, 25 percent; and (4) partial remission, 3 percent. The observation[8, 48, 266] that no progression of signs or symptoms may be found in a substantial number of patients over several years had led to difficulty in making the diagnosis and evaluating therapies.

Diagnostic Imaging Studies

Plain films of the cervical spine may show a dilated cervical canal and the craniocervical junction may show developmental abnormalities such as basilar impression, atlantoaxial dislocation, and oc-cipitalization of the atlas.[334] For example, McRae[245] was able to demonstrate bony abnormalities in the region of the foramen magnum in 38 percent of patients with a clinical diagnosis of syringomyelia. Occasionally, fused vertebrae, bifid spinous processes, Klippel-Feil deformity, and other vertebral anomalies may be seen, as well as anomalies in the thoracic and lumbosacral spines.[318]

The cystic cavitation of syringomyelia may change in shape and size and thus has been difficult in many cases to demonstrate myelographically.[284] Its appearance may vary depending upon whether air or positive contrast is used and whether the patient is in a sitting or reclining position. This phenomenon has given rise to the so-called collapsing cord sign and presents difficulties in the diagnosis of syringomyelia with myelography.[79, 80]

In 1975, Di Chiro and colleagues[98] described the value of CT scanning in the diagnosis of syringomyelia. The administration of intrathecal contrast material revealed the cystic cavity filled with contrast. Since that time, the criteria for the CT diagnosis of syringomyelia have evolved.[125, 148, 163] On CT scanning the transverse diameter of the spinal cord may be small, normal, or expanded.[125]

MRI (Fig. 4–11) has been found exceedingly sensitive in the diagnosis of intramedullary spinal cord disease.[81] MRI is equivalent or superior to CT myelography in the diagnosis of many cases of syringomyelia,[60, 189] and it may be able to differentiate intramedullary neoplasms from intramedullary cysts.[374] In addition, arachnoid cysts associated with syringomyelia recently have been reported using MRI.[15]

Therapy

Complications of syringomyelia such as burns and decubiti may be prevented if patients are aware of these risks. Neuropathic pain is a common problem, which may respond to routine analgesics, amitriptiline, or carbamazepine. Because this is a chronic disorder, the use of narcotic analgesics should be limited or avoided.

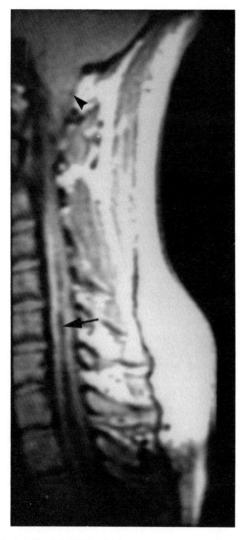

Figure 4—11. MRI of the craniocervical junction demonstrating an Arnold-Chiari malformation and associated syringomyelia (arrow). Note the cerebellar tonsils (arrowhead), which are abnormally low. (Courtesy of Dr. Helmuth Gehbauer)

Baclofen or diazepam may be effective for spasticity.[242]

Since the temporal course of neurologic function is frequently variable, with long periods of stabilization, the efficacy of surgical therapy is difficult to establish. Nonetheless, surgical intervention has been advocated in selected patients with: (1) early and/or rapid neurologic deterioration; (2) progressive motor deficit; (3) Arnold-Chiari malformation associated with hydrocephalus and/or neurologic de-

terioration; or (4) patients who previously benefited from surgery and have suddenly deteriorated. Alternatively, nonsurgical management is usually selected in patients with: (1) advanced, longstanding neurologic deficits, (2) progressive arachnoiditis, (3) no significant motor deficit or mild nonprogressive neurologic deficit, (4) no response to cyst puncture, or (5) high surgical risk.[242] There are a variety of surgical procedures (e.g., foramen magnum decompression, ventriculoperitoneal shunt, syringo-peritoneal shunt[325, 343]) that have been used in patients with syringomyelia and associated problems.[32, 218, 376] When syringomyelia is associated with neoplasm, the treatment is that of the underlying neoplasm. Because management decisions in patients with syringomyelia are usually difficult, patients should be treated by physicians with a wide experience with this disorder.

ARACHNOID CYSTS

Arachnoid cysts are leptomeningeal diverticula that may occur in the extradural, intradural, or perineural location. They are often asymptomatic and seen incidentally on radiological studies or at postmortem; they are rare causes of spinal cord or root compression.[1] Most arachnoid cysts communicate with the subarachnoid space and represent diverticula rather than closed cavities.[132, 136] Arachnoid cysts in the extradural, intradural, and perineural locations share a common pathogenesis, the location depending upon local abnormalities of tissue and hydrodynamic factors.[126] Their histopathology, which consists of arachnoidal tissue, is also similar in these different locations.[126]

Extradural Arachnoid Cysts

Arachnoid cysts extend into the extradural space through a defect in the dura mater that may be congenital or secondary to a rent from trauma or previous surgical intervention.[136] A communication may be found between the cyst and the subarachnoid space. In a surgical series of extradural arachnoid cysts,[77] a communication was seen in 58 percent of cases and was demonstrated on myelography in 46 percent. Congenital extradural arachnoid cysts preferentially occur at the junction of the radicular dural sheath and the spinal dura mater or more laterally along the radicular dural sheath.[136]

Extradural arachnoid cysts are usually single. Although the age of clinical presentation may vary enormously, symptoms frequently begin in adolescence. Arachnoid cysts are much more common in men than in women. The most commonly involved region is the thoracic spine posterior to the spinal cord.[15] In one review,[77] 65 percent of cases were found in the thoracic region.

The clinical symptoms and signs are similar to those of other space-occupying lesions of the spine and include pain, radicular dysfunction, and myelopathic manifestations. They may change dramatically in relation to postural movements. For example, one patient developed transient paraplegia during the exertion of defecation.[87] Transient paraplegia was also described in a pilot after a dive.[156] At times, the history of remissions and exacerbations may mimic multiple sclerosis. In some cases, periods of transient neurologic disturbance last weeks or months.

Lumbar puncture may reveal normal results or show nonspecific elevation of protein. At times, a block may be encountered. Some patients seem to show improvement following lumbar puncture, which may be due to reduction in CSF pressure with secondary emptying of a communicating cyst.

Extradural arachnoid cysts may cause erosion of the pedicles at the level of the cyst and enlargement of the adjacent intervertebral foramen if the cyst extends into the paravertebral area; these findings may be seen on plain films of the spine. If the cyst extends into the paravertebral region, it may be seen radiologically. CT scanning and MRI may also reveal these abnormalities. Kyphoscoliosis has been reported to occur with greater frequency in patients with extradural arachnoid cysts.[136] Myelography usually reveals evidence of an extradural mass. The treatment of spinal cord compression from an extradural arachnoid cyst is surgery if feasible.

Intradural Arachnoid Cysts

Intradural arachnoid cysts are frequently encountered as asymptomatic findings on spinal imaging studies. One study[347] reported a 10 percent frequency of these diverticula incidentally found in patients undergoing myelography. However, because these lesions are usually posteriorly located, myelography may not identify them unless the procedure is performed with the patient in a supine position and the posterior region of the intradural space is imaged.[73, 136]

Intradural arachnoid cysts may be congenital, post-traumatic, familial, or associated with intramedullary cysts.[1, 15, 132, 389] They may occur at any level of the spinal axis but are most commonly seen in the thoracic region. Unlike extradural arachnoid cysts, they are often multiple in number. They often become symptomatic in middle age.[126, 136]

The clinical manifestations of intradural arachnoid cysts are similar to those of their extradural counterparts. Although not always present, the most characteristic feature is the fluctuation of symptoms in relation to changes in posture. Clinical symptoms and signs often worsen with muscular exertion and increased thoracic and abdominal pressure.[136] The symptoms may fluctuate and thereby suggest multiple sclerosis. The clinical course may be acute or extend over several years.

Plain films of the spine are usually unrevealing. Due to mixing of the dye with CSF, myelography with water-soluble agents may fail to demonstrate the cyst if it freely communicates with the subarachnoid space.[132] CT scanning may be very helpful, especially when performed following the administration of intrathecal contrast material.[390] MRI also is a sensitive imaging modality of these lesions.[15]

The treatment of intradural arachnoid cysts depends upon their clinical manifestations, since many are asymptomatic. Some authors advocate rest in a recumbent position several times daily to alleviate minor symptoms.[136] The most definitive treatment of spinal cord compression from intradural arachnoid cysts is surgery. If the location and circumstances permit, resection of the cyst may be performed.

Alternatively, if resection is considered too hazardous, some advocate marsupialization or shunting of the cyst.[132]

PYOGENIC INFECTIONS CAUSING SPINAL CORD COMPRESSION

Bacterial infections of the spinal cord and its coverings (meningitis excluded) may be classified according to location. An abscess may occur in the epidural space or may be subdural or intramedullary.[84, 358] Epidural abscesses are responsible for approximately two thirds of surgically significant infections of the spine.[84] Spinal subdural abscesses are rare and often clinically indistinguishable from epidural abscesses.[166] Pachymeningitis may also occur in the setting of epidural and subdural abscess.[84, 180] Rarely, hypertrophic spinal pachymeningitis may occur and cause spinal cord and root compression.[144, 149, 271]

The symptoms of spinal cord compression from spinal abscesses are nonspecific, thus making diagnosis difficult.[43] As discussed below, in some cases of acute epidural abscess, the systemic symptoms and signs dominate the clinical picture. Alternatively, in chronic cases, there may be few if any signs of infection and a neoplasm may be considered. Thus in order to make the diagnosis in the early and most treatable stages, a high index of suspicion must be maintained. Epidural and intramedullary spinal abscesses are discussed separately.

Epidural Abscess

Early diagnosis and treatment of spinal epidural abscess is imperative for a successful outcome.[84, 88, 144] The diagnostic challenge is daunting because this is a rare disorder that may mimic other more commonly encountered diseases.[14]

Spinal epidural abscess is infrequently encountered in both community and referral hospitals.[27, 358] In a recent series of nontuberculous bacterial infections of the spinal epidural space reported from The New York Hospital, the overall incidence was one case per 12,720 admissions.[90]

The disease affects both sexes but men are more commonly represented in several series.[84, 144] Any age may be affected. In The New York Hospital series, the average age of patients was 58 years, with a range of 8 to 81.[90]

PATHOGENESIS AND PATHOLOGY

The infection spreads to the epidural space either through hematogenous dissemination from an infected remote site or by direct extension from a primary infection in the region of the spine.[27, 90, 138, 146, 167] When due to direct extension, the primary infection may be primary vertebral osteomyelitis[315] or extension from perinephric, retropharyngeal, or other paraspinal location. Direct extension to the epidural space may also occur following an infected spinal surgical wound, lumbar puncture, or epidural catheter placement for anesthesia.[90, 144, 217, 358] Rarely, an abscess may form from extension of an infected dermal sinus.

Hematogenous dissemination to the epidural space from an identified distant primary infection occurs in 25 to 50 percent of cases (Table 4–8). Skin and soft tissue infections are the most common sites of remote primary infection; other primary sources reported include urinary tract infection, upper respiratory infection, periodontal abscess, infected intravenous lines, or intravenous drug abuse.[90, 358] No identifiable source may be found in approximately 20–40 percent of patients.[90] The route of hematogenous spread to the epidural space and vertebral column is probably via the arterial supply[300] and Batson's plexus.[34, 315]

Anatomically, the epidural abscess usually resides in the posterior epidural space, with the lower thoracic and lumbar regions most frequently involved.[27, 167, 209] Among several series shown in Table 4–9, the thoracic spine was the most common level of involvement, followed by the lumbar and cervical levels, possibly due to the larger epidural space in the caudal half of the spine. In a series from the Massachusetts General Hospital, the average rostrocaudal extent of the abscess was 4 to 5 vertebral segments; in 3 patients, it ex

Table 4–8 PRIMARY SOURCES OF INFECTION IN PATIENTS
WITH EPIDURAL ABSCESS*

Source of Infection	No. of Patients (%) at Indicated Facility During Indicated Period					
	Boston City Hospital 1930–1948	Stoke Mandeville Hospital 1945–1968	Massachusetts General Hospital 1947–1974	Montefiore Hospital 1968–1978	New York Hospital 1971–1982	Total No. of patients (%)
Skin and soft tissue	9 (45)		7 (18)	4 (21)	8 (23)	28 (21)
Bone or joint†	4 (20)		11 (28)		3 (9)	18 (13)
Spinal surgery or procedures	0		9 (23)		5 (14)	14 (10)
Abdomen	1 (5)		1 (3)	2 (11)	1 (3)	5 (4)
Upper respiratory tract	0		4 (10)		4 (11)	8 (6)
Urinary tract	1 (5)		0		2 (6)	3 (2)
IV Drug abuse	0		0§	4 (21)	2 (6)	6 (4)
Specific source not identifiable‡		26 (53)				
No source identified	5 (25)	23 (47)	7 (18)	9 (47)	10 (29)	54 (40)
Total	20 (100)	49 (100)	39 (100)	19 (100)	35 (100)	136 (100)

*From Danner, RL and Hartman, BJ,[90] p 266 , with permission.

†Vertebral osteomyelitis was considered as a primary source by most authors when it was present without any other identifiable focus of infection. In The New York Hospital series, patients with vertebral osteomyelitis without a known antecedent infection were classified as *no source identified*. The three New York Hospital patients with a bone or joint source had a distant osteomyelitis, a hip infection, and an infection of the olecranon bursa, respectively.

‡These patients had an identifiable source that was not specified by the authors. These patients are not included in the calculations for the totals of all the series.

§Two patients were reported to be IV drug abusers.

tended 11 to 26 vertebrae.[27] In the transverse plane, the majority of abscesses in several series were located posteriorly (Table 4–9). Osteomyelitis occurred more frequently with anterior than posterior abscesses.[90]

The pathological findings of epidural abscess vary widely, including acute puru-

Table 4–9 LOCATION OF ABSCESS IN PATIENTS
WITH SPINAL EPIDURAL ABSCESS*

Location of Abscess	No. of Patients at Indicated Facility During Indicated Period							
	Boston City Hospital 1930–1948	Stoke Mandeville Hospital 1945–1968	Massachusetts General Hospital 1947–1974	The Royal Infirmary 1957–1973	Pinderfields General Hospital 1958–1978	Montefiore Hospital 1968–1978	New York Hospital 1971–1982	Total No. of Patients
Anterior	1	13	7	—	—	—	17	28
Posterior	19	36	32	—	—	—	18	105
Cervical	3	—	7	0	1	3	6	20
Thoracic	13	Commonest site	20	6	10	12	10	71
Lumbar	4	—	12	8	1	4	19	48
Total	20	49	39	14	12	19	35	188
Mean No. of Vertebrae Involved (Range)								
	3.6 (1–7)	—	4.5 (1–26)	4.4 (1–15)	—	1.8 (1–5)	3.8 (2–10)	3.8 (1–26)

*From Danner, RL and Hartman, BJ,[90] p 269, with permission.

lent material in some patients and chronic granulomatous findings in others. Vertebral osteomyelitis appears much more common among patients with chronic epidural abscess than in those with an acute condition.[27, 144]

The pathogenesis of neurologic dysfunction involves both neural compression and disturbances of spinal cord circulation without direct neural compression. The latter may be secondary to arterial compression and/or venous thrombosis and thrombophlebitis.[12, 244] Direct extension of the inflammatory cells into the spinal cord is unusual; the dura typically represents an effective barrier to the extension of infection into the central nervous system.[180]

CLINICAL FEATURES

Spinal epidural abscesses may be classified as either acute or chronic on the basis of duration of symptoms. Such a distinction is important because patients with a chronic abscess generally present less dramatically. Danner and Hartman[90] classified acute abscesses as those in which symptoms were present for less than 16 days. Using such a distinction, those with chronic abscesses were less likely to be febrile (average temperature $37.4° \pm 0.5°C$ in chronic cases, compared with $38.4° \pm 1.0°C$ in patients with acute abscesses). Moreover, the mean WBC count was $7.1 \pm 1.9 \times 10^3$ in chronic cases as compared with an average of $12.3 \pm 3.8 \times 10^3$ per cubic millimeter in acute abscesses.

In both chronic and acute spinal epidural abscesses, the most characteristic clinical course progresses through four stages: (1) local pain; (2) radicular pain; (3) motor weakness and sphincter disturbance; and (4) paralysis.[299] A sensory level may also be seen as transverse myelopathy develops. The tempo of progression of these symptoms and signs is quite variable, ranging from hours to several weeks.[90] Cases that commence as vertebral osteomyelitis may evolve slowly in the first two phases, and thus be classified as chronic, only to accelerate rapidly into the final phases.[144] In cases of rapid neurologic deterioration, an erroneous diagnosis of acute transverse myelitis may be considered.[14]

Patients with acute epidural abscess typically are acutely ill with signs of toxicity of systemic infection and fever. The early course is characterized by fever and back pain, often followed by radicular pain. Spasm of paraspinal muscles may occur. Headache is often present and neck stiffness may be marked. Percussion tenderness over the spine may be pronounced. There may be a history of a recent or remote infection elsewhere.

Despite this characteristic course, the clinical presentation of acute spinal epidural abscess is highly variable, resulting in a delayed diagnosis in many cases. In one series the diagnosis of spinal epidural abscess was considered initially in only one fourth of patients.[27] For example, when the abscess arises from a distant focus of infection that disseminates to the spine hematogenously, the clinical presentation may be dominated by the systemic illness. The patient may not complain of pain, and if lethargic or confused, he or she may fail to complain of weakness. However, once infection of the epidural space occurs, symptoms of local and radicular pain usually ensue rapidly.[358] At that time, the clinical presentation may mimic spinal tumor or disc disease.

In chronic cases (defined as symptoms present for longer than 16 days), the epidural abscess often arises from an adjacent vertebral osteomyelitis.[358] (Spinal epidural abscess is reported to develop in up to 20 percent of cases of vertebral osteomyelitis[310].) The progression of symptoms and signs beyond pain, fever, and weakness may evolve over weeks or even months before signs of neural dysfunction occur. Alternatively, the clinical evolution of an indolent chronic abscess may suddenly and unpredictably change, with the rapid development of paraplegia. In most (but not all) cases of both chronic and acute epidural abscess, symptoms and signs of spinal cord/cauda equina dysfunction develop following the onset of local and radicular pain.[299]

The clinical setting often provides clues helpful in diagnosis. In addition to remote and local infection, several other factors may be associated with spinal epidural abscess. Among them are diabetes mellitus, nonpenetrating or penetrating back trauma, pregnancy, cancer or spinal tumor, intravenous drug abuse, alcoholism, and degenerative joint disease of the spine.[27, 90] The possible association with cancer is especially important to recognize because the symptoms and signs of epidural abscess may be difficult to distinguish clinically from epidural spinal metastasis. As discussed below, even radiographic studies may not definitively establish the diagnosis of spinal epidural abscess or differentiate it from metastatic cancer.

In summary, *although the constellation of fever, back and radicular pain, and percussion tenderness over the spine is characteristic of both chronic and acute epidural abscess, fever and other constitutional symptoms may be entirely absent, particularly in chronic cases.*[90, 172] Furthermore, although local and radicular pain and spinal tenderness occur in over 90 percent of cases,[358] in occasional patients these findings have been absent.[154, 157] Thus whenever paraparesis develops without a well-defined cause, the clinician must think of epidural abscess. Even prior to the development of weakness, the development of back and/or radicular pain, or spinal tenderness, in the setting of systemic illness should alert the clinician to the possibility. The difficulty encountered in arriving at a correct diagnosis is demonstrated by the reported series of epidural abscess in Table 4–10. In The New York Hospital series, 43 percent of patients had an initial diagnosis unrelated to the spine; in many instances, patients were incoherent and therefore could not offer an accurate history.

Spinal subdural empyema is a rare cause of spinal cord compression. It is difficult on clinical grounds to differentiate from spinal epidural abscess; however, vertebral tenderness is usually lacking in subdural empyema.[127, 278] The myelogram may dis-

Table 4–10 INITIAL DIAGNOSIS FOR PATIENTS WITH SPINAL EPIDURAL ABSCESS*

Initial Diagnosis	No. of Patients at Indicated Facility				
	Boston City Hospital	Massachusetts General Hospital	Pinderfields General Hospital	New York Hospital	Total No. of Patients
Spinal epidural abscess	1	10	1	7	19
Vertebral osteomyelitis or infected disk	4	1	0	1	6
Spinal tuberculosis	0	0	0	1	1
Cholecystitis, pyelonephritis, or intraabdominal abscess	0	4	0	2	6
Meningitis	3	1	0	0	4
Dental infection	0	1	0	0	1
Bacterial infection, other sites	0	0	1	6	7
Herpes zoster	0	1	0	1	2
Viral syndrome	0	1	0	1	2
Infectious polyneuritis or transverse myelitis	1	1	1	1	4
Spinal tumor or metastatic cancer	4	1	0	6	11
Spinal hematoma	0	0	0	1	1
Extruded disk	0	5	3	3	11
Musculoskeletal pain, arthritis, neuritis	3	6	5	2	16
Fibrositis	0	0	1	0	1
Myocardial infarction	0	1	0	0	1
Cerebrovascular accident or subdural hematoma	0	2	0	1	3
Hysteria	2	2	0	0	4
Anemia	0	1	0	0	1
Benign prostatic hypertrophy	0	0	0	1	1
Drug fever	0	0	0	1	1
None	2	1	0	0	3
Total	20	39	12	35	106

*From Danner, RL and Hartman, BJ,[90] p 272, with permission.

tinguish between subdural and epidural collections of pus. Surgical intervention will differentiate between them.

LABORATORY STUDIES

Microbiology

Staphylococcus aureus is the most common bacterium isolated in cases of spinal epidural abscess (Table 4–11). Although *Mycobacterium tuberculosis* has been excluded from many series, it has been responsible for as many as one fourth of the cases in some reports.[190] In addition, fungal infections (e.g., *Cryptcoccus neoformans* and *Coccidioides immitis*) and several other organisms have been reported.[141, 212, 332, 358] In cases of tuberculosis and fungal infections, there may be a granulomatous mass or abscess.[296] Infrequently, multiple organisms are found.[144]

Blood cultures are often positive; among those patients with *Staphylococcus aureus*, results were positive in 18 (95 percent) of 19 patients reported from The New York Hospital series.[90] CSF cultures appear to yield positive results in far fewer

cases; only 2 were positive out of 31 cases in which the procedure was performed. In the same series, cultures of the abscess were positive in 84 percent of cases; patients who had been on antibiotics for longer than one week were unlikely to have positive cultures of the abscess.

Routine and CSF Studies

The peripheral white blood cell count is usually elevated. Although the erythrocyte sedimentation rate (ESR) is usually high, four patients in the series from The New York Hospital had a normal ESR.[90]

Blood glucose levels may reveal diabetes, and blood chemistries should be scrutinized for signs of renal disease. The cerebrospinal fluid typically shows evidence of a parameningeal infection with elevated protein, moderate pleocytosis (usually lower than 150 white cells per cubic millimeter) and normal sugar.[144, 358] The CSF can be xanthochromic, especially in cases of a subarachnoid block.

If there is suspicion of an epidural abscess, the lumbar puncture should be done cautiously to avoid entering the abscess

Table 4–11 BACTERIOLOGY OF SPINAL EPIDURAL ABSCESS*

Characteristic	No. of Patients (%) at Indicated Facility During Indicated Period					
	Boston City Hospital 1930–1948	Stoke Mandeville Hospital 1945–1968	Massachusetts General Hospital 1947–1974	Montefiore Hospital 1968–1978	New York Hospital 1971–1982	Total No. of Patients
Organism†						
Staphylococcus aureus	19 (95)	31 (63)	22 (52)	12 (60)	19 (54)	103 (62)
Aerobic streptococci	0		6 (14)	3 (15)	5 (15)	14 (8)
Staphylococcus epidermidis	0		1 (2)	0	3 (9)	4 (2)
Aerobic gram-negative rods	0	18 (37)	5 (12)	4 (20)	3 (9)	30 (18)
Anaerobes	0		3 (7)	0	0	3 (2)
Other	0		0	0	2 (6)	2 (1)
Unknown	1 (5)		5 (12)	1 (5)	3 (9)	10 (6)
Total	20 (100)	49 (100)	42 (100)	20 (100)	35 (100)	166 (100)
Culture site‡						
Blood, all organisms	6/14 (43)	NA	NA	6/12 (50)	24/34 (69)	36/60 (60)
Blood, *S. aureus*	6/14 (43)	NA	NA	3/7 (43)	18/19 (95)	27/40 (68)
CSF	NA	NA	8/38 (21)	5/18 (28)	2/31 (6)	15/88 (17)
Abscess	19/19 (100)	NA	34/39 (87)	17/19 (89)	27/32 (84)	97/107 (89)

*From Danner, RL and Hartman, BJ,[90] p 267, with permission.
†In some series the total number of organisms isolated exceeds the number of patients because of mixed infections.
‡In fractions, the numerator is the number of positive cultures, and the denominator is the number of patients from whom samples for culture were taken.

and contaminating the CSF. Lumbar puncture should not be performed at the site of a suspected abscess; if epidural abscess is suspected over the lumbar region, a cisternal tap may be performed. If lumbar puncture is performed in a patient with a possible abscess, gentle suction should be applied to the needle because the abscess may have extended to lumbar areas; aspiration of pus is diagnostic of epidural abscess. It is essential in such cases that the arachnoid not be penetrated by the needle. Furthermore, in the case of spinal block, the myelopathy may worsen following lumbar puncture; therefore, routine lumbar puncture should not be performed if epidural abscess is suspected.[144, 289]

Diagnostic Imaging Studies

Plain spinal radiographs may show evidence of osteomyelitis, discitis, compression fracture, or paravertebral mass, but it is common to find no specific abnormalities. Routine radiographs demonstrated osteomyelitis in 37 percent of patients in The New York Hospital series.[90] Radionuclide bone scanning often shows evidence of abnormality, but a substantial number of patients have normal bone scans.

Until the advent of MRI, myelography was considered the most sensitive technique for identifying epidural abscess.[103, 122, 358] The myelogram is nearly always abnormal, demonstrating an epidural mass.[358] It may show the longitudinal extent of the abscess and its anteroposterior relationship to the spinal cord.

Although CT scanning of the spine has recently been shown to be sensitive in identifying osteomyelitis, paravertebral infections, and epidural abscesses,[52, 139, 240] some authors have found it less accurate than myelography.[90] CT may be able to detect involvement of the spongy vertebral bone and intervertebral disc before changes are seen on plain radiographs. When combined with myelography, CT may be very sensitive for evaluating bony and epidural tissues.[53, 123, 139, 293] The paravertebral structures are seen more readily on CT than with plain films or myelography.

The role of MRI scanning has yet to be fully defined. Recent studies suggest that MRI is excellent for assessing vertebral osteomyelitis and epidural abscess, and it has been reported to be more sensitive than CT scanning.[122, 257, 259] MRI is said to be superior to myelography in demonstrating the extension of the lesion in disc spaces, bone, and paravertebral regions[122] (except, perhaps, in those cases accompanied by bacterial meningitis).[103] It may therefore supplant myelography in the future, avoiding the associated risk of lumbar puncture[122] (Fig. 4–12).

Preliminary surgical experience suggests that MRI may identify noncompressive epidural inflammatory tissue that is not an abscess and yet may be radiologically indistinguishable from one.[103] This may create a management dilemma (see below).

THERAPY

The treatment of spinal epidural abscess includes urgent surgical drainage and administration of intravenous antibiotics.[26, 90, 144, 358] Some authors[144] recommend initiating antibiotic therapy before surgery when a presumptive diagnosis can be made. Since *Staphylococcus aureus* is the most common offending organism, initial treatment includes a first-line antistaphylococcal agent.[90] When there are known sources of infection, antibiotic therapy should include coverage for these. For example, epidural abscesses due to gram-negative organisms are more common in the setting of intravenous drug abuse and following spinal operation. *S. epidermidis* infection is also more frequent following spinal procedures. Antibiotic therapy is modified based on the results of Gram stain and other special stains and laboratory culture results of operative specimens. The duration of antibiotic therapy is determined in part by the presence or absence of associated osteomyelitis. Recent reviews[26, 358] have suggested 6 to 8 weeks of parenteral antibiotic therapy if osteomyelitis is present, and some suggest oral antibiotics following this in selected cases.[90] The prognosis for neurologic recovery is good if treatment is begun before symptoms and signs of myelopathy occur; although patients with paraparesis may be restored to normal neurologic function, the presence of paraplegia for longer

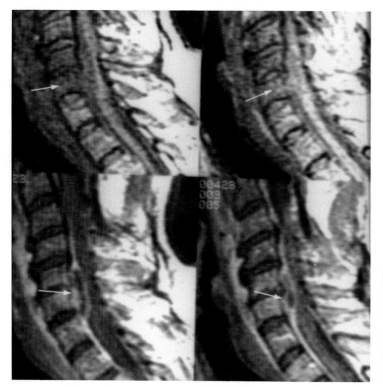

Figure 4–12. Multiple sagittal MR images of the cervical spine demonstrating a pyogenic epidural abscess (arrows) in a patient with AIDS. (Upper panels, noncontrast study. Lower panels, postcontrast study.) Note the anterior location and compression of the spinal cord. (Courtesy of Dr. Helmuth Gehbauer)

than 48 hours carries a very poor prognosis for recovery.[358]

As mentioned above, MRI is exceptionally sensitive in detecting small epidural inflammatory lesions or areas (for example, secondary to adjacent infections) that are not true abscesses. These infections might be successfully managed with antibiotics alone, without surgical drainage. However, early studies using MRI often have not been able to distinguish between the different stages of inflammatory tissue,[103] creating a management dilemma. In cases in which the MRI identifies a small noncompressive inflammatory lesion that is not considered to be a true abscess, some surgeons have been reluctant to attempt urgent open surgical drainage in neurologically intact patients who can be followed with repeated clinical and laboratory examinations and MRI scanning. In some of these patients, treatment with antibiotics alone has been successful, [227a] whereas in others, surgical drainage has been required after an unsuccessful trial of antibiotics.[90] With more experience using MRI and carefully performed clinical stud-

ies, criteria may be established to identify those patients not requiring urgent surgical drainage, but standard infectious disease references have recommended a combination of surgery and antibiotic therapy as the treatment of choice for spinal epidural abscess.[26, 90, 144, 358]

Case Illustration

A 61-year-old former housepainter with a history of alcoholism was admitted to the medical service after being found in his hotel room in a confused state, attributed to a withdrawal syndrome. The patient had a fever of 38 to 38.5°C. No focal neurologic signs were noted. The patient exhibited witzelsucht and did not complain of back pain, but said he was weak and could not get out of bed. A lumbar puncture yielded CSF showing mild xanthochromia, a moderate pleocytosis, protein of about 110 mg per dl, and normal glucose. The patient was treated with antibiotics but, because he remained confined to bed, neurologic consultation was obtained.

The consultant found the patient confused and uncooperative. He denied having any pain. He stated that he was weak and could not walk, but would not attempt to ambulate. The neck was supple and there was no paravertebral spasm, but percussion tenderness was present over the spine at T9–T10. Motor examination revealed flaccid paraparesis. Patellar and ankle jerks could not be obtained but the plantar responses were extensor. The patient was not cooperative for testing of vibratory or position sensation. Although he denied feeling a pin as painful over any part of his body, when the examiner watched for a facial wince on pinprick, a sensory level at the T5–T6 level could be appreciated.

Myelography revealed epidural abscess and the patient was taken to surgery. The abscess was found to extend over five vertebral segments. The confusional state resolved postoperatively, but the patient remained paraparetic.

Comment. This case illustrates some of the difficulties that can be encountered in the diagnosis of epidural abscess. While back pain and neck stiffness are usually encountered, they did not appear to be present in this patient, possibly being masked by his confusional state. While this patient complained of weakness, a careful neurologic examination was not initially carried out and the paraparesis was not appreciated. The initial work-up did not include percussion of the vertebral column to determine whether tenderness was present. It is essential for the spinal column to be examined carefully in any patient with back pain, radicular signs or symptoms, or weakness that includes the legs. In retrospect, the patient's confusional state may have been partially due to the meningitis that accompanied his epidural abscess. This case illustrates that an associated confusional state may make this diagnosis difficult.

Intramedullary Spinal Cord Abscess

Intramedullary spinal cord abscess is a rare but devastating infection. It usually occurs in the setting of systemic infection and multiple septic foci elsewhere[180] but occasionally there is no history of prior infection.[40] Chiari's[74] well-studied case of a metastatic spinal cord abscess associated with meningitis and cerebellar abscess secondary to bronchiectasis increased the awareness of this clinical syndrome and described its clinical constellation. A report[378] of a child who recovered following surgical drainage of a staphylococcal abscess of the thoracic cord demonstrated the value of early recognition.

Between the original descriptions and 1977, only 54 cases had been reported.[102, 250] Courville[82] found only one case among 40,000 postmortem examinations. Intramedullary abscess may occur at any age; one review cited 27 percent of cases during the first decade of life and 40 percent before the age of 21.[102] The male-female ratio was 3:2.[250]

Among other routes, the abscess may arise from a remote site by hematogenous spread, infected dermal sinus, or trauma. In most cases, intramedullary spinal cord abscesses have been metastatic from a pyogenic infection elsewhere. Bronchiectasis and endocarditis are common sources. Less commonly, intramedullary abscesses arise from an adjacent infection;[180, 289] for example, they have been reported to follow a stab wound[380] and high lumbar puncture.[305] In those cases in which no source can be identified, the abscesses are called primary. One review[250] found 20 percent to be primary, with the remainder secondary to known infection. The most common organism found to cause intramedullary spinal cord abscesses is *Staphylococcus aureus*; *Streptococcus*, *Actinomyces*, gram-negative organisms, and others were isolated less frequently.[106, 250] Multiple organisms may also be isolated.

The abscesses may be classified as single or multiple, and acute, subacute, or chronic. Among 55 reported cases,[250] 42 were single and 13 were multiple. The thoracic region was the most common location, with 80 percent located in this area. Most extend over several segments in the rostro-caudal axis. The entire spinal cord occasionally may be involved.[250]

On pathological examination, intramedullary abscesses may be centrally located but often the posterior horns are more involved than the anterior region.[289] The spinal cord is usually swollen and this may be visualized on radiological studies. The margins of the abscess may be poorly defined and there may be little fibroglial reaction.[191]

In most cases, the time between onset of symptoms and diagnosis ranges from days to months. One report[102] found the interval between onset and diagnosis to be less than 2 weeks in 43 percent, 1 to 3 months in 33 percent, and 4 months to 3 years in 24 percent. When myelopathy develops over a few days and the radiological studies are nondiagnostic, an erroneous diagnosis of acute transverse myelopathy or multiple sclerosis may be made. Subacute and chronic presentations, with radiological studies that usually are nondiagnostic or show enlarged spinal cords, may mimic intramedullary tumors.

The clinical presentation of intramedullary spinal cord abscess varies according to the location of involvement and the chronicity of infection. Fever and signs of infection are usually present. Pain is a common presenting complaint regardless of the site and chronicity.[250] In one review,[102] incontinence was present in 88 percent, paraplegia in 72 percent, and anesthetic sensory loss in 61 percent at the time of diagnosis. In chronic cases, the progression of symptoms may be slow and, at times, stuttering in nature.[250]

There is usually leukocytosis on the complete blood count and other signs of infection on laboratory studies. The cerebrospinal fluid may be nonspecifically abnormal or may suggest meningitis.[180, 289] Myelography may demonstrate an intramedullary expansion of the spinal cord consistent with an intraspinal mass.[240] CT scanning following intrathecal injection of contrast material and MRI may be helpful in demonstrating the intramedullary expansion of the spinal cord.

Treatment of intramedullary spinal cord abscess includes prompt surgical drainage and appropriate parenteral antibiotic therapy.[40, 250]

OTHER INFECTIOUS AND INFLAMMATORY DISEASES

Tuberculosis

Mycobacterium tuberculosis may injure the spinal cord and cauda equina through involvement of the epidural and intradural locations.[83, 142, 232, 360] The most common spinal involvement is tuberculous spondylitis, which classically consists of destruction of vertebral bodies and intervening disc space, and a paravertebral abscess, combining to cause spinal cord or cauda equina compression from its anterior aspect.[133, 180, 228] Percival Pott[145] called attention to curvature of the spine and the resulting paraplegia due to tuberculous involvement that now bears his name. Less commonly, compression may occur secondary to neural arch involvement or extension into the epidural space without radiographic changes of the vertebral bodies and intervening disc space.

Tuberculous meningitis may cause a subacute myelopathy secondary to granulomatous meningitis.[359] Intramedullary spinal tuberculomas have been reported[91, 92, 214] and may cause myelopathy in patients with AIDS.[379] Rarely, an intramedullary spinal cord tuberculoma may represent a primary focus of infection within the central nervous system.[314]

Epidural compression of the spinal cord and nerve root(s) may be due to granuloma formation, abscess, pathological subluxation, or collapse of a vertebral body.[142] Thrombosis of spinal blood vessels may also occur.[142] The pathological anatomy and clinical features of tuberculosis involving the nervous system have been reviewed.[142, 145]

Most commonly, spinal involvement follows a primary tuberculous infection elsewhere, with either a short or long latency period. The vertebral column usually is seeded hematogenously, immediately from the primary infection, or later from that site or from another extraosseus secondary site.[83]

Although in developing countries, younger patients appear to be at greater risk for spinal involvement than older individuals, in industrialized nations, the age of presentation is usually in the fifth and sixth decades.[83, 142, 362] Although tuberculous involvement of the spine has not been seen commonly in developed countries, the use of immunosuppressive therapy and the AIDS epidemic may increase the frequency of this disease.[227, 265]

CLINICAL FEATURES

The clinical presentation of tuberculous spondylitis may be very similar to that of other infectious or neoplastic processes in the same location.[133, 180, 223, 279] Patients typically complain of pain and tenderness in the region of the infected vertebrae. They often have a low-grade fever, chills, weight loss, and other constitutional symptoms.[142] The average duration of symptoms prior to diagnosis is one year but may range from weeks to years.[142, 213] Local and radicular pain as well as motor, sensory, and sphincter disturbances caudal to the lesion progresses if the disease is not recognized and treated.[24, 213] According to a recent review of tuberculous spondylitis, paraplegia occurred with a frequency ranging from 4 to 38 percent. [142]

Skin testing for tuberculosis has been reported negative in up to 20 percent of patients in some series.[142, 213] The chest radiograph has been negative for active or inactive pulmonary tuberculosis in one half of patients with osteoarticular tuberculosis.[142] Thus some patients may not have evidence of tuberculosis elsewhere when they present with tuberculous spondylitis.

The thoracic spine or thoracolumbar region are favored levels of involvement, with the cervical spine much less frequently represented.[83, 138, 213] Plain films often show features that resemble pyogenic infections and abscess formation[146, 198, 362] or metastatic cancer.[228] The kyphosis that develops from vertebral body and disc involvement may approach 90°. The radionuclide bone scan has been reported negative in 35 percent and the gallium scan negative in 70 percent of cases.[213] When epidural neural compression occurs secondary to extension of a paravertebral mass, the bone scan may be negative. Both CT and MRI may be helpful in demonstrating the vertebral destruction and paravertebral mass associated with tuberculous spondylitis[94] (Fig. 4–13).

Biopsy of bone, often performed as needle biopsy under fluoroscopy or CT, is important in the confirmation of the diagnosis. Specimens should be sent for studies for Acid-fast bacilli, fungi, bacteria, and neoplastic disease. Culture of the bone has been reported to yield acid-fast bacilli in only 60 to 80 percent of cases.[142] When cultures are negative, histological studies of the involved bone or other involved tissue may confirm the diagnosis or establish an alternative diagnosis.[232] Superinfection of tuberculous osteomyelitis with pyogenic organisms has been reported.[232] If the diagnosis is not established by needle biopsy or aspirate, extraspinal disease should be sought and, if necessary, an open biopsy and culture obtained.

THERAPY

Because the benchmark of microbiologic diagnosis of infection with *Mycobacterium tuberculosis* is culture of the organism from biopsy or tissue fluids, the therapy of tuberculous spondylitis must usually be initiated before culture results are available. Thus therapy usually is started on clinical and radiological grounds, supported by laboratory studies such as histologic evidence of granulomatous inflammation and lymphocytic reaction, when available. Recently, new techniques such as serologic tests for *Mycobacterium tuberculosis*–specific antigens[222, 301] and probes to identify *Mycobacterium tuberculosis* DNA[110] have been developed for diagnosis.[133]

With the advent of effective antituberculous chemotherapy, a controversy has developed over the need for surgical decompression in cases of tuberculous spondylitis with spinal cord compression.[142] For example, neurologic function may return following paraparesis due to tuberculous epidural infection with antituberculous chemotherapy alone.[358] One review[142] has recommended an antituberculous regimen consisting of three drugs. Decompression and spinal fusion would be reserved for those with: (1) severe loss of neurologic function when first seen; (2) progressive loss of neurologic function while on adequate antituberculous chemotherapy; and (3) no improvement of neurologic function after 4 to 6 weeks of adequate antituberculous chemotherapy. Alternatively, despite the apparent success of nonsurgical management, another recent review[358] generally recommends sur-

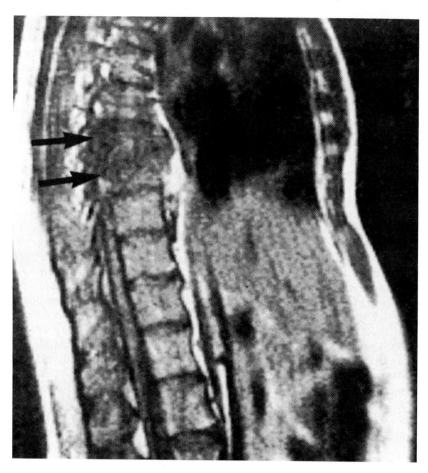

Figure 4–13. MRI of tuberculous spondylitis. (From Gandy, SE, [133] with permission.)

gery for suspected tuberculous epidural abscess with neurologic abnormalities, for both diagnostic and therapeutic reasons. A short course of corticosteroids may be helpful in cases of progressing myelopathy, with the concurrent administration of antituberculous chemotherapy. Prolonged antituberculous chemotherapy is required when spondylitis is present. The prognosis for neurologic recovery is good for 75 to 95 percent of appropriately treated patients with tuberculous spondylitis.[133]

Fungal Infections

Several different fungi may involve the spinal cord either as a primary infection or as a manifestation of disseminated disease. As with bacterial infections, fungal infections may involve the intramedullary spinal cord or the leptomeninges, or they may cause epidural spinal cord compression. In the spine, many fungal infections behave as masses compressing the spinal cord or cauda equina.[180] The radiographic appearance of spinal fungal infections may be similar to pyogenic and tuberculous infection.[198]

Cryptococcal involvement of the spine usually occurs as a necrotic granulomatous mass in the intradural location,[180, 331] but may occur secondary to osteomyelitis.[233] *Coccidioides*,[97, 239] *Blastomyces*,[180, 272] *Aspergillus*,[123, 237, 243] and *Nocardia*[121, 366] have been found to cause myelopathy or cauda equina compression due to granulomas in both intradural and extradural locations. Candidiasis may also rarely involve the spine.[164, 173] Spinal involvement from actinomycosis is considered rare, but may occur due to extension from a paravertebral site or, less commonly, from a vertebra.[198]

Parasitic Disease

Although parasitic disease involving the spine is rare in North America and Europe, it is occasionally seen in patients who have visited endemic areas or who are immunosuppressed.[246] The parasitic diseases most commonly seen are cysticercosis, hydatid disease, and schistosomiasis.[180]

Cysticercosis is a disease that results from ingestion of the pork tapeworm, *Taenia solium.* Involvement of the central nervous system results from dissemination of embryos to the brain and, occasionally, the spinal cord in the form of cysts, or occurs as the racemose form in the cerebral ventricles and subarachnoid space, in which multiple cysts are grouped together. A case of cysticercosis was reported involving the posterior spinal cord.[171]

Hydatid disease results from the larval form of the parasite *Taenia echinococcus.* It is rarely encountered in North America. The liver is most often involved;[180] the central nervous system may be involved as a primary site or as a metastatic cyst. The most common cause of spinal dysfunction is vertebral involvement with secondary spinal canal encroachment. According to a 1955 study by Fischer,[180] there had been a dozen cases of cysts involving the spinal cord, but over 200 reports of vertebral column involvement.

Schistosomiasis arises from infection with one of three trematode parasites: *Schistosoma haematobium,* found mainly in Africa; *S. mansoni,* present primarily in Africa and South America; and *S. japonicum,* seen in the Far East.[180] Involvement of the central nervous system is rare with any of the three parasites, yet each reveals a different pattern of CNS invasion. For example, *S. haematobium* primarily affects the spinal cord, while *S. japonicum* may involve the brain and almost never invade the spinal cord. *S. mansoni* causes lesions in the brain and spinal cord with similar frequency and is the most common cause of spinal schistosomiasis.[169]

Back pain and leg pain that may be present for a few weeks are often part of the initial clinical presentation. These symptoms give way to weakness, sensory loss, and sphincter dysfunction.[229, 295] Although the clinical presentation may evolve over several months, the myelopathic signs may develop acutely over several hours or days.[39] Schistosomiasis is to be suspected in the patient who has been in an endemic area. The pathological findings are those of arterial and venous infarction secondary to ova in these blood vessels.[180]

In addition to the above parasitic diseases, myelopathy may rarely be due to toxoplasmosis, paragonimiasis, gnathostomiasis, trichinosis, and malaria.[180, 246, 248, 251]

Sarcoidosis

Neurologic involvement has been reported in 5 percent of sarcoidosis cases.[96] Involvement of the spinal cord is considered rare; 17 cases had been reported at the time of Delaney's 1979 review.[96] Radiculopathy may also occur secondary to sarcoid involvement of the spine.[21] Furthermore, the spinal manifestations may be the presenting features of neurologic sarcoidosis in some cases.

Sarcoidosis may involve the spine or nerve roots secondary to intradural or epidural localization of granulomata. For example, there have been isolated reports of sarcoidosis causing the clinical syndrome of an expanding intramedullary mass.[30, 231, 322] Alternatively, clinical and myelographic findings may be consistent with arachnoiditis. The sarcoid granulomata may cause vascular compression with secondary ischemic changes of the spinal cord.[180] Sarcoid may infrequently involve the skeletal system.[198, 316] Pulmonary involvement may be seen radiographically in 80 to 90 percent of patients with osseous sarcoidosis.[198] When the vertebral column is involved, the thoracic and lumbar regions are the most common sites;[58] in such cases, roentgenograms of the spine may show a variable appearance.[36, 83, 96, 387] Corticosteroids have been used in the treatment of systemic and neurologic manifestations of sarcoidosis.[231, 337] It is important to evaluate the patient for active or prior exposure to tuberculosis and manage accordingly, especially if steroids are used.

Rheumatoid Arthritis

Rheumatoid arthritis (RA), an inflammatory disease affecting synovial joints as well as periarticular tissues, is an infrequent but well defined cause of spinal cord compression.[197] While the upper cervical spine is the most common level involved, the lower spinal cord and roots are occasionally involved.[197] For example, rheumatoid pachymeningitis of the spinal dura[152] and involvement of the epidural space with rheumatoid nodules and granulation tissue[129, 201] may cause spinal cord or nerve root compression. Furthermore, the vertebral bodies[23, 219] or intervertebral discs[65] may infrequently be the site of rheumatoid involvement, resulting in subluxation and neural compression.

A recent review[249] reported that the cervical spine is clinically affected in 44 to 88 percent of patients with RA. The most common form of rheumatoid involvement of the cervical spine is atlantoaxial subluxation (AAS),[197, 298, 333] because the odontoid is bordered anteriorly and posteriorly by synovial joints, and posteriorly by the transverse atlantal ligament, which may be involved.

In adults, the most common abnormality found is anterior C1−C2 subluxation.[226] Posterior subluxation is a less frequent cause of compressive myelopathy.[215] Involvement of the occipito-atlantoaxial complex may also permit the skull to settle on the cervical spine, resulting in upward migration of the dens through the foramen magnum. This abnormality has been reported to occur in 5 to 8 percent of patients with RA and has been variously termed cranial settling,[111, 249, 364] atlantoaxial impaction,[302, 304] and pseudobasilar invagination.[230] Brainstem compression may occur secondary to this vertical migration.

CLINICAL FEATURES AND DIAGNOSTIC IMAGING STUDIES

Symptoms and signs of AAS are diverse. Paresthesias, crepitation, and pain are commonly seen early symptoms. The pain may radiate to the occiput if the second cervical root is compressed. Lhermitte's sign suggests spinal cord compression. Pyramidal signs and posterior column dysfunction are also early clinical features.

Radiographs of the spine show a variety of abnormalities in patients with RA.[56, 198, 249, 304]. Anterior AAS, considered the most common radiographic abnormality, is found in approximately 25 to 35 percent of patients in some series.[198, 230, 283] It may not be apparent if flexion and extension views are not obtained, underscoring the importance of obtaining these films.[198, 216, 304] Since such subluxation may cause spinal cord compression, flexion-extension studies must be performed with caution to avoid neurologic injury. AAS may occur secondary to a variety of other causes, including Down's syndrome,[64, 93, 182, 260] trauma, neoplasms,[162] Behçet's syndrome,[196] psoriatic arthritis,[195] achondroplasia,[150] and neurofibromatosis.[85] (See Chaper 2.)

In addition to plain radiographs, CT scanning has been used to delineate the spinal deformities associated with RA.[55, 349] CT myelography has also been used in the radiological evaluation of AAS.[202] MRI appears to be an excellent imaging modality for the evaluation of AAS because the anatomical relationship between the spinal cord and the vertebrae may readily be demonstrated;[56, 63, 304] pannus formation may also be visualized.[309] In addition to the C1−2 level, subluxation may occur at other levels of the spine and radiographic abnormalities associated with spinal cord compression at lower levels are occasionally seen.[198]

NATURAL HISTORY AND THERAPY

Cervical spine involvement and AAS due to RA are commonly seen early in the course of the disease, and correlate with its severity elsewhere. Many patients who develop anterior AAS will do so within a few years of onset of RA. In a postmortem study, anterior AAS was found in 11 to 46 percent of cases.[216] Neurologic signs are noted in up to one third of patients with cervical spine involvement, and neurologic progression may occur in 2 to 36 percent of cases.[216] Mortality is high among patients with cervical myelopathy, with some fatalities due to spinal cord/medullary compression.

The management of rheumatoid AAS must be individualized and includes both medical and surgical options. Medical therapy, often successful, includes treatment of the overall disease process, a collar, anti-inflammatory agents, and an exercise program.[41] Surgical intervention, not uniformly successful, must be considered in patients with progressive neurologic impairment due to compression or those with incapacitating pain.[205, 311] Several surgical procedures for AAS have been recently reviewed.[216] Because many patients requiring surgery have debilitating intercurrent problems associated with their underlying disease and are thus susceptible to infection and poor wound healing, they represent a major surgical challenge.[216] According to Bland,[41] 5 to 10 percent of patients with rheumatoid arthritis of the cervical spine require surgical fusion and the prognosis is good for 85 percent of cases.[41]

Ankylosing Spondylitis

Ankylosing spondylitis (AS) is a rheumatologic disorder that is the prototype of the seronegative spondyloarthropathies.[67, 68, 287] It frequently presents with back pain and may compromise spinal cord, cauda equina, or nerve root function. As it is also to be distinguished from diffuse idiopathic skeletal hyperostosis (Forestier's disease), a noninflammatory ossifying disorder affecting the spine, which may also cause spinal cord compression.

A full discussion of the diagnostic criteria for AS is beyond the scope of this book. An inflammatory disorder involving the sacroiliac joints, spine, and larger peripheral joints,[348, 381] it usually presents between the ages of 20 and 40 years. The male-female ratio is approximately 3:1.[67] There is a strong association with the presence of HLA-B27.[184] Extra-articular manifestations often occur and may include anterior uveitis, aortic insufficiency, and pulmonary fibrosis. Back pain, which may be nocturnal, is the most common presenting complaint of AS.[67] Patients often report morning stiffness that improves with activity; a flexed posture is often assumed to alleviate pain.

In addition, major neurologic complica-tions such as vertebral fracture due to minor trauma,[158, 263, 363] spinal epidural hematoma,[151, 174] spinal cord and root compression, and cauda equina dysfunction[33, 234, 369] may occur. Several reports have emphasized the extreme vulnerability of the vertebral column to trauma in patients with AS.[263] The cervical spine appears especially prone to fracture. Although not as common as in rheumatoid arthritis, subluxation of the atlantoaxial joint is not an infrequent finding in patients with AS.[327, 369] Epidural hematomas may result from trauma and also have been found following spinal anesthesia.[151, 174]

CLINICAL FEATURES

Spinal root pain, usually thoracic or lumbar, is the most common neurologic manifestation of AS.[369] Such radiculopathies may or may not be associated with abnormal neurologic signs. In a retrospective series of 54 patients, 7 described symptoms typical of sciatica.[234] In addition, thoracic radiculopathy may cause girdle pain. Spinal cord compression due to granulomatous tissue and dural thickening may be a potential cause of myelopathy,[234] and multiple sclerosis has been reported at an increased frequency among patients with AS.[348]

A progressive cauda equina syndrome is an infrequent and obscure but well described complication of AS.[46] Its pathogenesis is poorly understood; pathological studies have typically shown arachnoid diverticula. Although evidence of arachnoiditis is not routinely seen, the arachnoid cysts and cauda equina syndrome may be late sequelae of arachnoiditis.[234]

The cauda equina syndrome appears to be a late complication of AS and is often seen years after the disease has become quiescent. The shortest interval reported between diagnosis of AS and the development of cauda equina syndrome was 4 years, with one third of patients suffering from the disease for over 30 years before the syndrome evolved.[369] Fourteen patients with the cauda equina syndrome secondary to AS were reported from the Mayo clinic;[33] the interval ranged from 17 to 53 years, with an average of 35 years. Furthermore, the AS had burned out in 10 of the 14 patients prior to the onset of neurologic symptoms. Once diagnosed, the cauda equina syndrome is usually slowly progressive.[33]

The clinical manifestations of the syndrome secondary to AS are typical of cauda equina syndrome due to other causes: sphincter disturbances, impotence, a lax anal sphincter, pain, loss of sensation over the sacral and lower lumbar dermatomes, and weakness and wasting of muscles innervated by the cauda equina. In the Mayo Clinic series,[33] the most common finding on neurologic examination was sensory loss, usually symmetrical, in the distribution of multiple nerve roots at and below the L5, S1, S2, S3 level. In the same series, weakness (often asymmetric) was found in the distribution of the L5 and sacral roots. Deep tendon reflexes are depressed routinely at the ankles, and occasionally at the knees.

LABORATORY STUDIES AND DIAGNOSTIC IMAGING STUDIES IN THE CAUDA EQUINA SYNDROME

The electromyogram commonly shows evidence of denervation of muscles innervated by multiple lumbar and sacral nerve roots. The cerebrospinal fluid findings usually do not show typical signs of arachnoiditis; rather, normal or modestly elevated protein is commonly found.[33] Conventional radiography usually shows involvement of the sacroiliac joints, which are almost always affected.[99, 208, 303] Spinal inflammation accompanies this involvement, and eventually may result in the appearance of the so-called bamboo spine.[303] The changes found on plain films of the spine have been recently reviewed.[198]

Myelography may be normal, especially if the procedure is done with the patient in a prone position. However, if the patient is in the supine position, myelography often reveals multiple arachnoid diverticula,[234] which usually erode the adjacent vertebrae. The thecal sac may be widened in the lumbosacral region.

Lumbar puncture is difficult to perform in patients with AS, and there is a risk of transient neurologic worsening after myelography.[33, 386] In some patients, CT scanning may eliminate the need for myelography. Among other abnormalities, CT scanning may show scalloping of the laminae, multiple posterior diverticula, and calcification of ligaments and discs associated with dural ectasia and posterior diverticula.[33, 147, 199] The complete role of MRI with CT in evaluating these patients has yet to be determined; they may supplant the need for myelography.

THERAPY

The treatment of AS includes the use of anti-inflammatory agents and strengthening exercises.[306] Extension exercises, hydrotherapy, and swimming appear very effective. Bartleson and colleagues[33] report no effective therapy for the cauda equina syndrome secondary to longstanding AS and advise that surgical intervention be avoided.

SPINAL HEMORRHAGE

Spinal hemorrhage may occur in the spinal cord itself, the subarachnoid space, the subdural space, or the epidural space. In each setting, the clinical presentation is typically sudden pain followed by neurologic symptoms and signs determined by the level of the hematoma. Some cases are due to trauma, but in many the etiology is a coagulopathy, anticoagulant therapy, or a vascular malformation.[235, 275, 317]

Intramedullary Hemorrhage

Although commonly secondary to trauma, nontraumatic hematomyelia is encountered rarely. It may occur secondary to bleeding from a spinal arteriovenous malformation (AVM), venous infarction, AVM with aneurysm, neoplasm, syrinx, or bleeding diathesis such as hemophilia, anticoagulant therapy, or coagulopathy.[61, 275, 317] According to Buchan and Barnett,[61] neither congophilic hemorrhage nor hypertensive hemorrhage, sometimes seen in intracerebral hemorrhages, has been reported.

The clinical presentation most commonly is that of sudden severe back pain with or without a radicular component. The neurologic symptoms and signs will largely depend upon the level and extent of the hemorrhage. The hemorrhage may cause a central cord syndrome; a complete cord transection may develop in massive hemorrhage. The CSF usually demonstrates evidence of hemorrhage. The myelogram may show an enlarged spinal cord. MRI may be significant in evaluating these patients.

Treatment of nontraumatic hematomyelia depends upon the underlying cause. Drainage of the hematoma may be beneficial in appropriately selected patients.[61]

Spinal Subarachnoid Hemorrhage

Spontaneous spinal subarachnoid hemorrhage, as distinguished from hemorrhage related to major trauma, is a rare disorder, accounting for less than 1 percent of all cases of subarachnoid hemorrhage.[61, 360] While aneurysm is a frequent cause of intracranial subarachnoid hemorrhage, spontaneous spinal subarachnoid hemorrhage is commonly associated with arteriovenous malformations, coagulopathy, neoplastic and infectious meningitis, extreme physical exertion, collagen vascular disease, and lumbar puncture.[61, 168, 308, 341]

Among these diverse etiologies, the most common cause appears to be an AVM of the spinal cord.[168, 341] Nearly 10 percent of spinal AVMs present with a spinal subarachnoid hemorrhage; these AVMs may be associated with spinal artery aneurysms.[341] Spinal tumor appears to be a less common cause. A 1984 review[308] found that only 55 cases of spinal subarachnoid hemorrhage attributable to spinal neoplasm had been reported; 89 percent were in the region of the conus medullaris and cauda equina. Although several different histological types have been reported, ependymomas are the most frequent tumor responsible.[308, 341]

The clinical presentation of spinal subarachnoid hemorrhage is usually that of sudden severe back or neck pain.[288, 308]

Michon[254] termed the presenting complaint le coup de poignard (the strike of the dagger). The pain may be localized to the spine or may radiate into the legs or trunk and thereby suggest a visceral catastrophe.[341] There may be a history of prior, repeated, less severe pain suggesting earlier hemorrhage. When nerve roots or spinal cord are involved, there is associated radiculopathy or myelopathy. Auscultation of the spine may reveal a bruit in patients with an AVM.[178] Intracranial symptoms and signs may develop as the blood circulates over the cerebral hemispheres.[70]

The CSF typically demonstrates evidence of hemorrhage. The bleeding may be diluted by CSF, but occasionally a hematoma may form due to massive hemorrhage resulting in mass effect that may be seen on imaging studies. Subarachnoid hemorrhage may be associated with a subdural hematoma.[341] When a spinal AVM is the cause, they also may be seen radiographically.

The treatment of spinal subarachnoid hemorrhage depends upon the cause. Patients with a bleeding diathesis are treated with appropriate measures. Those with a spinal AVM are evaluated for definitive treatment of this lesion.[61, 253] If a subarachnoid hematoma is found to cause spinal cord compression, evacuation of the clot may be necessary.[61]

Spinal Subdural Hemorrhage

Spinal subdural hematoma unrelated to major trauma is a rarely described clinical entity, with only about 60 reported cases noted in a 1987 review.[235] It usually occurs in the setting of coagulopathies such as hemophilia, anticoagulant therapy, or thrombocytopenia, and/or following lumbar puncture, spinal surgery, or vascular malformation.[107, 329, 384] Lumbar puncture as an etiology of spinal subdural hemorrhage in the setting of a coagulation disturbance is an important etiology to emphasize.[107, 193, 235]

Because the subdural space harbors few blood vessels, the source of bleeding in spinal subdural hematomas has been a source of conjecture and debate.[193] The greater frequency of spinal epidural hemorrhage than subdural hemorrhage may reflect the greater density of blood vessels in the epidural space.[107] Spinal subdural hematomas occur most commonly in the thoracic and thoracolumbar regions.[312]

The clinical presentation of spinal subdural hematoma is usually acute in onset and evolution. Patients usually present with severe back or neck pain with or without a radicular component. Paraplegia, sensory loss, and bowel/bladder dysfunction may rapidly ensue over several minutes, hours, or (less commonly) days.[235] Although less frequent, chronic subdural hematomas have been described.[61, 193] These patients may show fluctuating neurologic signs.[193]

The cerebrospinal fluid may show blood if there is an associated subarachnoid hemorrhage. A complete block due to a hematoma may result in a dry tap. Myelography may demonstrate a filling defect from a hematoma in the subdural space. CT scanning may show a clot if the level of the hematoma is imaged. If found to be a sensitive imaging technique for these lesions, the use of MRI would avoid the risks of lumbar or cisternal puncture in many of these patients with a bleeding diathesis.

mon spinal subdural hemorrhage.[61] Although an epidural hematoma rarely may develop without pain,[323] patients nearly always complain of axial pain, which may radiate in a radicular distribution.[235] The motor, sensory, and sphincter functions disrupted generally depend upon the level of the spinal axis involved. Symptoms and signs of spinal cord and/or cauda equina dysfunction generally follow within minutes, hours, or (less commonly) days.[235] The thoracic and thoracolumbar areas are the most commonly involved regions; the hematoma may extend over several segments and is usually in the posterior epidural space.[35, 235]

The CSF may be clear, have an elevated protein, or be bloody. The most useful laboratory studies are imaging techniques. Myelography has been used to demonstrate the presence and extent of spinal epidural hemorrhage.[235] CT scanning may show a convex, hyperdense mass,[165, 203, 211] but the rostral-caudal extent of the hematoma may be difficult to determine accurately with CT alone.[235] MRI may be a valuable imaging technique that could avert the need for lumbar and cisternal puncture in patients with bleeding diatheses.

Spinal Epidural Hemorrhage

Since first described in 1869 by Jackson, there have been approximately 250 cases of nontraumatic spinal epidural hematoma reported up to 1987.[235] Most traumatic cases share similar predisposing factors as those seen in spinal subdural hemorrhage. For example, many patients are receiving anticoagulant therapy[329] or have a bleeding diathesis for a reason such as thrombocytopenia or liver disease. Many cases occur in such patients following lumbar puncture or epidural anesthesia.[151] Patients with ankylosing spondylitis are reported to be at increased risk,[174] and vascular malformations also may be responsible. Occasionally no explanation can be found other than possible exertion or Valsalva maneuver.

Spinal epidural hemorrhage has a clinical presentation similar to the less com-

Differential Diagnosis of Spinal Hematoma

At the time that patients have only local and/or radicular pain, the differential diagnosis of spinal hematoma is exceedingly broad, including diseases of the spine as well as visceral diseases such as myocardial infarction and dissecting aortic aneurysm. When neurologic symptoms and signs of spinal cord or cauda equina dysfunction develop, the differential diagnosis includes those diseases that may cause rapidly evolving paraparesis or tetraparesis, such as herniated discs, neoplasm (extradural, intradural-extramedullary, and intramedullary), abscess, as well as sequelae of trauma. Intramedullary diseases such as acute and subacute transverse myelitis, demyelinating disease, spinal cord infarction, and infectious diseases also need to be considered.[235]

Therapy

Spinal cord compression secondary to nontraumatic spinal subdural and epidural hematoma is a neurologic and neurosurgical emergency. Patients with impaired hemostasis due to thrombocytopenia should receive platelet transfusions. In patients receiving anticoagulation, fresh frozen plasma and, when indicated, phytonadione should be administered urgently to correct the bleeding diathesis.[235] Prompt surgical decompression of the compressed spinal cord and/or cauda equina is recommended because the prognosis for neurologic recovery depends upon the preoperative neurologic status and the duration of neurologic dysfunction.[61, 235] In patients with noncorrectable bleeding disorders, however, the risks of surgical intervention may outweigh the benefits.[107]

The prognosis for neurologic recovery depends upon several factors. Many patients with incomplete motor and sensory paralysis preoperatively can be expected to enjoy a good recovery, whereas those with complete sensorimotor paralysis have less than a 50 percent chance of successful recovery.[235] Other prognostic factors include the time-course of sensorimotor paralysis and the rostrocaudal location of the hematoma. Those with a rapid deterioration of neurologic function have a worse prognosis than those with slow progression. Those with hematomas at the cervical and thoracic levels fare more poorly than those with lumbar hematomas.[235]

REFERENCES

1. Aarabi, B, Pasternak, G, Hurko, O, and Long, DM: Familial intradural arachnoid cysts: Report of two cases. J Neurosurg 50:826–829, 1979.
2. Adams, C: Cervical spondylotic radiculopathy and myelopathy. In Vinken, PJ and Bruyn, GW (eds): Handbook of Clinical Neurology, Vol 26. North-Holland Publishing, Amsterdam, 1976, pp 97–112.
3. Adams, CBT and Logue, V: Studies in cervical spondylotic myelopathy. I. Movement of the cervical roots, dura and cord and their relation to the course taken by extrathecal roots. Brain 94:557–568, 1971.
4. Adams, CBT and Logue, V: Studies in cervical spondylotic myelopathy. II. Observations on the movement and contour of the cervical spine in relation to the neural complications of cervical spondylosis. Brain 94:569–586, 1971.
5. Adams, CBT and Logue, V: Studies in cervical spondylotic myelopathy. III. Some functional effects of operations for cervical spondylotic myelopathy. Brain 94:587–594, 1971.
6. Adams, RD and Victor, M: Pain in the back, neck, and extremities. In Adams, RD and Victor, M (eds): Principles of Neurology, ed 3. McGraw-Hill, New York, 1985, pp 149–172.
7. Adams, RD and Victor, M: Diseases of the spinal cord. In Adams, RD and Victor, M (eds): Principles of Neurology, ed 3. McGraw-Hill, New York, 1985, pp 665–698.
8. Adelstein, LJ: The surgical treatment of syringomyelia. Am J Surg 40:384–395, 1938.
9. Al-Mefty, O, Harkey, LH, Middleton, TH, et al: Myelopathic cervical spondylotic lesions demonstrated by magnetic resonance imaging. J Neurosurg 68:217–222, 1988.
10. Alexander, E Jr: Significance of the small lumbar spinal canal: Cauda equina compression syndromes due to spondylosis: Achondroplasia. J Neurosurg 31:513–519, 1969.
11. Allen, KL: Neuropathies caused by bony spurs in the cervical spine with special reference to surgical treatment. J Neurol Neurosurg Psychiatry 15:20–36, 1952.
12. Allen, SS and Kahn, EA: Acute pyogenic infection of the spinal epidural space. JAMA 98:875–878, 1932.
13. Altman, RD, Brown, M, and Gargano, F: Low back pain in Paget's disease of bone. Clin Orthop 217:152–161, 1987.
14. Altrocchi, PH: Acute spinal epidural abscess vs. acute transverse myelopathy. Arch Neurol 9:17–25, 1963.
15. Andrews, BT, Weinstein, PR, Rosenblum, ML, and Barbaro, NM: Intradural arachnoid cysts of the spinal canal associated with intramedullary cysts. J Neurosurg 68:544–549, 1988.
16. Anton, HA and Schweigel, JF: Posttraumatic syringomyelia: The British Columbia experience. Spine 11:865–868, 1986.
17. Arce, CA and Dohrmann, GJ: Thoracic disc herniation: Improved diagnosis with computerized tomographic scanning and a review of the literature. Surg Neurol 23:356–361, 1985.
18. Arnoldi, CC, Brodsky, AE, Cauchoix, J, et al: Lumbar spinal stenosis and nerve root entrapment syndromes: Definition and classification. Clin Orthop 115:4–5, 1976.
19. Arroyo, IL, Barron, KS, and Brewer, EJ: Spinal cord compression by epidural lipomatosis in juvenile rheumatoid arthritis. Arthritis and Rheumatology 31:447–451, 1988.
20. Arseni, C and Nash, F: Protrusion of thoracic intervertebral discs. Acta Neurochir (Wien) 31:3–33, 1963.
21. Atkinson, R, Ghelman, B, Tsairis, P, et al:

Sarcoidosis presenting as cervical radiculo-pathy: A case report and literature review. Spine 7:412–416, 1982.

22. Badami, JP, Norman, D, Barbaro, NM, et al: Metrizamide CT myelography in cervical myelopathy and radiculopathy: Correlation with conventional myelography and surgical findings. AJR 144:675–680, 1985.
23. Baggenstoss, AH, Bickel, WH, and Ward, LE: Rheumatoid granulomatous nodules as destructive lesions of vertebrae. J Bone Joint Surg 34:601–609, 1952.
24. Bailey, HL, Gabriel, M, Hodgson, AR, et al: Tuberculosis of the spine in children: Operative findings and results in one hundred consecutive patients treated by removal of the lesion and anterior grafting. J Bone Joint Surg 54A:1633–1657, 1972.
25. Bailey, P and Casamajor, L: Osteo-arthritis of the spine as a cause of compression of the spinal cord and its roots. J Nerv Ment Dis 38:588–609, 1911.
26. Baker, AS: Spinal epidural abscess. In Braude, AI, Davis, CE, and Fierer, J (eds): Infectious Disease and Medical Microbiology, ed 2. WB Saunders, Philadelphia, 1986, pp 1101–1103.
27. Baker, AS, Ojemann, RJ, Swartz, NM, et al: Spinal epidural abscess. N Engl J Med 293:463–468, 1975.
28. Ball, MJ and Dayan, AD: Pathogenesis of syringomyelia. Lancet 2:799–801, 1972.
29. Banna, M: Clinical Radiology of the Spine and Spine Cord. Aspen, Rockville, Md, 1985.
30. Bannerjee, T and Hunt, WE: Spinal cord sarcoidosis. J Neurosurg 36:490–493, 1972.
31. Barnett, GH, Hardy, RW, Little, JR, Bay, JW, and Sypert, GW: Thoracic spinal canal stenosis. J Neurosurg 66:338–344, 1987.
32. Barnett, HJM, Foster, JB, and Hudgson, P: Syringomyelia. WB Saunders, Philadelphia, 1973.
33. Bartleson, JO, Cohen, MD, and Harrington, TM: Cauda equina syndrome secondary to long-standing ankylosing spondylitis. Ann Neurol 14:662–669, 1983.
34. Batson, OV: The function of the vertebral veins and their role in the spread of metastases. Ann Surg 112:138–148, 1940.
35. Beatty, RM and Winston, KR: Spontaneous cervical epidural hematoma. Consideration of etiology. J Neurosurg 61:143–148, 1984.
36. Beck, RN and Brower, TD: Vertebral sarcoidosis. Radiology 82:660–663, 1964.
37. Bernard, TN and Kirkaldy-Willis, WH: Recognizing specific characteristics of nonspecific low back pain. Spine 217:266–280, 1987.
38. Bhole, R and Gilmer, RE: Two-level thoracic disc herniation. Clin Orthop 190:129–131, 1984.
39. Bird, AV: Acute spinal schistosomiasis. Neurology 14:647–656, 1964.
40. Blacklock, JB, Hood, TW, and Mazwell, RE: Intramedullary cervical spinal cord abscess: Case report. J Neurosurg 57:270–273, 1982.
41. Bland, JH: Disorders of the Cervical Spine:

Diagnosis and Medical Management. WB Saunders, Philadelphia, 1987.
42. Blau, JN and Logue, V: The natural history of intermittent claudication of the cauda equina. Brain 101:211–222, 1978.
43. Boharas, S and Koskoff, YD: The early diagnosis of acute spinal epidural abscess. JAMA 117:1085–1088, 1941.
44. Bohlman, HH and Emery, SE: The pathophysiology of cervical spondylosis and myelopathy. Spine 13:843–846, 1988.
45. Bolender, NF, Schonstrom, NSR, and Spengler, DM: Role of computed tomography and myelography in the diagnosis of central spinal stenosis. J Bone Joint Surg 67A:240–246, 1985.
46. Bowie, EA and Glasgow, GL: Cauda equina lesions associated with ankylosing spondylitis. Br Med J 2:24–27, 1961.
47. Bradley, WG and Banna, M: The cervical dural canal: A study of the "tight dural canal" and of syringomyelia by prone and supine myelography. Br J Radiol 41:608–614, 1968.
48. Brain, R and Wilkinson, M: Cervical arthropathy in syringomyelia, tabes dorsalis and diabetes. Brain 81:275–289, 1958.
49. Brain, WR: Rupture of the intervertebral disc in the cervical region. Proc R Soc Med 49:509–511, 1948.
50. Brain, WR, Northfield, D, and Wilkinson, M: The neurological manifestations of cervical spondylosis. Brain 75:187–225, 1952.
51. Brain, WR and Wilkinson, M: Cervical Spondylosis and Other Disorders of the Cervical Spine. Heinemann, London, 1967.
52. Brant-Zawadzski, M, Burke, VD, and Jeffrey, RB: CT in the evaluation of spine infection. Spine 9:358–364, 1983.
53. Brant-Zawadzki, M, Miller, EM, and Federle, MP: CT in the evaluation of spine trauma. AJR 136:369–375, 1981.
54. Braun, IF, Hoffman, JC, Davis, PC, et al: Contrast enhancement in CT differentiation between recurrent disc herniation and postoperative scar: Prospective study. AJR 145:785–790, 1985.
55. Braunstein, EM, Weissman, BN, Seltzer, SE, et al: Computed tomography and conventional radiographs of the craniocervical region in rheumatoid arthritis. Arthritis and Rheumatology 27:26–31, 1984.
56. Breedveld, FC, Algra, PR, Vielvoye, CJ, and Cats, A: Magnetic resonance imaging in the evaluation of patients with rheumatoid arthritis and subluxation of the cervical spine. Arthritis and Rheumatology 30:624–630, 1987.
57. Brish, A, Lerner, MA, and Braham, J: Intermittent claudication from compression of cauda equina by a narrowed spinal canal. J Neurosurg 21:207–211, 1964.
58. Brodey, PA, Pripstein, S, Strange, G, et al: Vertebral sarcoidosis: A case report and review of the literature. AJR 126:900–902, 1976.
59. Brooker, AE and Barter, AW: Cercical spondylosis. Clinical study with comparative radiology. Brain 88:925–936, 1965.

60. Brunberg, JA, Latchaw, RE, Kanal, E, et al: Magnetic resonance imaging of spinal dysraphism. Radiol Clin North Am 26:181–205, 1988.
61. Buchan, AM and Barnett, JM: Vascular malformations and hemorrhage of the spinal cord. In Barnett, HJM, Mohr, JP, Stein, BM and Yatsu, FM (eds): Stroke: Pathophysiology, Diagnosis and Management. Churchill Livingstone, New York, 1986, pp 721–730.
62. Bull, JWD: Discussion on rupture of the intervertebral disc in the cervical region. Proc R Soc Med 41:513–516, 1948.
63. Bundschuch, CV, Modic, MT, Kearny, F, and others: Rheumatoid arthritis of the cervical spine. Surface-coil MR imaging. AJNR 9:565–571, 1988.
64. Burke, SW, French, HG, Roberts, JM, et al: Chronic atlanto-axial instability in Down's syndrome. J Bone Joint Surg 67A:1356–1360, 1985.
65. Bywaters, EGL: Thoracic intervertebral discitis in rheumatoid arthritis due to costovertebral joint involvement. Rheumatol Int 1:83–97, 1981.
66. Cahan, LD and Bentson, JR: Considerations in the diagnosis and treatment of syringomyelia and the Chiari malformation. J Neurosurg 57:24–31, 1982.
67. Calabro, JJ: The seronegative spondyloarthropathies: A graduated approach to management. Postgrad Med 80:173–188, 1986.
68. Calin, A: The spondyloarthropathies. In Wyngaarden, JB and Smith, LK (eds): Cecil: Textbook of Medicine, ed 17. WB Saunders, Philadelphia, 1985, pp 1917–1922.
69. Caron, JP. Djindjian, R, Julian, H, et al: Les hernies discales dorsales. Ann Med Interne 67:675–688, 1971.
70. Caroscio, JT, Brannan, T, Budabin, M, et al: Subarachnoid hemorrhage secondary to spinal arteriovenous malformation and aneurysm. Report of a case and review of the literature. Arch Neurol 37:101–103, 1980.
71. Castillo, M, Quencer, RM, Green, BA, and Montalvo, BM: Syringomyelia as a consequence of compressive extramedullary lesions: Postoperative clinical and radiological manifestations. AJR 150:391–396, 1988.
72. Chafetz, N, Genant, HK, Gillespy, T, and Winkler, M: Magnetic resonance imaging. In Kricun, ME (ed): Imaging Modalities in Spinal Disorders. WB Saunders, Philadelphia, 1988, pp 478–502.
73. Chan, RC, Thompson, GB, and Bratty, PJA: Symptomatic anterior spinal arachnoid diverticulum. Neurosurgery 16:663–665, 1985.
74. Chiari, H: Uber myelitis suppurativa bei bronchiektasie. Z Heilk 1:351–372, 1900.
75. Ciapetta, P, Delfini, R, and Cantore, GP: Intradural lumbar disc hernia: Description of three cases. Neurosurgery 8:104–107, 1981.
76. Clarke, E and Robinson, PK: A complication of cervical spondylosis. Brain 79:483–507, 1956.
77. Cloward, RB: Congenital extradural cysts: Case report with a review of the literature. Ann Surg 168:851–864, 1968.
78. Coin, CB and Coin, JT: Computed tomography of cervical disk disease: Technical considerations with representative case reports. J Comput Assist Tomogr 5:275–280, 1981.
79. Conway, LW: Radiographic studies of syringomyelia. Transactions of the American Neurological Association 86:205–206, 1961.
80. Conway, LW: Hydrodynamic studies in syringomyelia. J Neurosurg 27:501–514, 1967.
81. Council, Scientific Affairs: Magnetic resonance imaging of the central nervous system. JAMA 259:1211–1222, 1988.
82. Courville, CB: Pathology of the Central Nervous System. Mountainview, Calif, 1950, pp 191–192.
83. CPC: A 34 year-old man with a destructive sacral lesion and a left gluteal mass. N Engl J Med 318:306–312, 1988.
83a. CPC: A 79-year-old woman with an osteolytic lesion of the spine and increasing paraparesis after a fall. N Engl J Med 321:1178–1187, 1989.
84. D'Angelo, CM and Whisler, WW: Bacterial infections of the spinal cord and its coverings. In Vinken, PJ and Bruyn, GW (eds): Handbook of Clinical Neurology, Vol 33. North-Holland Publishing, Amsterdam, 1978, pp 187–194.
85. D'Aprile, P, Krajewska, G, Perniola, T, et al: Congenital dislocation of dens of the axis in a case of neurofibromatosis. Neuroradiology 26:405–440, 1984.
86. Dagi, TF, Tarkington, MA, and Leech, JJ: Tandem lumbar and cervical spinal stenosis. Natural history, prognostic indices, and results after surgical decompression. J Neurosurg 66:842–849, 1987.
87. Dandy, W: A sign and symptom of spinal cord tumors. Archives of Neurology and Psychiatry 16:435–441, 1920.
88. Dandy, WE: Abscesses and inflammatory tumors in the spinal epidural space (so-called pachymeningitis externa). Arch Surg 13:447–494, 1926.
89. Daniels, DL, Grogan, JP, Johansen, JG, et al: Cervical radiculopathy: Computed tomography and myelography compared. Radiology 151:109–113, 1984.
90. Danner, RL and Hartman, BJ: Update of spinal epidural abscess: 35 cases and review of the literature. Rev Infect Dis 9:265–274, 1987.
91. Dastur, DK and Lalitha, VS: The many facets of neurotuberculosis: An epitome of neuropathology. In Zimmerman, HM (ed): Progress in Neuropathology. Grune & Stratton, New York, 1973, pp 351–408.
92. Davison, C and Keschner, M: Myelitic and myelopathic lesions (a clinico-pathologic study): I. Myelitis. Archives of Neurology and Psychiatry 29:332–343, 1933.
93. Dawson, EG and Smith, L: Atlanto-axial subluxation in children due to vertebral anomalies. J Bone Joint Surg 61A:582–587, 1979.
94. de Roos, A, van Persijn van Meerten, E, Bloem, JL, and Bluemm, RG: MRI of tuberculous spondylitis. AJR 146:79–82, 1986.
95. Dejerine, J: Sur la claudication intermittente de la moelle epiniere. Rev Neurol 14:341–350, 1906.

96. Delaney, P: Neurologic manifestations in sarcoidosis: Review of the literature, with a report of 23 cases. Ann Intern Med 87:336–345, 1977.

97. Delaney, P and Niemann, B: Spinal cord compression by Coccidioides immitis abscess. Arch Neurol 39:255–256, 1982.

98. Di Chiro, G, Axelbaum, SP, Schellinger, D, et al: Computerized tomography in syringomyelia. N Engl J Med 292:13–16, 1975.

99. Dihlmann, W: Current radiodiagnostic concept of ankylosing spondylitis. Skeletal Radiol 4:179–188, 1979.

100. Dillon, WP, Kaseff, LG, Knackstedt, VE, et al: Computed tomography and differential diagnosis of the extruded lumbar disc. J Comput Assist Tomogr 7:969–975, 1983.

101. Dinakar, I and Balaparameswararao, I: Lumbar disc prolapse. Study of 300 surgical cases. Int Surg 57:299–302, 1972.

102. Ditulio, MV: Intramedullary spinal abscess: A case report with a review of 53 previously described cases. Surg Neurol 7:351–354, 1977.

103. Donovan Post, MJ, Quencer, RM, Montalvo, BM, et al: Spinal infection: Evaluation with MR imaging and intraoperative ultrasound. Radiology 169:765–771, 1988.

104. Douglas, DI, Duckworth, T, Kanis, JA, et al: Spinal cord dysfunction in Paget's disease of bone. Has medical treatment a vascular basis? J Bone Joint Surg 63B:495–503, 1981.

105. Dreyfus, P, Six, B, Dorfman, H, and De Seze, S: Thoracic disc hernia. In Vinken, PJ and Bruyn, GW (eds): Handbook of Clinical Neurology, Vol 20. North-Holland Publishing, Amsterdam, 1976, pp 565–571.

106. Dutton, JEM and Alexander, GL: Intramedullary spinal abscess. J Neurol Neurosurg Psychiatry 17:303–307, 1954.

107. Edelson, RN, Chernik, NL, and Posner, JB: Spinal subdural hematomas complicating lumbar puncture. Occurrence in thrombocytopenic patients. Arch Neurol 31:134–137, 1974.

108. Edwards, WC and LaRocca, SH: The developmental segmental diameter in combined cervical and lumbar spondylosis. Spine 10:42–49, 1985.

109. Efird, TA, Genant, HK, and Wilson, CB: Pituitary giantism with cervical spinal stenosis. AJR 134:171–173, 1980.

110. Eisenach, KD, Crawford, JT, and Bates, JH: Genetic relatedness among strains of Mycobacterium tuberculosis complex. Am Rev Respir Dis 133:1065–1068, 1986.

111. El-Khoury, GY, Wener, MH, Menezes, AH, et al: Cranial settling in rheumatoid arthritis. Radiology 137:637–642, 1980.

112. Elisevich, K, Fontaine, S, and Bertrand, G: Syringomyelia as a complication of Paget's disease. Case report. J Neurosurg 66:611–613, 1987.

113. Elster, AD: Quadriplegia after minor trauma in the Klippel-Feil syndrome: A case report and review of the literature. J Bone Joint Surg 66A:1473–1474, 1984.

114. Epstein, B, Epstein, JA, and Jones, MD: Lumbar spinal stenosis. Radiol Clin North Am 15:227–239, 1977.

115. Epstein, BS and Epstein, JA: Cervical spinal stenosis. Radiol Clin North Am 15:215–226, 1977.

116. Epstein, BS, Epstein, JA, and Lavine, L: The effect of anatomic variations in the lumbar vertebrae and spinal canal on cauda equina and nerve root syndromes. AJR 91:1055–1063, 1964.

117. Epstein, JA: The surgical management of cervical spinal stenosis, spondylosis, and myeloradiculopathy by means of the posterior approach. Spine 13:864–869, 1988.

118. Epstein, JA, Janin, Y, Carras, R, and Lavine, LS: A comparative study of the treatment of cervical spondylotic myeloradiculopathy. Acta Neurochir 61:89–104, 1982.

119. Epstein, NE, Epstein, JA, Carras, R, et al: Coexisting cervical and lumbar spinal stenosis: Diagnosis and management. Neurosurgery 15:489–496, 1984.

120. Epstein, NE, Epstein, JA, and Zilkha, A: Traumatic myelopathy in a seventeen-year-old child with cervical spinal stenosis (without fracture or dislocation) and a C2–C3 Klippel-Feil fusion: A case report. Spine 9:344–347, 1984.

121. Epstein, S, Holden, M, Feldshuh, J, and Singer, JM: Unusual cause of spinal cord compression: Nocardiosis. New York J Med 63:3422–3427, 1963.

122. Erntell, M, Holtas, S, Norlin, K, et al: Magnetic resonance imaging in the diagnosis of spinal epidural abscess. Scand J Infect Dis 20:323–327, 1988.

123. Ferris, B and Jones, C: Paraplegia due to aspergillosis: Successful conservative treatment of two cases. J Bone Joint Surg 67B:800–803, 1985.

124. Finlayson, AI: Syringomyelia and related conditions. In Baker, AB and Baker, LH (eds): Clinical Neurology, Vol 3. Harper & Row, Hagerstown, Md, 1980.

125. Fitz, CR: The pediatric spine. In Gonzalez, CF, Grossman, CB, and Masdeu, JC (eds): Head and Spine Imaging. John Wiley & Sons, New York, 1985, pp 759–780.

126. Fortuna, A, La Torre, E, and Ciapetta, P: Arachnoid diverticula: A unitary approach to spinal cysts communicating with the subarachnoid space. Acta Neurochir 39:259–268, 1977.

127. Fraser, RAR, Ratzan, K, Wolpert, SM, et al: Spinal subdural empyema. Arch Neurol 28:235–238, 1973.

128. Freidenberg, ZB and Miller, WT: Degenerative disc disease of the cervical spine: A comparative study of asymptomatic and symptomatic patients. J Bone Joint Surg 45A:1171–1178, 1963.

129. Friedman, H: Intraspinal rheumatoid nodule causing nerve root compression. Case report. J Neurosurg 32:689–691, 1970.

130. Frymoyer, JW: Back pain and sciatica. N Engl J Med 318:291–300, 1988.

131. Frymoyer, JW, Newberg, A, Pope, MH, Wilder,

DG, Clements, J, and MacPherson, B: Spine radiographs in patients with low-back pain. J Bone Joint Surg 66A:1048–1055, 1984.

132. Galzio, RJ, Zenobil, M, Lucantoni, D, and Cristuib-Grizzi, L: Spinal intradural arachnoid cyst. Surg Neurol 17:388–391, 1981.

133. Gandy, SE: Tuberculosis of the central nervous system: Recent experience and reappraisal. In Plum, F (cd): Advances in Contemporary Neurology. FA Davis, Philadelphia, 1988, pp 153–184.

134. Gardner, WJ: The Dysraphic States from Syringomyelia to Anencephaly. Excerpta Medica, Amsterdam, 1973.

135. Gathier, JC: Radicular disorders due to lumbar discopathy (hernia nuclei puplosi). In Vinken, PJ and Bruyn, GW (eds): Handbook of Clinical Neurology, Vol 20. North-Holland Publishing, Amsterdam, 1976, pp 573–604.

136. Gimeno, A: Arachnoid, neurenteric and other cysts. In Vinken, PJ and Bruyn, GW (eds): Handbook of Clinical Neurology, Vol 32. North Holland Publishing, Amsterdam, 1978, pp 393–447.

137. Godersky, JC, Erickson, DL, and Seljeskog, EL: Extreme lateral disc herniation: Diagnosis by computed tomographic scanning. J Neurosurg 14:549–552, 1984.

138. Goldman, AB and Freiberger, RH: Localized infectious and neuropathic diseases. Skeletal Radiol 14: 19–32, 1979.

139. Golimbu, C, Firoonzia, H, and Rafil, M: CT of osteomyelitis of the spine. AJR 142:159–163, 1984.

140. Good, DC, Couch, Jr, and Wacasar, L: "Numb, clumsy hands" and high cervical spondylosis. Surg Neurol 22:285–291, 1984.

141. Goodhart, SP and Davison, C: Torula infection of the nervous system. AMA Archives of Neurology and Psychiatry 37:435–439, 1937.

142. Gorse, GJ, Pais, MJ, Kusske, JA, and Cesario, TC: Tuberculous spondylitis: A report of six cases and review of the literature. Medicine (Baltimore) 62:178–193, 1983.

143. Gowers, WR: Diseases of the Nervous System. Vol. I, Spinal Cord and Nerves, ed 1. J & A Churchill, London, 1886.

144. Greenlee, JE: Epidural abscess. In Mandell, GL, Douglas, RG, and Bennett, JE (eds): Principles and Practice of Infectious Diseases, ed 2. John Wiley & Sons, New York, 1985, pp 594–596.

145. Griffiths, D, Seddon, HJ, and Roaf, R: Pott's Paraplegia. Oxford University Press, London, 1956.

146. Griffiths, HED and Jones, DM: Pyogenic infection of the spine: A review of 28 cases. J Bone Joint Surg 53B:383–391, 1971.

147. Grosman, H, Gray, R, and St Louis, EL: CT of longstanding ankylosing spondylitis with cauda equina syndrome. AJNR 4:1077–1080, 1983.

148. Grossman, CB and Post, MJD: The adult spine. In Gonzalez, CF, Grossman, CB and Masdeau, JC (eds): Head and Spine Imaging. John Wiley & Sons, New York, 1985, pp 781–858.

149. Guidetti, B and LaTorre, E: Hypertrophic spinal pachymeningitis. J Neurosurg 26:496–503, 1967.

150. Gulati, DR and Rout, D: Atlantoaxial dislocation with quadriparesis in achondroplasia: Case report. J Neurosurg 40:394–396, 1974.

151. Gustafson, H, Rutberg, H, and Bengtsson, M: Spinal haematoma following epidural analgesia. Report of a patient with ankylosing spondylitis and a bleeding diathesis. Anesthesia 43:220–222, 1988.

152. Guttmann, L and Hable, K: Rheumatoid pachymeningitis. Neurology 13:901–905, 1963.

153. Hadley, LA: The Spine: Anatomico-Radiographic Studies, Development and the Cervical Region. Charles C Thomas, Springfield, Ill, 1956.

154. Hakin, RN, Burt, AA, and Cook, JB: Acute spinal epidural abscess. Paraplegia 17:330–336, 1979.

155. Hall, SH, Bartleson, JD, Onofrio, BM, et al: Lumbar spinal stenosis: Clinical features, diagnostic procedures, and results of surgical treatment in 68 patients. Ann Intern Med 103:271–275, 1985.

156. Hamlin, H, Garrity, RW, and Golden, JB: Extradural spinal cyst. A case report. J Neurosurg 6:260–263, 1949.

157. Hancock, DO: A study of 49 patients with acute spinal extradural abscess. Paraplegia 10:285–288, 1973.

158. Harding, JR, McCall, IW, Park, WM, and Jones, BF: Fracture of the cervical spine in ankylosing spondylitis. Br J Radiol 58:3–7, 1985.

159. Harkelius, A and Hindmarsh, J: The comparative reliability of preoperative diagnostic methods in lumbar disc surgery. Acta Orthop Scand 43:234–238, 1972.

160. Harsh, GR, Sypert, GW, Weinstein, PR, et al: Cervical spine stenosis secondary to ossification of the posterior longitudinal ligament. J Neurosurg 67:349–357, 1987.

161. Hashizume, Y, Iljima, S, Kishimoto, H, et al: Pencil-shaped softening of the spinal cord. Pathological study in 12 autopsy cases. Acta Neuropathol 61:219–224, 1983.

162. Hastings, DE, Macnab, I, and Lawson, V: Neoplasms of the atlas and axis. Can J Surg 11:290–296, 1968.

163. Haughton, VM and Williams, AL: Computed Tomography of the Spine. CV Mosby, St Louis, 1982.

164. Hayes, WS, Berg, RA, and Dorfman, HD: Candida discitis and vertebral osteomyelitis at L1–L2 from hematogenous spread. Case report 291. Skeletal Radiol 12:184–287, 1984.

165. Haykal, HA, Wang, A-M, Zamani, AA, and Rumbaugh, CL: Computed tomography of spontaneous acute cervical epidural hematoma. J Comput Assist Tomogr 8:229–231, 1984.

166. Heindell, CC, Ferguson, JP, and Kumarasamy, T: Spinal subdural empyema complicating pregnancy. Case report. J Neurosurg 40:654–656, 1974.

167. Hensner, AP: Nontuberculous spinal epidural infections. N Engl J Med 239:845–854, 1948.

168. Henson, RA and Croft, PB: Spontaneous spinal subarachnoid hemorrhage. Q J Med 25:53–66, 1956.

169. Herskowitz, A: Spinal cord involvement with Schistosoma mansoni. J Neurosurg 36:494–498, 1972.

170. Herzberg, L and Bayliss, E: Spinal cord syndrome due to non-compressive Paget's disease of bone: A spinal artery steal phenomenon reversible with calcitonin. Lancet 2:13–15, 1980.

171. Hesketh, KT: Cysticercosis of the dorsal cord. J Neurol Neurosurg Psychiatry 28:445–448, 1965.

172. Heusner, AP: Nontuberculous spinal epidural infections. N Engl J Med 239:845–854, 1948.

173. Hirschmann, JV and Everett, ED: Candida vertebral osteomyelitis: Case report and review of the literature. J Bone Joint Surg 58A:573–575, 1976.

174. Hissa, E, Boumphrey, F, and Bay, J: Spinal epidural hematoma and ankylosing spondylitis. Clin Orthop 208:225–227, 1986.

175. Hitselberger, WE and Witten, RM: Abnormal myelograms in asymptomatic patients. J Neurosurg 28:204–206, 1968.

176. Ho, EKW and Leong, JCY: Traumatic tetraparesis: A rare neurologic complication in ankylosing spondylitis with ossification of posterior longitudinal ligament of the cervical spine. A case report. Spine 12:403–405, 1987.

177. Hochman, MS and Pena, C: Calcified herniated thoracic disc diagnosed by computerized tomography: Case report. J Neurosurg 52:722–723, 1980.

178. Hook, O and Lidvall, H: Arteriovenous aneurysms of the spinal cord. A report of two cases investigated by vertebral angiography. J Neurosurg 15:84–91, 1958.

179. Hughes, JT: Diseases of the spinal cord. In Blackwood, W and Corsellis, JAN (eds): Greenfield's Neuropathology. Year Book Medical Publishers, Chicago, 1976, pp 652–687.

180. Hughes, JT: Pathology of the Spinal Cord. WB Saunders, Philadelphia, 1978.

181. Hughes, JT and Brownell, B: Cervical spondylosis complicated by anterior spinal artery thrombosis. Neurology 14:1073–1077, 1964.

182. Hungerford, GD, Akkaraju, V, Rawe, SE, et al: Atlanto-axial dislocations with spinal cord compression in Down's syndrome: A case report and review of the literature. J Radiol 54:758–761, 1981.

183. Iwasaki, Y, Abe, H, Isu, T, et al: CT myelography with intramedullary enhancement in cervical spondylosis. J Neurosurg 63:363–366, 1985.

184. Jajic, I, Kerhin, V, and Kastelen, A: Ankylosing spondylitis in patients without HLA-B27. Br J Rheum (Suppl 2)22:136, 1983.

185. Jellinger, K and Neumayer, E: Claudication of the spinal cord and cauda equina. In Vinken, PJ and Bruyn, GW (eds): Handbook of Clinical Neurology, Vol 12. North-Holland Publishing, Amsterdam, 1972, pp 507–547.

186. Jinkins, JR, Bashir, R, Al-Mefty, O, et al: Cystic necrosis of the spinal cord in compressive cervical myelopathy: Demonstration by io-pamidol CT-myelography. AJNR 7:693–701, 1986.

187. Johnsson, K-E, Rosen, I, and Uden, A: Neurophysiologic investigation of patients with spinal stenosis. Spine 12:483–487, 1987.

188. Jungreis, CA and Cohen, WA: Spinal cord compression induced by steroid therapy: CT findings. J Comput Assist Tomogr 11:245–247, 1987.

189. Kanaze, MG, Gado, MH, Sartor, KJ, and Hodges, FJ: Comparison of MR and CT myelography in imaging the cervical and thoracic spine. AJR 150:397–403, 1988.

190. Kaufman, DM, Kaplan, JG, and Litman, N: Infectious agents in spinal epidural abscesses. Neurology 30:844–850, 1980.

191. Keener, EB: Abscess formation in the spinal cord. Brain 78:394–400, 1955.

192. Keyes, DC and Compere, EL: The normal and pathological physiology of the nucleus pulposus of the intervertebral disc. An anatomical, clinical, and experimental study. J Bone Joint Surg 14:897–939, 1932.

193. Khosla, VK, Kak, VK, and Mathuriya, SN: Chronic spinal subdural hematomas. Report of two cases. J Neurosurg 63:636–639, 1985.

194. Kikaldy-Willis, WH, Paine, KWE, Cauchoix, J, et al: Lumbar spinal stenosis. Clin Orthop 99:30–50, 1974.

195. Killebrew, K, Gold, RH, and Sholkoff, SD: Psoriaticspondylitis.Radiology108:9–16,1973.

196. Koss, JC and Dalinka, MA: Atlantoaxial subluxation in Behçet's syndrome. AJR 134:392–393, 1980.

197. Krane, SM and Simon, LS: Rheumatoid arthritis: Clinical features and pathogenetic mechanisms. Advances in Rheumatology 70:263–284, 1986.

198. Kricun, ME: Conventional radiography. In Kricun, ME (ed): Imaging Modalities of Spinal Disorders. WB Saunders, Philadelphia, 1988, pp 59–288.

199. Kricun, R and Kricun, ME: Computed tomography. In Kricun, ME (ed): Imaging Modalities in Spinal Disorders. WB Saunders, Philadelphia, 1988, pp 376–467.

200. Kristoff, FV and Odom, GL: Ruptured intervertebral disk in the cervical region. Arch Surg 54:287–304, 1947.

201. Kudo, H, Iwano, K, and Yoshizawa, H: Cervical cord compression due to extradural granulation tissue in rheumatoid arthritis. A review of five cases. J Bone Joint Surg 66B:426–430, 1984.

202. Laasonen, EM, Kankaanpaa, U, Paukku, P, et al: Computed tomographic myelography (CTM) in atlanto-axial rheumatoid arthritis. Neuroradiology 27:119–122, 1985.

203. Lanzieri, CF, Sacher, M, Solodnik, P, and Moser, F: CT myelography of spontaneous spinal epidural hematoma. J Comput Assist Tomogr 9:393–394, 1985.

204. LaRocca, H: Cervical spondylotic myelopathy: Natural history. Spine 13:854–855, 1988.

205. Larsson, S-E and Toolanen, G: Posterior fusion for atlanto-axial subluxation in rheumatoid arthritis. Spine 11:525–530, 1986.

206. Lee, SH, Coleman, PE, and Hahn, FJ: Magnetic resonance imaging of degenerative disk disease of the spine. Radiol Clin North Am 26:949–964, 1988.

207. Lees, F and Turner, JWA: Natural history and prognosis of cervical spondylosis. Br Med J 2:1607–1610, 1963.

208. Lehtinen, K, Kaarela, K, Antilla, P, et al: Sacroiliitis in inflammatory joint diseases. Rheumatol 52:19–22, 1984.

209. Leibowitz, U, Halpern, L, and Alter, M: Clinical studies of multiple sclerosis in Israel. V. Progressive spinal syndromes and multiple sclerosis. Neurology 17:988–992, 1967.

210. Lestini, WF and Wiesel, SW: The pathogenesis of cervical spondylosis. Clin Orthop 239:69–93, 1989.

211. Levitan, LH and Wiens, CW: Chronic lumbar extradural hematoma: CT findings. Radiology 148:707–708, 1983.

212. Lifeso, RM, Harder, E, and McCorkell, SJ: Spinal brucellosis. J Bone Joint Surg 67B:345–351, 1985.

213. Lifeso, RM, Weaver, P, and Harder, EH: Tuberculous spondylitis in adults. J Bone Joint Surg 67A:1405–1413, 1985.

214. Lin, TH: Intramedullary tuberculoma of the spinal cord. J Neurosurg 17:497–499, 1960.

215. Lipson, S: Cervical myelopathy and posterior atlanto-axial subluxation in patients with rheumatoid arthritis. J Bone Joint Surg 67A:593–597, 1985.

216. Lipson, SJ: Rheumatoid arthritis in the cervical spine. Clin Orthop 239:121–127, 1989.

217. Loarie, DJ and Fairley, HB: Epidural abscess following spinal anesthesia. Anesth Anal 57:351–353, 1978.

218. Logue, V and Edwards, MR: Syringomyelia and its surgical treatment—an analysis of 75 cases. J Neurol Neurosurg Psychiatry 44:273–284, 1981.

219. Lorber, A, Pearson, CM, and Rens, RM: Osteolytic vertebral lesions as a manifestation of rheumatoid arthritis and related disorders. Arthritis and Rheumatology 4:514–532, 1961.

220. Love, JG and Schorn, VS: Thoracic disc protrusions. JAMA 191:627–631, 1965.

221. Lucci, B, Reverberi, S, and Greco, G: Syringomyelia and syringomyelic syndrome by cervical spondylosis. Report of three cases presenting with neurogenic osteoarthropathies. J Neurosurg Sci 25:169–172, 1981.

222. Ma, Y, Wang, Y-M, and Daniel, TM: Enzyme-linked immunosorbent assay using Mycobacterium tuberculosis Antigen 5 for the diagnosis of pulmonary tuberculosis in China. Am Rev Respir Dis 134:1273–1275, 1986.

223. MacKay, AD and Cole, RB: The problems of tuberculosis in the elderly. QJ Med 212:497–510, 1984.

224. Madsen, JR and Heros, RC: Spinal arteriovenous malformations and neurogenic claudication. Report of two cases. J Neurosurg 68:793–797, 1988.

225. Mair, WGP and Folkerts, JF: Necrosis of the spinal cord due to thrombophlebitis (sub-acute necrotic myelitis). Brain 76: 563–575, 1953.

226. Makela, A-L, Lang, H, and Sillinpas, M: Neurological manifestations of rheumatoid arthritis. In Vinken, PJ and Bruyn, GW (eds): Handbook of Clinical Neurology, Vol 38. North-Holland Publishing, Amsterdam, 1979, pp 479–503.

227. Mallolas, J, Gatell, JM, Rovira, M, et al. Vertebral arch tuberculosis in two human immunodeficiency virus-seropositive heroin addicts. Arch Intern Med 148:1125–1127, 1988.

227a. Mampalam, TJ, Rosegay, H, Andrews, et al: Nonoperative treatment of spinal epidural infections. J Neurosurg 71:208-210, 1989.

228. Mann, JS and Cole, RB: Tuberculous spondylitis in the elderly: A potential diagnostic pitfall. Br Med J 294:1149–1150, 1987.

229. Marcial-Rojas, RA and Fiol, RE: Neurological complications of schistosomiasis. Ann Intern Med 59:215, 1963.

230. Martel, W: The occipito-atlanto-axial joints in rheumatoid arthritis and ankylosing spondylitis. AJR 86:223–240, 1961.

231. Martin, CA, Murall, R, and Trasi, SS: Spinal cord sarcoidosis: Case report. J Neurosurg 61:981–982, 1984.

232. Martini, M, Adjrad, A, and Boudjemaa, A: Tuberculous osteomyelitis: A review of 125 cases. Int Orthop 10:201–207, 1986.

233. Matsushita, T and Suzuki, K: Spastic paraparesis due to cryptococcal osteomyelitis. Clin Orthop 196:279–284, 1985.

234. Matthews, WB: The neurological complications of ankylosing spondylitis. J Neurol Sci 6:561–573, 1968.

235. Mattle, H, Sieb, JP, Rohner, M, and Mumenthaler, M: Nontraumatic spinal epidural and subdural hematomas. Neurology 37:1351–1358, 1987.

236. Mawhinney, R, Jones, R, and Worthington, BS: Spinal cord compression secondary to Paget's disease of the axis: Case reports. Br J Radiol 58:1203–1206, 1985.

237. Mawk, JR, Erickson, DL, Chou, SN, and Seljeskog, EL: Aspergillus infections of the lumbar disc spaces: Report of three cases. J Neurosurg 58:270–271, 1983.

238. McCallister, VL and Sage, MR: The radiology of thoracic disc protrusion. Clin Radiol 27:291–299, 1976.

239. McGahan, JP, Graves, DS, and Palmer, PES: Coccidioidal spondylitis: Usual and unusual radiographic manifestations. Radiology 136:5–9, 1980.

240. McGeachie, RE, Ford, WJ, Nelson, MJ, et al: Neuroradiology case of the day. AJR 148:1053–1058, 1987.

241. McIlroy, WJ and Richardson, JC: Syringomyelia: A clinical review of cases. Can Med Assoc J 93:731–734, 1965.

242. McIlroy, WJ and Stowe, RM: Syringomyelia. In Johnson, RT (ed): Current Therapy in Neurologic Disease—2. BC Decker, Toronto, 1987, pp 94–97.

243. McKee, DF, Barr, WM, Bryan, CS, et al: Primary aspergillosis of the spine mimicking Pott's

paraplegia. J Bone Joint Surg 66A:1481–1483, 1984.

244. McLaurin, RL: Spinal suppuration. Clin Neurosurg 14:314–336, 1967.

245. McRae, DL: Bony abnormalities in the region of the foramen magnum: Correlation of the anatomic and neurologic findings. Acta Radiol 40:335–354, 1953.

246. Mehren, M, Burns, PJ, Mamani, F, et al: Toxoplasmic myelitis mimicking intramedullary spinal cord tumor. Neurology 38:1648–1650, 1988.

247. Melmon, KG and Rosen, SW: Lindau's disease. Am J Med 36:695–703, 1964.

248. Meltzer, LE and Bockman, AA: Trichinosis involving the nervous system: Treatment with corticotrophin (ACTH) and cortisone. JAMA 164:1566–1569, 1957.

249. Menezes, A, VanGilder, JC, Clark, CR, and El-Khoury, G: Odontoid upward migration in rheumatoid arthritis. An analysis of 45 patients with "cranial settling." J Neurosurg 63:500–509, 1985.

250. Menezes, AH, Graf, CJ, and Perret, GE: Spinal cord abscess: A review. Surg Neurol 8:461–467, 1977.

251. Merritt, HH and Rosenbaum, M: Involvement of the nervous system in trichinosis. JAMA 106:1646–1649, 1936.

252. Meyer, GA, Stein, J, and Pappel, MW: Rapid osseous changes in syringomyelia. Radiology 69:415–418, 1957.

253. Michelsen, WJ: Arteriovenous malformation of the brain and spinal cord. In Johnson, RT (ed): Current Therapy in Neurologic Disease—2. BC Decker, Toronto, 1987, pp 170–173.

254. Michon, P: Le coup de poignard rachidien symptome initial de certaines hemorragies sous-arachnoidennes. Essai sur les hemorragies meningees spinales. Presse Med 36:964–966, 1928.

255. Mixter, WJ and Ayer, JB: Herniation or rupture of the intervertebral disc into the spinal canal. Report of thirty-four cases. N Engl J Med 213:385–393, 1935.

256. Mixter, WJ and Barr, JS: Rupture of the intervertebral disc with involvement of the spinal canal. N Engl J Med 211:210–215, 1934.

257. Modic, MT, Feiglin, DH, Piraino, DW, et al: Vertebral osteomyelitis: Assessment using MR. Radiology 151:157–166, 1985.

258. Modic, MT, Masaryk, T, Boumphrey, F, et al: Lumbar herniated disk disease and canal stenosis: Prospective evaluation by surface coil MR, CT and myelography. AJR 147:757–765, 1986.

259. Modic, MT, Pflanze, W, Feiglin, DH, and Belhobek, G: Magnetic resonance imaging of musculoskeletal infections. Radiol Clin North Am 24:247–258, 1986.

260. Moore, RA, McNicholas, KW, and Warran, SP: Atlantoaxial subluxation with symptomatic spinal cord compression in a child with Down's syndrome. Anesth Analg 66:89–90, 1987.

261. Morgan, DF and Young, RF: Spinal neurological complications of achondroplasia: results of

surgical treatment. J Neurosurg 52:463–472, 1980.

262. Mulder, DW and Dale, AJD: Spinal cord tumors and disks. In Baker, AB and Baker, LH (eds): Clinical Neurology. Harper & Row, Hagerstown, Md, 1975, pp 1–28.

263. Murray, GC and Persellin, RH: Cervical fracture complicating ankylosing spondylitis: Report of eight cases and review of the literature. Am J Med 70:1033–1041, 1981.

264. Naidich, TP, McLone, DG, and Harwood-Nash, DC: Systemic malformations. In Newton, TH and Potts, DG (eds): Computed Tomography of the Spine and Spinal Cord. Clavadell Press, San Anselmo, CA, 1983, pp 367–381.

265. Nemir, RL and Krasinki, K: Tuberculosis in children and adolescents in the 1980's. Pediatr Infect Dis J 7:375–379, 1988.

266. Netsky, MG: Syringomyelia. Arch Neurol Psychiatry 70:741–777, 1953.

267. Nurick, S: The pathogenesis of the spinal cord disorder associated with cervical spondylosis. Brain 95:87–100, 1972.

268. O'Connell, JEA: Involvement of the spinal cord by intervertebral disk protrusions. Br J Surg 43:225–247, 1955.

269. O'Connell, JEA: Cervical spondylosis. Proc Roy Soc Med 49:202–208, 1956.

270. Ogino, H. Tada, K, Okada, K, et al: Canal diameter, anteroposterior compression ratio, and spondylotic myelopathy of the cervical spine. Spine 8:1–15, 1983.

271. Oonishi, T, Ishiko, T, Arai, M, and others: Pachymeningitis cervicalis hypertrophica. Acta Pathol Jpn 32:163, 1982.

272. Osmond, JD, Schweitzer, G, Dunbar, JM, and Villet, W: Blastomycosis of the spine with paraplegia. S Afr Med J 45:431–434, 1971.

273. Paine, KWE: Clinical features of lumbar spinal stenosis. Clin Orthop 115:77–82, 1976.

274. Pallis, C, Jones, AM, and Spillane, JD: Cervical spondylosis. Brain 77:274–289, 1954.

275. Papo, I and Luongo, A: Massive intramedullary hemorrhage in a patient on anticoagulants. J Neurosurg Sci 18:268, 1974.

276. Parfitt, AM and Duncan, H: Metabolic bone disease affecting the spine. In Rothman, RH and Simeone, FA (eds): The Spine. WB Saunders, Philadelphia, 1982, pp 775–905.

277. Parikh, M, Iyer, K. Elias, AN, and Gwinup, G: Spinal stenosis in acromegaly. Spine 12:627–628, 1987.

278. Patronas, NJ, Marx, WJ, and Duda, EE: Radiographic presentation of spinal abscesses in the subdural space. American Journal Radiology 132:138–139, 1979.

279. Pattison, PRM: Pott's paraplegia: An account of the treatment of 89 consecutive patients. Paraplegia 24:77–91, 1986.

280. Payne, EE and Spillane, JD: Cervical spine. An anatomico-pathological study of 70 specimens using a special technique with particular reference to the problem of cervical spondylosis. Brain 80:571–596, 1957.

281. Peerless, SJ and Durward, QJ: Management of syringomyelia: A pathophysiological ap-

proach. Clin Neurosurg 30:531–576, 1983.

282. Peet, MM and Echols, DH: Herniation of the nucleus pulposus. A cause of compression of the spinal cord. Archives of Neurology and Psychiatry 32:924–932, 1934.

283. Pellicci, PM, Ranawat, CS, Tsairas, P, et al: A prospective study of the progression of rheumatoid arthritis of the cervical spine. J Bone Joint Surg 63A:342–350, 1981.

284. Pendergrass, EP, Schaeffer, JP, and Hodes, PJ: The Head and Neck in Roentgen Diagnosis, ed 2. CC Thomas, Springfield, Ill, 1956.

285. Pennes, DR, Martel, W, and Ellis, CN: Retinoid-induced ossification of the posterior longitudinal ligament. Skeletal Radiol 14:191–193, 1985.

286. Perot, P, Feindel, W, and Lloyd-Smith, D: Hematomyelia as a complication of syringomyelia. Gowers syringal haemorrhage. J Neurosurg 25:447–451, 1966.

287. Petty, RE and Malleson, P: Spondyloarthropathies of childhood. Pediatr Clin North Am 33:1079–1096, 1986.

288. Plotkin, R, Ronthal, M, and Froman, C: Spontaneous spinal subarachnoid hemorrhage. Report of 3 cases. J Neurosurg 25:443–446, 1966.

289. Plum, F and Olson, ME: Myelitis and Myelopathy. In Baker, AB and Baker, LH (eds): Clinical Neurology. Harper & Row, Hagerstown, Md, 1973, pp 1–52.

290. Poser, CM: The Relationship Between Syringomyelia and Neoplasm. CC Thomas, Springfield, Ill, 1956.

291. Poser, S, Hermann-Gremmeis, I, Wikstrom, J, and Poser, W: Clinical features of the spinal form of multiple sclerosis. Acta Neurol Scand 57:151–158, 1978.

292. Postacchini, F, Massobrio, M, and Ferro, L: Familial lumbar stenosis: Case report of three siblings. J Bone Joint Surg 67A:321–323, 1985.

293. Price, AC, Allen, JH, Eggers, FM, et al: Intervertebral disc-space infection: CT changes. Radiology 149:725–729, 1983.

294. Prusick, VR, Samberg, LC, and Wesolowski, DP: Klippel-Feil syndrome associated with spinal stenosis. A case report. J Bone Joint Surg 67:161–164, 1985.

295. Queiroz, LD, Nucci, A, Facure, NO, and Facure, JJ: Massive spinal cord necrosis in schistosomiasis. Arch Neurol 36:517–519, 1979.

296. Rahman, NU: Atypical forms of spinal tuberculosis. J Bone Joint Surg 62:162–165, 1980.

297. Ram, Z, Findler, G, Spiegelman, R, et al: Intermittent priapism in canal stenosis. Spine 12:377–378, 1987.

298. Rana, NA, Hancock, DO, and Hill, AGS: Atlantoaxial subluxation in rheumatoid arthritis. J Bone Joint Surg 55B:458–470, 1973.

299. Rankin, RM and Flothow, PG: Pyogenic infection of the spinal epidural space. Western Journal of Surgery, Obstetrics and Gynecology 54:320–323, 1946.

300. Ratcliffe, JF: Anatomic basis for the pathogenesis and radiologic features of vertebral osteomyelitis and its differentiation from discitis: a microarteriographic investiga-

tion. Acta Radiol (Diagn) 26:137–143, 1985.

301. Raymond, CA: Ushering in a new generation of diagnostics. JAMA 256:3330, 1986.

302. Redlund-Johnell, I and Pettersson, H: Radiographic measurements of the cranio-vertebral region; designed for evaluation of abnormalities in rheumatoid arthritis. Acta Radiol (Diagn) 25:23–28, 1984.

303. Resnick, D: Radiology of seronegative spondyloarthropathies. Clin Orthop 143:38–45, 1979.

304. Reynolds, H, Carter, SW, Murtaugh, FR, and Rechtine, GR: Cervical rheumatoid arthritis: Value of flexion and extension views in imaging. AJR 164:215–218, 1987.

305. Rifaat, M, ElShafei, I, Samra, K, and Sorour, O: Intramedullary spinal abscess following spinal puncture. J Neurosurg 38:366–367, 1973.

306. Roberts, WN, Larson, MG, Liang, MH, et al: Sensitivity of anthropometric techniques for clinical trials in ankylosing spondylitis. Br J Rheumatol 28:40–45, 1989.

307. Rodriguez, HA and Berthrong, M: Multiple intracranial tumors in von Recklinghausen's neurofibromatosis. Arch Neurol 14:467–475, 1966.

308. Roscoe, MWA and Barrington, TW: Acute spinal subdural hematoma. A case report and review of literature. Spine 9:672–675, 1984.

309. Ross, JS: Inflammatory Disease. In Modic, MT, Masaryk, TJ, and Ross, JS (eds): Magnetic Resonance Imaging of the Spine. Year Book Medical Publishers, Chicago, 1988, pp 167–182.

310. Ross, PM and Fleming, JL: Vertebral body osteomyelitis. Clin Orthop 118:190–198, 1976.

311. Rothman, RH and Simeone, FA: The Spine. WB Saunders, Philadelphia, 1982.

312. Russell, NA and Benoit, BG: Spinal subdural hematoma: A review. Surg Neurol 20:133–137, 1983.

313. Rybock, JD: Acute back pain and disc herniation. In Johnson, RT (ed): Current Therapy in Neurological Disease—2. BC Decker, Toronto, 1987, pp 48–50.

314. Sahs, AL and Joynt, RT: Meningitis. In Baker, AB and Baker, LH (eds): Clinical Neurology. Harper & Row, Hagerstown, Md, 1962.

315. Sapico, FL and Montgomerie, JZ: Pyogenic vertebral osteomyelitis: Report of nine cases and review of the literature. Rev Inf Dis 1:754–776, 1979.

316. Saroris, DJ, Resnick, D, Resnick, C, et al: Musculoskeletal manifestations of sarcoidosis. Semin Roentgenol 20:376–386, 1985.

317. Schenk, VWD: Hemorrhages in spinal cord with syringomyelia in a patient with hemophilia. Acta Neuropathol (Berlin) 2:306–308, 1963.

318. Schliep, G: Syringomyelia and syringobulbia. In Vinken, PJ and Bruyn, GW (eds): Handbook of Clinical Neurology, Vol 32. North-Holland Publishing, Amsterdam, 1978, pp 255–326.

319. Schmidek, HH: Neurologic and neurosurgical sequelae of Paget's disease of bone. Clin Orthop 127:70–77, 1977.

320. Schmiel, S and Deeb, ZL: Herniated thoracic intervertebral disks. J Comput Tomogr 9:141–143, 1985.

321. Scotti, G, Scialfa, G, Pieralli, S, et al: Myelopathy and radiculopathy due to cervical spondylosis: Myelographic-CT correlations. AJNR 4:601–603, 1983.

322. Semins, H, Nugent, GR, and Chou, SM: Intramedullary spinal cord sarcoidosis. J Neurosurg 37:233–236, 1972.

323. Senelick, RC, Norwood, CW, and Cohen, CH: Painless spinal epidural hematoma during anticoagulant therapy. Neurology 26:213–215, 1976.

324. Shannon, FT and Hopkins, JS: Paget's sarcoma of the vertebral column with neurological complications. Acta Orthop Scand 48:385–390, 1977.

325. Shannon, N, Simon, L, and Logue, V: Clinical features, investigation, and treatment of post-traumatic syringomyelia. J Neurol Neurosurg Psychiatry 44:35–42, 1981.

326. Shapiro, R: Myelography, ed 4. Year Book Medical Publishers, Chicago, 1984.

327. Sharp, J and Purser, DW: Spontaneous atlanto-axial dislocation in ankylosing spondylitis and rheumatoid arthritis. Ann Rheum Dis 20:47–77, 1961.

328. Sherman, JL, Barkovich, AJ, and Citrin, CM: The MR appearance of syringomyelia: New observations. AJR 148:381–391, 1987.

329. Silverstein, A: Neurological complications of anticoagulation therapy. A neurologist's review. Arch Intern Med 139:217–220, 1979.

330. Singer, FR: Paget's disease of bone (osteitis deformans). In Wyngaarden, JB and Smith, LH (eds): Cecil Textbook of Medicine, ed 17. WB Saunders, Philadelphia, 1985, pp 1461–1463.

331. Skulety, FM: Cryptococci granuloma of the dorsal spinal cord. Neurology 11:1066–1070, 1961.

332. Smith, FB and Crawford, JS: Fatal granulomatosis of the central nervous system due to a yeast (Torula). J Path Bact 33:291–296, 1930.

333. Smith, PH, Benn, RT, and Sharp, J: Natural history of rheumatoid cervical subluxations. Ann Rheum Dis 31:431–439, 1972.

334. Spillane, JD, Pallis, C, and Jones, AM: Developmental abnormalities in the region of the foramen magnum. Brain 80:11–48, 1957.

335. Spiller, WG: Syringomyelia, extending from the sacral region of the spinal cord through the medulla oblongata, right side of the pons and right cerebral peduncle to the upper part of the right internal capsule (syringobulbia). Br Med J 2:1017, 1906.

336. Spiller, WG: Central pain in syringomyelia and dysesthesia and overreaction to sensory stimuli in lesions below the optic thalamus. AMA Archives of Neurology and Psychiatry 10:491–499, 1923.

337. Stern, BJ and Krumholz, A: Neurosarcoidosis. In Johnson, RT (ed): Current Therapy in Neurologic Disease—2. BC Decker, Toronto, 1987, pp 135–137.

338. Stoltman, HF and Blackwood, W: The role of ligamenta flava in the pathogenesis of myelopathy in cervical spondylosis. Brain 87:45–50, 1964.

339. Stookey, B: Compression of the spinal cord due to ventral extradural cervical chondromas. Diagnosis and surgical treatment. AMA Archives of Neurology and Psychiat 20:275–291, 1928.

340. Stookey, B: Compression of spinal cord and nerve roots by herniation of the nucleus pulposus in the cervical region. Arch Surg 40:417–432, 1940.

341. Swann, KW, Ropper, AH, New, PJF, and Poletti, CE: Spontaneous spinal subarachnoid hemorrhage and subdural hematoma. J Neurosurg 61:975–980, 1984.

342. Taggart, HMcA and Tweedyie, DR: Spinal cord compression: Remember osteoporosis. Br Med J 294:1148–1149, 1987.

343. Tator, CH, Meguro, K, and Rowed, DW: Favorable results with syringosubarachnoid shunts for treatment of syringomyelia. J Neurosurg 56:517–523, 1982.

344. Taylor, AR: Mechanism and treatment of spinal cord disorders associated with cervical spondylosis. Lancet 264:717–720, 1953.

345. Taylor, AR: Vascular factors in the myelopathy associated with cervical spondylosis. Neurology 14:62–68, 1964.

346. Taylor, J and Collier, J: The occurrence of optic neuritis in lesions of the spinal cord. Injury, tumour, myelitis (an account of twelve cases and one autopsy). Brain 24:532–553, 1901.

347. Teng, P and Rudner, N: Multiple arachnoid diverticula. Arch Neurol 2:348–356, 1960.

348. Thomas, D, Kendall, MJ, and Whitfield, AGW: Nervous system involvement in ankylosing spondylitis. Br Med J 1:148–150, 1974.

349. Toolanen, G, Garsson, S-E, and Fagerlund, M: Medullary compression in rheumatoid atlanto-axial subluxation evaluated by computerized tomography. Spine 11:191–194, 1986.

350. Tsuyama, N: Ossification of the posterior longitudinal ligament of the spine. Clin Orthop 84:71–78, 1984.

351. van Ameyden van Duym, FC and van Wiechen, PJ: Herniation of calcified nucleus puposus in the thoracic spine: Case report. J Comput Assist Tomogr 7:1122–1123, 1983.

352. Van Gelderen, C: Ein orthotisches (lordotisches) Kaudasyndrom. Acta Psychiat Scand 23:57–68, 1948.

353. Veidlonger, OF, Colwill, JC, Smyth, HS, and Turner, D: Cervical myelopathy and its relationship to cervical stenosis. Spine 6:550–552, 1981.

354. Verbiest, H: A radicular syndrome from developmental narrowing of the lumbar vertebral canal. J Bone Joint Surg 26B:230–237, 1954.

355. Verbiest, H: Neurogenic intermittent claudica-

tion—lesions of the spinal canal and cauda equina, stenosis of the vertebral canal, narrowing of intervertebral foramina and entrapment of peripheral nerves. In Vinken, PJ and Bruyn, GW (eds): Handbook of Clinical Neurology, Vol 20. North-Holland Publishing, Amsterdam, 1976, pp 611–804.

356. Verbiest, H: Results of surgical treatment of idiopathic developmental stenosis of the lumbar vertebral canal. J Bone Joint Surg 59B:181–188, 1977.

357. Verbiest, H: The significance and principles of computerized axial tomography in idiopathic developmental stenosis of the lumbar vertebral canal. Spine 4:369–378, 1979.

358. Verner, EF and Musher, DM: Spinal epidural abscess. Med Clin North Am 69:375–384, 1985.

359. Vleck, B, Burchiel, KJ, and Gordon, T: Tuberculous meningitis presenting as an obstructive myelopathy. J Neurosurg 60:196–199, 1984.

360. Walton, JN: Subarachnoid hemorrhage of unusual etiology. Neurology 3:517–543, 1953.

361. Waltz, TA: Physical factors in the production of the myelopathy of cervical spondylosis. Brain 90:395–404, 1967.

362. Weaver, P and Lifeso, RM: The radiological diagnosis of tuberculosis of the adult spine. Skeletal Radiol 12:178–186, 1984.

363. Weinstein, PR, Karpman, RR, Gall, EP, and Pitt, M: Spinal cord injury, spinal fracture and spinal stenosis in ankylosing spondylitis. J Neurosurg 57:609–616, 1982.

364. Weissman, BNW, Aliabadi, P, Weinfeld, MS, et al: Prognostic features of atlantoaxial subluxation in rheumatoid arthritis patients. Radiology 144:745–751, 1982.

365. Weisz, GM: Lumbar canal stenosis in Paget's disease. The staging of the clinical syndrome, its diagnosis, and treatment. Clin Orthop 206:223–227, 1986.

366. Welsh, JD, Rhoades, ER, and Jaques, W: Disseminated nocardiosis involving spinal cord. Arch Intern Med 108:73–79, 1961.

367. White, AA and Panjabi, MM: The basic kinematics of the human spine. A review of past and current knowledge. Spine 3:12–20, 1978.

368. Whitecloud, TS: Anterior surgery for cervical spondylotic myelopathy. Smith-Robinson, Cloward, and vertebrectomy. Spine 13:861–863, 1988.

369. Whitfield, AGW: Neurological complications of ankylosing spondylitis. In Vinken, PJ and Bruyn, GW (eds): Handbook of Clinical Neurology, Vol 38. North-Holland Publishing, Amsterdam, 1979, pp 505–520.

370. Wiesel, SW, Tsourmas, N, Feffer, HL, et al: A study of computer-assisted tomography. 1. The incidence of positive CAT scans in an asymptomatic group of patients. Spine 9:549–551, 1984.

371. Wilkinson, M: The morbid anatomy of cervical spondylosis and myelopathy. Brain 83:589–617, 1960.

372. Wilkinson, M: Cervical Spondylosis. Its Early Diagnosis and Treatment. Heinemann, London, 1970.

373. Williams, AL, Haughton, VM, Daniels, DL, et al: Differential CT diagnosis of extruded nucleus pulposus. Radiology 146:141–146, 1983.

374. Williams, AL, Haughton, VM, Pojunas, KW, et al: Differentiation of intramedullary neoplasms and cysts by MR. AJR 149:159–164, 1987.

375. Williams, B: On the pathogenesis of syringomyelia: A review. Royal Society of Medicine 73:798–806, 1980.

376. Williams, B and Fahy, G: A critical appraisal of "terminal ventriculostomy" for the treatment of syringomyelia. J Neurosurg 58:188–197, 1983.

377. Wilson, CB: Significance of the small lumbar spinal canal. Cauda equina compression syndromes due to spondylosis. 3. Intermittent claudication. J Neurosurg 31:499–506, 1969.

378. Woltman, HW and Adson, AW: Abscess of the spinal cord: Functional recovery after operation. Brain 49:193–206, 1926.

379. Woolsey, RM, Chambers, TJ, Chung, HD, and McGarry, JD: Mycobacterial meningomyelitis associated with human immunodeficiency virus infection. Arch Neurol 45:691–693, 1988.

380. Wright, RL: Intramedullary spinal cord abscess: Report of a case secondary to stab wound with good recovery following operation. J Neurosurg 23:208–210, 1965.

381. Wu, PC, Fang, D, Ho, EKW, and Leong, JCY: The pathogenesis of extensive discovertebral destruction in ankylosing spondylitis. Clin Orthop 230:154–161, 1988.

382. Wyburn-Mason, R: Vascular Abnormalities and Tumors of the Spinal Cord and Its Membranes. Kimpton, London, 1943.

383. Yamamoto, I, Matsumae, M, Ikeda, A, et al: Thoracic spinal stenosis: Experience with seven cases. J Neurosurg 68:37–40, 1988.

384. Yomarken, JL: Spinal subdural hematoma. Ann Emerg Med 14:261–263, 1985.

385. Yoss, RE, Corbin, KB, MacCarty, CS, and Love, JG: Significance of symptoms and signs in localization of involved root in cervical disc protrusion. Neurology 7:673–683, 1957.

386. Young, A, Dixon, A, Getty, J, et al: Cauda equina syndrome complicating ankylosing spondylitis: Use of electromyography and computerised tomography in diagnosis (case report). Ann Rheum Dis 40:317–322, 1981.

387. Zener, JC, Alpert, M, and Klainer, LM: Vertebral sarcoidosis. Arch Intern Med 111:696–702, 1963.

388. Zlatkin, MR, Lander, PH, Hadjipaviou, AG, and Levine, JS: Paget disease of the spine: CT with clinical correlation. Radiology 160:155–159, 1986.

389. Zuccarello, M, Powers, G, Tobler, WB, et al: Chronic posttraumatic lumbar intradural arachnoid cyst with cauda equina compression: Case report. Neurosurgery 20:636–637, 1987.

Chapter 5

NEOPLASTIC CAUSES OF SPINAL CORD COMPRESSION: EPIDURAL TUMORS

Epidural neoplasms are classified as either primary or metastatic. In the former case, several different benign or malignant tumors may arise from those cells that form the vertebral column and associated supporting structures; the most common are osteogenic, chondrogenic, vascular, fibrous, hematopoietic, lipomatous, and undifferentiated mesenchymal elements.

Neoplasms not originating from spinal structures differ in their propensity to metastasize to the spine. However, any malignancy with metastatic potential may metastasize to the spine and cause epidural spinal cord compression (ESCC). (The term spinal cord compression is used to include cauda equina compression unless otherwise noted.)

The diagnosis of epidural neoplasms can be difficult. Pain is usually the first symptom of both primary and metastatic epidural spinal tumors.[6, 32, 57] However, as discussed in Chapter 3, pain is a common manifestation of many non-neoplastic spinal disorders as well, making clinical history alone rarely sufficient to establish the cause with certainty. Rather, a meticulous history and physical examination supplemented, when indicated, with appropriate laboratory and diagnostic imaging studies often are necessary to identify the cause.

Even when diagnostic imaging studies demonstrate an epidural neoplasm, one still must distinguish between a primary and a metastatic tumor. If there is a history of a malignancy with a propensity to metastasize to the spine, the epidural tumor is usually considered metastatic; rarely, a metastasis from a second unknown primary or even a primary spinal tumor may be the cause. When a malignancy has not been previously diagnosed, one must still consider the possibility of a metastasis from an unknown primary, since metastatic epidural spinal tumors are much more frequent than primary tumors of the spine. Certain clues help the physician locate a primary tumor:

1. The patient's sex and age may suggest the most likely histological types to consider. For example, whereas breast, lung, and prostate cancers are frequent sources of spinal metastases in adults,[7, 63, 153, 173] in children, sarcomas and neuroblastoma are common causes.[107]

2. The general physical examination and laboratory screening may help in establishing leads.

3. The frequency of certain primary tumors in adults to metastasize to the spine guides the work-up for a primary tumor.

4. The appearance of the neoplasm on imaging studies of the spine and elsewhere may be very helpful in suggesting the etiology.

The reasons one searches for a nonspinal primary tumor are twofold: First, metastases (even from occult primaries) are much more common than primary spinal tumors. Second, an accurate diagnosis of the neoplasm causing ESCC is necessary for most effective treatment. When indicated, histological confirmation may be essential for further management, if the diagnosis is in doubt.

This chapter first reviews in detail the

clinical features and imaging studies frequently encountered in the evaluation of metastatic spinal neoplasms. A brief review of some of the clinical features of primary epidural tumors follows.

METASTATIC NEOPLASMS

Epidemiology

Much of the epidemiological information on spinal tumors is obtained from neurosurgical series. These series often underrepresent the frequency of metastatic cancer because such patients may not be considered good surgical candidates and may not, therefore, be referred. Thus, it is quite difficult to determine accurately the relative frequency of intramedullary, extramedullary-intradural, and epidural spinal tumors from surgical series. One review[3] cites several neurosurgical studies that report that extramedullary-intradural tumors (e.g., neurofibroma and meningioma) are the most common tumor types, but spinal metastases from systemic cancer appear to have been excluded from the analysis.

When epidural tumors are considered alone, metastatic tumors are found to be more common than primary spinal neoplasms; this has been the experience even in some neurosurgical series.[6, 137] For example, in one study of vertebral tumors,[6] 66 percent of 350 tumors were metastatic, whereas only 30 percent were primary. The remaining 4 percent were paravertebral tumors that invaded the spinal column. An extensive review of the literature of primary and secondary tumors of the vertebral column[137] concluded that metastatic tumors are three to four times more frequent than primary malignant neoplasms. In a neurosurgical series of 413 solitary tumors of the vertebral column,[32] 121 were metastatic in origin, thus emphasizing that even apparently solitary vertebral lesions are often metastatic.

The enormous clinical impact of metastatic cancer to the vertebral column and epidural space in the general population is supported by several large autopsy series[1, 137, 174, 197] that report vertebral metastases in 15 to 41 percent of patients dying of cancer. Furthermore, the frequency of skeletal metastases was much higher for some tumors: 84 percent of cases of prostatic cancer; 74 percent of breast cancer. Moreover, among skeletal metastases, the vertebral column has been found to be the most common site.[58, 122]

All patients with vertebral metastasis are at potential risk of developing spinal cord compression. The frequency of spinal cord compression from metastases to the vertebral column is unknown, but one autopsy study[7] estimated that approximately 5 percent of patients dying of cancer have spinal cord compression, the great majority arising from vertebral metastases. Thus among the nearly 400,000 individuals dying of cancer annually in the United States, between 60,000 and 160,000 have spinal metastases and 20,000 develop ESCC. These figures, although only estimates, underscore the magnitude of the clinical problem of spinal metastases in the cancer population. It must be emphasized that vertebral metastases are not confined to patients dying of cancer; this treatable complication occurs even in patients whose primary malignancy is treatable, and in about 8 percent of patients, it may be the only symptom.

Concepts of Cancer Metastasis

Cancer metastasis implies the release of cells from one site and passage of these cells through lymphatics or blood vessels to a distant site where there is invasion and growth into a secondary neoplasm.[134] The mechanism of passage of these shed cancer cells has been a source of debate.[13] Although both organ and tumor cell properties are probably important in the metastatic cascade,[136] the predominant view has been that anatomic and hemodynamic factors play a primary role in the dissemination of cancer.

The hemodynamic theory explains the metastatic cascade on the basis of anatomy of the draining veins. In a series of elegant experiments using human cadavers, Batson[8] showed that injection of radiopaque material into the dorsal vein of the penis and the draining breast veins resulted in opacification of the vertebral venous system. Furthermore, in living primates, abdominal straining augmented the venous flow from the pelvic viscera to the vertebral veins (Fig. 5–1). Batson demonstrated that because the vertebral venous system is valveless and of low intraluminal pressure, coughing, sneezing, and straining allow venous effluent from the breast, intrathoracic, intraabdominal and pelvic organs to enter and move in a rostral or caudal direction unimpeded.

Batson noted in 1956 that he had rediscovered this plexus of veins, first described by Breschet in the first half of the 19th century and then overlooked for over a century.[9] In recognition of Breschet's contribution, Batson generously stated, "Eponymically, the veins in the vault of the skull are known as Breschet's veins. We commonly forget that the veins in the bodies of the vertebrae are likewise Breschet's veins." Figure 5–2 illustrates the pathways available for spread to the axial skeleton from pelvic, abdominal, thoracic, and breast malignancies.

In a series of experiments,[34] suspensions of tumor cells were injected into the veins of rats and rabbits. The pattern of metastases in the animals (experimental group) in which intra-abdominal pressure was elevated transiently during the injection was compared with the pattern in which there was no increase in pressure (control group). The results of these studies confirmed Batson's hypothesis. In nearly all of the control animals, the metastases were localized to the lungs alone; the majority of experimental animals demonstrated spinal metastases. Furthermore, the spinal metastases arose from emboli to

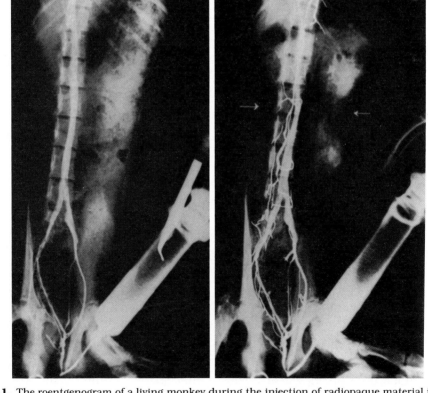

Figure 5–1. The roentgenogram of a living monkey during the injection of radiopaque material into the deep dorsal vein of the penis. (A) The injected material passes into the inferior vena cava without entering the vertebral veins. (B) The same animal is shown, but the abdomen has been compressed with a towel, mimicking a Valsalva maneuver. The contrast material passes upward through the vertebral venous system. (From Batson,OV, [8] with permission.)

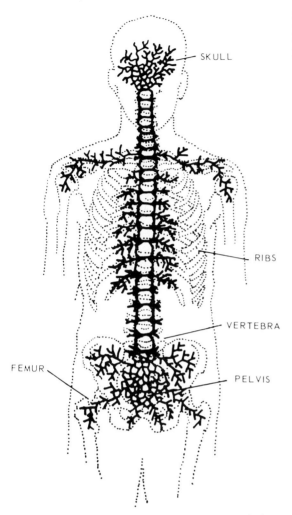

Figure 5–2. This figure illustrates some of the anastomoses of the vertebral venous system with other venous systems. Neoplasms from the pelvis, abdomen, breast, and elsewhere show collaterals with the vertebral venous system. (From del Regato, JA,[40] with permission.)

the thin-walled vertebral veins, not the arterial system.

Although the system of vertebral veins that has come to be called Batson's plexus could explain many cases of aberrant metastasis, it is now recognized that patterns of metastases are not explained by hemodynamic factors alone. Although the hemodynamic model may explain the arrest of tumor embolus in a specific organ, it may not predict the ultimate pattern of metastasis, which requires invasion and growth of the tumor cells.[54] Thus ulti-

mately both Paget's seed-and-soil hypothesis[136] and Ewing's anatomic and hemodynamic factors[53] may have a role in the metastatic spread of cancer.[13]

Location of Epidural Tumor in Relation to Spinal Cord

Malignant ESCC usually results from metastasis to one of three sites: the vertebrae, the paravertebral tissues, or the epidural space itself. By extending into the adjacent vertebral canal, tumor in any of these locations may impinge on the neural structures. An understanding of these different mechanisms of compression is helpful in recognizing the pathogenesis of spinal cord compression and interpreting imaging studies.

The vertebral column is the most frequent site from which metastases may cause ESCC. The regions involved most often are the vertebral body (especially subchondral areas) and the pedicles (Fig. 5–3), probably because of the extensive vascular supply of these areas.[75, 96]

Eighty-five percent of patients with metastatic ESCC at Memorial Sloan-Kettering Cancer Center (MSKCC) were found to have vertebral involvement.[144] In a neurosurgical series,[35] review of the radiological findings of 600 cases of spinal cord compression from metastatic cancer showed the vertebral column involved in 94 percent; of those cases with vertebral metastases, 86 percent showed more than one vertebral body was involved. Isolated bone lesions without extension of tumor into the epidural space was found in 10 percent of the 600 cases; in this setting, vertebral body collapse with resulting cord compression was considered responsible for neurologic abnormalities. These findings not only explain the pathogenesis of many cases of metastatic ESCC, but also place in perspective the value of performing radiological procedures on the vertebral column. Based on these data, one must conclude that a negative plain radiograph of the spine or a negative radionuclide bone scan does not entirely exclude metastatic ESCC, because a few patients will have no vertebral involvement. Although radionuclide bone scanning is far

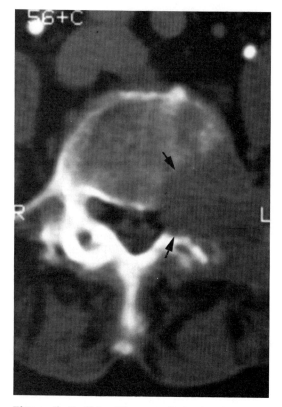

Figure 5–3. This CT scan of the lumbar spine demonstrates a metastasis from lung cancer (arrows) to a pedicle, which extends into the vertebral body, vertebral canal, and paravertebral tissues.

more sensitive than plain films in the detection of bone metastases,[31, 120] false-negative radionuclide bone scans remain a problem.[36]

Paravertebral tumors that extend into the vertebral canal through the intervertebral foramina constitute another important cause of ESCC. Plain films of the spine and radionuclide bone scan are often unrevealing if the vertebrae are not involved by tumor. While any paravertebral neoplasm may be responsible, this phenomenon seems to be commonly seen in renal cell cancer, superior sulcus tumors (Pancoast syndrome[138]), neuroblastoma, and lymphoma, especially if the paravertebral regions are not included in the radiotherapy port[63] (Fig. 5–4A). Lymphoma has been considered a neoplasm especially prone to cause cord compression by invading the epidural space through the intervertebral foramina from paravertebral

lymph nodes rather than via the more commonly encountered vertebral metastasis[144] (Fig. 5–4B). Among all cases of metastatic ESCC, the precise frequency in which paravertebral tumors are responsible is unknown but has been estimated to be approximately 10 percent.[144] With the advent of high-resolution CT scanning and MRI that can adequately study the paravertebral soft tissues, these lesions may be more frequently recognized.

Pure epidural lesions alone are rare. In the neurosurgical series above,[35] the incidence of epidural tumor alone was 5 percent (Fig. 5–5).

Pathology

The evolution of spinal cord symptoms and signs may be better appreciated in light of the pathological findings within the spinal cord, including areas of demyelination, infarction, and cystic necrosis.

Over 30 years ago, McAlhany and Netsky[119] performed a clinicopathological study on a series of patients with extramedullary spinal cord compression. Of the 19 cases reported, 15 were epidural, predominantly from metastatic cancer; the remaining 4 were intradural-extramedullary meningiomas. These authors found no correlation between the location of the neoplasm in the transverse plane of the spinal cord and the presenting neurologic complaint of their patients. For example, in a laterally placed epidural mass, corticospinal dysfunction initially might not be ipsilateral, nor loss of pain and temperature contralateral to the lesion. This clinical observation was explained by the pathological finding that both ipsilateral and/or contralateral areas of demyelination were often seen; at times, the contralateral damage was more marked than the ipsilateral injury. Furthermore, the white matter was more severely affected than the gray matter. The white matter of the anterior funiculus was relatively spared in comparison to that of the lateral and posterior columns, even in anteriorly placed epidural masses. Thus the authors rejected the previously held belief that the dentate ligaments, which anchor the spinal cord in the vertical plane, play a significant role

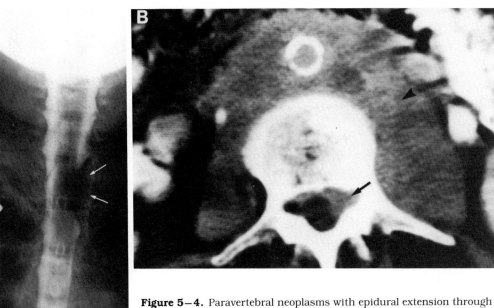

Figure 5—4. Paravertebral neoplasms with epidural extension through intervertebral foraminae without bone involvement. (A) This myelogram demonstrates an epidural metastatic breast cancer at the T1—2 level. The bone scan and plain films were negative, and MRI was interpreted as normal. The tumor had extended from a paravertebral mass through the intervertebral foramen. (B) This upper lumbar spine CT scan demonstrates a paravertebral lymphoma (arrowhead) extending into the epidural space (arrow).

in the evolution of spinal cord compression.[90] Moreover, distribution of pathology in the transverse plane did not reveal areas of demyelination that conformed to the arterial supply. In addition to demyelination, areas of infarction were also found, but the regions of infarction did not conform to the vascular distribution of any major radicular or sulcal blood vessel.

Pathologists have also reported pencil-shaped softenings of the spinal cord at the level of epidural tumors.[76] These softenings may extend longitudinally over several segments of the spinal cord in a cephalad or, less frequently, caudad direction. The necrotic cavity which forms the pencil-shaped softening is usually located in the anterior portion of the posterior column or posterior horn. This region, which corresponds to the region involved in cases of venous infarction,[78, 82] is also considered a watershed zone for arterial circulation.[78] Although circulatory disturbances have been considered important in the development of pencil-shaped softenings,[127] mechanical factors also have been cited.[76]

These cystic necrotic lesions have been imaged using delayed CT myelography and MRI.[2]

Pathophysiology of Neurologic Signs and Symptoms in Spinal Cord Compression

The mechanism of spinal cord injury induced by epidural tumors is complex and probably multifactorial. Neurosurgical experience showed venous engorgement and diminished arterial pulsation at operation.[49] Tarlov[184, 185] undertook a series of experiments producing acute or chronic ESCC in dogs. He inflated a balloon in the spinal canal for varying periods of time. If the balloon was rapidly inflated to a pressure just sufficient to produce motor paralysis and complete sensory loss below the compression, recovery could ensue if the compression was relieved within two hours. However, when the balloon was slowly inflated over a 48-hour period, a pressure just sufficient to cause complete

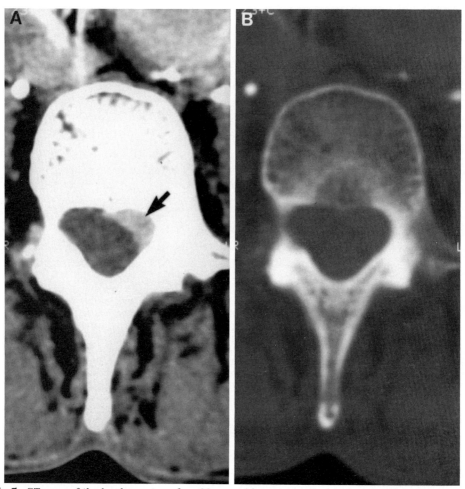

Figure 5–5. CT scan of the lumbar spine of an 82-year old woman with rectal carcinoma who complained of radiating pain into the left anterolateral thigh. Her left knee deep tendon reflex was absent. (A) CT scan of the lumbar spine using soft-tissue windows demonstrates a metastasis in the epidural space. (B) CT scan at the same level using bone windows shows no vertebral involvement.

paralysis and a sensory level at the level of compression could be maintained for one week before paralysis was irreversible. Tarlov considered that mechanical pressure on nervous tissue rather than ischemia was primarily responsible for paralysis.[183]

Several authors have studied the sequence of vascular, biochemical, pathological, and neurophysiological changes in experimental ESCC under conditions that simulate those of neoplastic cord compression. By injecting Walker 256 carcinoma into the epidural space of the rat, Ushio and colleagues[188] demonstrated that vasogenic edema of the spinal cord was an early pathological finding. A marker normally excluded from the spinal cord entered the cord at the site of compression, suggesting a breakdown of the blood–spinal cord barrier as a cause of edema. As vasogenic edema developed, animals manifested increasing hind-limb weakness. Improvement in spinal cord function following the administration of corticosteroids to the animals was paralleled by improvement in vasogenic edema.

These findings have been extended and confirmed.[84, 93] The pathophysiology of circulatory disturbances secondary to ESCC appears to follow a step-wise progression: (1) Compression of Batson's plexus by tumor causes venous congestion, white matter edema, and axonal swelling and is associated with clinical evidence of early myelopathy. Experimentally, these changes may occur in the absence of tumor within the spinal canal, suggesting that paravertebral masses may disturb venous drainage in the spinal cord, resulting in neurologic symptoms. At this early stage of cord compression, spinal cord blood flow is not diminished. (2) In the middle stage, direct tumor compression of the spinal cord is added to venous congestion of the cord. The white matter edema progresses and spinal cord blood flow in response to carbon dioxide inhalation, at the level of compression and caudal to compression, becomes altered. Clinical evidence of myelopathy also progresses. (3) In the final stage of cord compression, as the tumor compresses the spinal cord further, the blood flow drops precipitously, producing irreversible cord damage.

Siegal and colleagues[167] examined the role of prostaglandins and somatosensory-evoked responses in the evolution of pathological changes and myelopathy in ESCC.

Confirming an earlier report,[162] these authors found abnormalities in spinal somatosensory-evoked responses preceding neurologic signs of myelopathy in their experimental model. Myelin destruction was caused by both mechanical compression and ischemia as demonstrated by electron-microscopic studies. Elevation in prostanoid, PGE2, was found in paraplegic rats. This compound, which promotes vasodilatation and plasma exudation,[87] was found in parallel with the development of spinal cord edema.

Mechanical compression of spinal axons *per se* may also interfere with conduction. It is well established that focal compression of myelinated fiber tracts can cause damage to myelin[131] and conduction block.[157] As would be expected on the basis of biomechanics, larger fibers are more susceptible to the effects of compression.[14, 115] On the basis of careful morphological study, it is now clear that demyelination can occur at sites of spinal cord compression[15, 16, 193] (Fig. 5-6). There is, moreover, some evidence for

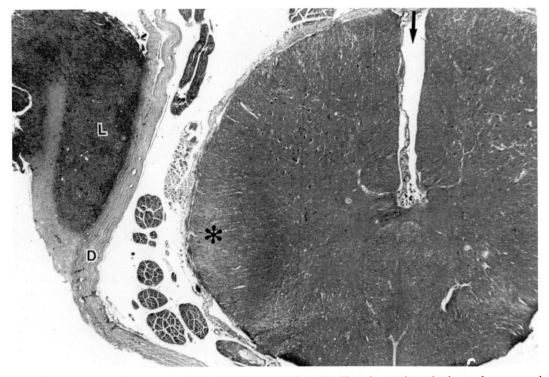

Figure 5-6. Extradural lymphoma (L) abutting the spinal dura (D). The adjacent lateral column shows a poorly defined area of subtle demyelination (asterisk). Arrow: anterior median fissure. Luxol fast blue stain. Magnification X14. (Courtesy of Dr. Jung Kim.)

remyelination after transient compression of the spinal cord,[65] providing a possible morphological correlate for recovery of function following prompt surgical relief of spinal cord compression.

Types of Primary Neoplasms Metastasizing to the Spine

Several studies report the relative frequency of primary tumors that metastasize to the spine and cause ESCC.[6, 7, 29, 32, 35, 63, 137, 173] As discussed earlier, such reports from neurosurgical series select patients who are considered candidates for surgical procedures. If patients who are not surgical candidates are excluded, much epidemiological data will be subject to bias. In an attempt to overcome selection bias, the studies reviewed in Table 5–1 and cited below are those that attempted to include all patients that presented to reporting institutions, irrespective of the therapy chosen.[7, 63, 153, 173]

The often-quoted autopsy study of 127 cases exhibiting symptomatic spinal cord compression by Barron and colleagues[7] provides a basis for epidemiological analysis of metastatic ESCC. A review of their findings indicates that epidural metastasis was found in all but three patients (two with intramedullary metastases and one with leptomeningeal metastases). The total number of autopsied cases with each primary tumor type during the same period (1950–1956) was also determined. Thus, the risk of developing spinal cord compres-

sion with each individual tumor type could be determined. Over 10 different primary tumors were found to be responsible for ESCC. In descending frequency, the five most common malignancies were lung (n = 31; 24 percent), breast (20; 16 percent), lymphoma (20; 16 percent), kidney (12; 9 percent), and myeloma (9; 7 percent). Recognizing a changing pattern of primary malignancies, these authors noted that neither the earlier series of Neustaedter[128] nor that of Elsberg[48] reported a case of lung cancer as a cause of spinal cord compression. Also unlike an earlier series,[21] in which spinal metastasis from prostate cancer was considered a rarity, Barron and colleagues[7] found it to be the fifth most common cause in males. The increasing frequency of spinal metastases from prostate cancer is discussed below.

The study of Gilbert and colleagues[63] from MSKCC found breast, lung, and prostate cancers to be the most frequent primary tumors causing ESCC, comprising over 40 percent (see Table 5–1). The relative frequencies of these primary tumors reflected that seen at MSKCC, except that gastrointestinal tumors did not cause cord compression as frequently as would have been expected based on their relative incidence. (A similar experience was reported by Barron and colleagues.[7]) Of further interest was that Gilbert and associates[63] found lymphomas less frequently represented in the later years of their study. They attributed this change to the modification of therapy to include total nodal

Table 5–1 TYPES OF PRIMARY TUMORS CAUSING METASTATIC EPIDURAL SPINAL CORD COMPRESSION IN VARIOUS SERIES (%)

Primary Tumor	Barron[7]	Gilbert[63]	Stark[173]	Rodichok[153]
Lung	24	13	33	31
Breast	16	20	28	24
Prostate	4	9	4	8
Kidney	9	7	3	1
Myeloma	7	4	excluded	1
Lymphoma	16	11	excluded	6
Melanoma	—	3	1	4
Sarcoma	6	9	1	4
Female reproductive	—	2	3	6
GI	5	4	5	9
Miscellaneous	13	18	22	8

— = insufficient data

irradiation, including the paravertebral regions.

The London Hospital study by Stark and colleagues[173] (see Table 5–1) reports a 10-year experience of spinal metastases from solid tumors (hematological malignancies were excluded). Although there are some differences in the relative frequencies of primary tumors in these various series, lung, breast, and prostate cancers are generally the most frequent offenders. Furthermore, lung cancer is much more likely to present initially as a spine metastasis than breast cancer; the latter usually causes spinal cord compression after the diagnosis of cancer is already established.[173] Although not a common cause of ESCC, leukemia is an occasional offender.

Table 5–2 demonstrates the relative frequency of primary malignancies causing ESCC for men and women separately.[173] This information is important in evaluating the patient who presents with the clinical and radiographic constellation of malignant ESCC.

As noted above, by comparing the number of autopsied cases of spinal cord compression secondary to a specific tumor with the total number of autopsied cases with the same neoplasm, Barron and colleagues[7] were able to estimate the risk of developing spinal metastasis with individual neoplasms. Multiple myeloma and prostate cancer had the highest risks, 14 percent and 10 percent, respectively; ovarian (0 percent) and stomach cancer (1 percent) were the least likely to cause spinal cord compression. Alternatively, the commonly encountered breast and lung malignancies had frequencies of approximately 5 percent each. The authors noted that these frequency figures should be considered as a minimum since some patients with spinal cord compression may not have been recognized clinically.

The changing pattern of spinal metastasis from prostate cancer deserves further comment. Barron and associates[7] noted that the incidence of spinal cord compression in their patients with prostate cancer, 10 percent, was significantly higher than the earlier experience of 1 percent.[21] They speculated that the increasing frequency of spinal metastases could be due to the advent of hormonal manipulation that might prolong life and could, thereby, increase the risk of metastases. Although some recent studies continue to show a low frequency of spinal metastasis from prostate cancer,[110] others have found that 80 percent of men dying of prostate cancer demonstrate vertebral metastases,[156] though in one recent series spinal cord compression was found in only 7 percent.[103] A similar experience of increasing neurologic involvement with more effective control of systemic malignancy continues to be reported for many different types of malignancy such as leukemia,[125, 146, 155, 200] lymphoma,[22, 24] small-cell bronchogenic carcinoma,[140] and others.[143]

Table 5–2 TYPES OF PRIMARY TUMORS CAUSING METASTATIC EPIDURAL SPINAL CORD COMPRESSION IN MEN AND WOMEN (%)

	Stark et al[173]		Barron et al[7]	
	Male	Female	Male	Female
Lung	53	12	32	14
Breast	0	59	0	39
Prostate	8	N/A	8	N/A
Kidney	3	3	12	6
Myeloma	Excluded		8	6
Lymphoma	Excluded		20	9
Melanoma	0	1	—	—
GI	5	3	5	5
Female reproductive	N/A	6	N/A	6
Miscellaneous	31	16	15	15

Interval from Primary Tumor Diagnosis to Epidural Spinal Cord Compression

The interval between the diagnosis of cancer and spinal cord compression is extremely variable. In the series from MSKCC, it was 0 to 19 years.[63] While only 10 patients in this series presented with cord compression as the initial manifestation of their malignancy, this may be explained by the fact that most patients in a cancer hospital already carry a diagnosis of malignancy. Alternatively, in the study from the London Hospital,[173] 62 of 131 patients had spinal cord compression as the presenting manifestation of cancer. The series reported by Barron and colleagues[7] from a general hospital similarly concluded that lung cancer often presents with spine metastasis, whereas this mode of presentation is atypical with breast cancer. These factors probably explain the greater frequency of breast cancer than lung primaries in the MSKCC series.[63]

Age and Sex Distribution

The age of patients with spinal metastases reflects the age at which the respective primary neoplasms occur. In many series, there is a peak at 50–70 years.[29, 63, 153, 173] Similarly, the sex ratio is dependent on the underlying neoplasms. Breast cancer has been much more frequently seen than lung cancer in women but this is expected to change as lung cancer becomes more common.

Level of Spinal Cord Compression

Most studies agree that the thoracic spine is the most frequent site of spinal cord compression.[7, 18, 63, 103, 145, 173] In the MSKCC series,[63] the cervical spine was the site of epidural tumor in 15 percent, the thoracic spine in 68 percent, and the lumbosacral spine in 16 percent. Lung and breast cancer tended to metastasize to the thoracic spine, whereas the spread of colon cancer was disproportionately more frequent to the lumbosacral spine.[63] In two other studies[103, 110] of genitourinary tumors alone, the thoracic spine was the most common site, followed by the lumbar and then the cervical spine.

In the London Hospital study,[173] breast metastases showed no predisposition to any single area of the spine. Pelvic tumors more often spread to the lumbar spine than tumors from elsewhere. Lung cancer demonstrated a slight tendency to spread to the thoracic spine.

Clinical Presentation of Epidural Metastasis

The dominant presenting clinical signs and symptoms of ESCC are pain, weak-ness, sensory loss, and autonomic disturbance; on rare occasions, ataxia is found. This pattern appears similar among patients with different primary tumors.[173] The time course of these signs and symptoms is important for diagnosis as well as for predicting outcome.

PAIN

Pain is the most common initial complaint of both vertebral metastasis and ESCC. In cancer patients with symptoms and signs of spinal metastases, it is often difficult to distinguish those patients with vertebral metastasis alone from those with spinal cord compression. In a study of patients with symptoms of spinal metastases who were suspected of ESCC,[12] no single clinical symptom or sign or index of symptoms and signs could accurately distinguish between patients with metastatic cord compression and those with vertebral metastasis alone. Thus each patient with symptoms or signs of spinal metastases must be viewed as at risk for ESCC.

Pain generally occurs at the stage of irritation of the innervated spinal structures, before spinal cord or cauda equina compression occurs. The prognosis for continued ambulation thus is optimal if the diagnosis is made at this stage.

In their autopsy study, where the patients were not examined directly by the authors, Barron and colleagues[7] reported back pain, radicular pain, or both preceding signs of neurologic deficit in 82 percent of patients. Chade[29] reported radicular pain in 96 percent of 172 cases referred to a neurosurgical clinic with ESCC. In the London Hospital,[173] a somewhat lower incidence of pain was reported as the presenting manifestation, with 69 percent describing this complaint preceding the neurological deficit. However, at the time of diagnosis of spinal cord compression, only 14 percent of patients denied pain. When pain was reported, it was described as axial (local) in 72 percent and radicular in 41 percent. There was no significant difference in the prevalence of pain between groups of patients with different primary tumor types.

In the MSKCC series,[63] pain was the first symptom in 96 percent of 130 cases of

ESCC (Table 5–3). Pain was of an axial and/or radicular type. Radicular pain was found in 79 percent of cervical lesions, 55 percent of thoracic lesions, and 90 percent of lumbosacral lesions, and was typically bilateral when it occurred in the thoracic region. Occasionally, local and radicular pain was misleading in localizing the level of spinal involvement. Of particular note is that vertebral tenderness was reported in only 42 of 130 patients.[63] The London Hospital study[173] found no spinal tenderness in over 25 percent of cases. These results are comparable to another study[130] in which findings on physical examination were correlated with spinal CT scanning. No spinal percussion tenderness was reported in 7 of 20 patients with epidural extension of tumor from a vertebral metastasis. Thus, although it is often sought by clinicians, spinal tenderness is absent in many patients ultimately proven to have ESCC.

Pain of epidural spinal metastasis is often reported to be exacerbated by Valsalva maneuver, neck flexion and, at times, straight leg raising.[63] In addition, recumbency provokes pain in many patients.[7, 63, 147] At times, because the pain appears intermittent and exacerbated by activity, it may be considered secondary to a musculoligamentous strain or bony instability. Often the diagnosis of spinal cord compression is delayed because the complaint of pain, in the absence of other neurological signs, is attributed to arthritis, rheumatism, or neurosis.[6, 7, 137] As emphasized in Chapter 3, the finding of

incidental osteoarthritis or degenerative joint disease on radiographs of the spine frequently confirms the incorrect clinical impression in these cases, and can result in a delay in diagnosis of several months.[137]

The duration of pain prior to diagnosis of the spinal cord compression from different primary tumors has been analyzed in the London Hospital series.[173] On average, pain was present for 5 months (range 3 days to 3.8 years) prior to diagnosis. This duration was significantly shorter for spine metastases from lung cancer (mean, 4 months) than for metastases secondary to breast cancer (mean, 7 months). In the MSKCC series,[63] the median duration of pain was 2 months for all patients irrespective of their primary tumor. Similar results have been reported by others.[137]

MOTOR DISORDERS

Although weakness may be the only complaint in patients with metastatic ESCC, it much more commonly follows pain. For example, as shown in Table 5–3, only 2 of 130 patients in the MSKCC series[63] had weakness as the initial manifestation of cord compression. However, at the time of diagnosis, these authors reported subjective weakness in over 76 percent and objective signs of weakness in 87 percent of patients.

In the London Hospital series,[173] leg weakness was reported in 82 percent of patients at the time of diagnosis. According to the Medical Research Council scale, at the time of diagnosis, 24 percent of all patients were graded as 0–1/5 strength. Among patients with spinal metastasis from lung cancer, 40 percent were grade 0–1/5, compared with 16 percent of those with metastasis secondary to breast cancer. As the severity of neurological deficit at the time of diagnosis affects outcome, this difference may account for the worse prognosis experienced by patients with spine metastases from lung cancer than from breast cancer.

SENSORY LOSS

Although often present at the time of diagnosis, sensory loss is rare as a sole

Table 5–3 SIGNS AND SYMPTOMS OF EPIDURAL SPINAL CORD COMPRESSION IN 130 PATIENTS*

Sign/Symptom	First Symptom		Symptoms at Diagnosis	
	No.	%	No.	%
Pain	125	96	125	96
Weakness	2	2	99	76
Autonomic dysfunction	0	0	74	57
Sensory complaints	0	0	66	51
Ataxia	2	2	4	3
Herpes zoster	0	0	3	2
Flexor spasms	0	0	2	1

*From Gilbert, RW et al,[63] p 42, with permission.

presenting manifestation of metastatic ESCC; it was not the presenting manifestation in any of the 600 patients with spinal metastasis reported by Constans and colleagues.[35] However, although sensory disturbance was not the presenting complaint in any of the 130 patients from MSKCC,[63] numbness and paresthesias were reported at the time of diagnosis by 51 percent of patients (Table 5–3). On examination, sensory loss was found in 78 percent of the MSKCC group. Loss of pinprick sensibility was as frequent as loss of vibration and position sense.

In the London Hospital series,[173] sensory symptoms were present in the form of radicular complaints in 17 percent and numbness or tingling below the level of the lesion in 44 percent of patients. A sensory level was found on physical examination in 72 percent. No difference was found in sensory symptoms or signs among different primary tumors metastatic to the spine. Although generally there was a good correlation between the sensory level and the level of cord compression, misleading sensory levels were seen in this study and have been reported by others. For example, Barron and colleagues[7] reported cases of sacral sensory sparing associated with extramedullary tumors, perhaps due to the collapse of intramedullary blood vessels as the tumor enlarges, causing patchy areas of infarction and demyelination, as has been shown pathologically.[119] The lamination of the lateral spinothalamic tracts is often responsible for an apparent ascending sensory level in patients with extramedullary neoplasms.

AUTONOMIC DISTURBANCES

As an initial and isolated finding, sphincter disturbances infrequently are the presenting manifestation of ESCC unless the lesion is located at the conus medullaris or cauda equina.[63, 106, 129, 154, 160] Among the series of 600 patients reported by Constans and colleagues,[35] sphincter disturbances were the sole presenting complaint in only 2 percent. Similarly, 1 of 127 patients reported by Barron and colleagues[7] presented with only incontinence of several weeks' duration.

In the MSKCC series,[63] no patients presented with sphincter dysfunction alone. At the time of diagnosis, however, sphincter disturbances were present in 57 percent (Table 5–3). The only patients with sphincter disturbances without motor or sensory loss were those with lesions at T10–T12 vertebral bodies. Sphincter disturbance was a poor prognostic indicator for continued ambulation after therapy. Alternatively, patients with caudal tumors may present with bladder difficulties and impotence.[106, 129] Large volumes of urine may be retained, with secondary overflow incontinence.

UNUSUAL CLINICAL MANIFESTATIONS

The Brown-Séquard syndrome (ipsilateral weakness and position/vibration loss and contralateral pain and temperature dysfunction) is rare among patients with metastatic ESCC.[29] Only 2 percent of cases in the London Hospital series had a true Brown-Séquard syndrome.

Herpes zoster is commonly seen in patients suffering from cancer. Some authors have claimed that an eruption of zoster frequently will presage an episode of cord compression at the same level. Among the 127 patients reported by Barron and colleagues,[7] seven had an eruption at the level of cord compression. In another series,[63] 3 of 130 patients were similarly affected, though others have not commented on the association.[35, 173] Some authors consider that the virus in the dorsal root ganglion is activated by tumor invasion.[7, 63]

Gait ataxia[92] and truncal ataxia[70] have been reported as a rare presenting manifestation. Ataxia was the sole presenting symptom in 2 percent of cases in the MSKCC series and was present in an additional seven patients on examination.[63] The mechanism of gait ataxia was not secondary to position sense abnormalities; these were not significantly impaired. It may be secondary to compression of the spinocerebellar tracts and, when not associated with pain or signs of myelopathy, may suggest cerebellar or cerebral disease.

Laboratory Studies

CEREBROSPINAL FLUID ANALYSIS AND LUMBAR PUNCTURE

CSF abnormalities in cases of malignant ESCC are nonspecific. Because the tumor is epidural, and not within the central nervous system *per se*, CSF findings differ from those in leptomeningeal cancer, in which malignant cells are present within the subarachnoid space. With ESCC, CSF is generally obtained at the time of myelography. The protein content is typically elevated, as expected in cases of partial or complete spinal block. In the detailed London Hospital report,[173] of 56 CSF analyses, the protein was below 40 mg per dl in 9 cases; between 41 and 100 mg per dl in 11 cases; and above 100 mg per dl in 36 cases. In the study of Barron and colleagues,[7] the lowest CSF protein in the setting of a complete manometric block was 48 mg per dl. The highest protein levels were found in cases of epidural tumor in the region of the cauda equina, with one case showing a protein greater than 2,000 mg per dl. At higher spinal levels, the CSF protein did not correlate with the level of spinal cord compression or the primary tumor type.

The cell count is usually normal; Barron and colleagues[7] found CSF pliocytosis in only one case, in a patient with an associated carcinomatosis of the leptomeninges. In the London Hospital[173] experience, there was CSF pleocytosis in 7 of 56, but only 2 had over 10 cells. This mild CSF pleocytosis may reflect inflammation from a parameningeal tumor or concomitant metastases involving the leptomeninges. Although these authors did not find malignant cells in the CSF of their patients, it is well known that the CSF cytology is positive in only approximately 60 percent of patients with leptomeningeal invasion on the initial lumbar puncture.[192, 198] The CSF glucose is typically normal in cases of malignant ESCC.

Lumbar puncture in the presence of increased intracranial pressure secondary to mass lesions may result in a cerebral and cerebellar herniation.[37, 121] There is concern over a similar risk of spinal herniation in patients harboring spinal tumors. Although not all investigators have had similar experiences,[7] some reports suggest that lumbar puncture may result in neurological deterioration in patients with extramedullary neoplasms.[45, 81] For instance, Elsberg[49] believed that radicular pain and neurological disturbances worsened after the removal of spinal fluid in some patients with spinal tumors. He particularly noted that occasionally an indefinite sensory level could become distinct after a lumbar puncture was performed.[49]

A recent study[81] reviewed the risk of neurological deterioration after lumbar puncture for myelography below the level of a complete spinal subarachnoid block. In this retrospective series, 14 percent of 50 patients had significant neurological deterioration after lumbar puncture. No deterioration was seen in patients undergoing myelography via a cervical (C1–2) puncture. The mechanism for neurological deterioration following lumbar puncture is uncertain but has been thought secondary to impaction of the spinal cord tumor, also known as spinal coning.[88] Elsberg[49] attributed it to removal of CSF, which acted as a buffer between the tumor and the spinal cord.

Despite these occasional reports, the risk is difficult to establish. Specific mention was made that there were no cases of clinical worsening that could be attributed to lumbar puncture in 72 patients reported in the series of Barron and colleagues.[7] Furthermore, no neurological worsening is reported after myelography in several series[63, 153, 173] composed of an accumulated several hundred patients. Thus, despite this concern, there have been several recent reports recommending myelography in patients suspected of harboring metastatic spinal cord compression.[25, 130, 142, 145, 153] Alternatively, the development of MRI may preclude the need for myelography in many patients.

There is no specific information to be gained from CSF analysis that assists in the diagnosis of malignant ESCC. Therefore, lumbar puncture should not be performed to rule in or rule out this diagnosis. If infectious or neoplastic meningitis is suspected, then CSF analysis is indicated, with close neurological observation following lumbar puncture and neurosurgical consultation when indicated.

DIAGNOSTIC IMAGING STUDIES

Radiological evaluation of patients with suspected spinal cord compression is changing because of rapid advances in imaging techniques. Plain radiography, radionuclide bone scanning, and myelography were the standard techniques reported in the large clinical studies that form the basis of our current understanding of the problem. More recently, though, CT and MRI have been reported to be helpful in evaluating these patients.[66, 124, 130, 159]

This section reviews selected reports concerning the value of various imaging techniques in the evaluation of metastatic spinal cord compression. At this time, myelography is still considered to be the gold standard against which all other imaging modalities should be compared, and for this reason, it has been recommended by many as the imaging technique of choice.[24, 142, 145, 153, 191] In the future, it may be replaced by the less invasive MRI in most cases. However, in those patients who cannot undergo MRI (such as those with aneurysm clips or pacemakers), those who cannot remain still during the procedure, or those patients in hospitals where MRI is not available, myelography remains the procedure of choice.

Plain Radiography

Plain radiography of the spine often is performed as an initial screening test in patients who may have metastatic ESCC because epidural metastases usually extend from metastasis in the vertebra. Some of the abnormalities seen with metastatic disease include osteolytic and/or osteoblastic lesions and collapse of vertebrae. Paravertebral soft tissue masses are also occasionally seen.

Plain radiographs of bone are very insensitive to the presence of metastatic disease because at least 50 percent of bone must be destroyed before a lesion is identified.[46] Furthermore, the radiological manifestations of metastatic disease are protean and require the interpretation of a skilled radiologist. *The physician who has examined the patient should review the films with the radiologist to provide clinical-radiological correlation.*

The series of metastatic neoplasms involving the spine reported by Barron and colleagues[7] provides information regarding the findings on plain films of the spine in an era prior to the development of many of the newer imaging modalities. Overall, these authors found that 83 percent of patients with spine metastases complaining of back or radicular pain alone had roentgenographic signs of metastatic disease. The frequency of roentgenographic involvement varied among different primary tumors. In cases of spine metastasis secondary to carcinoma of the prostate, breast cancer, and multiple myeloma, abnormal plain films were generally present even at the stage of pain before the development of neurological signs. Such was not the case, however, with lung cancer, lymphoma, and renal cancer, where normal plain films, although still in the minority, were more common.

In the same series,[7] among different primary tumor types, the frequency of solitary spinal metastasis was compared with multiple metastases. Carcinoma of the breast and multiple myeloma invariably were associated with several vertebral levels of involvement, whereas lung cancer, renal cancer, and lymphoma often demonstrated only a single level of metastasis on plain films. Of the 109 cases available for plain film analysis, it did not accurately predict the level of involvement in 15 (14 percent); in eight of these patients, the epidural lesion was distant from the site of metastasis seen on plain film, and in seven patients, the spine was too diffusely involved to define a level of epidural disease.

The London Hospital study[173] also includes an analysis of findings on plain films of the spine (Table 5–4); these findings largely corroborate those noted in the previous series.[111] Of all patients with spinal cord metastases, 16 percent had normal plain films, whereas 84 percent showed involvement by tumor. However, not all tumors demonstrated a similar frequency of plain film abnormalities; spinal metastases arising from carcinoma of the breast were much more likely to demonstrate abnormalities on plain films (94 percent) than those arising from carcinoma of the lung (74 percent). Moreover, metastases from carcinoma of the lung

Table 5−4 FINDINGS ON PLAIN RADIOGRAPH OF THE SPINE IN PATIENTS WITH METASTATIC SPINAL CORD COMPRESSION (%)*

| Primary Tumor | Plain Radiograph | | Number of Vertebrae Involved (as percent of abnormal cases) | | |
	Normal	Abnormal	One	Multiple Contiguous	Multiple Separate
Lung	26	74	52	38	10
Breast	6	94	18	32	50
Miscellaneous	10	90	68	15	18

*Adapted from Stark, RJ et al, [173] p 212.

were much more likely to involve only a single vertebral level (52 percent) than those from carcinoma of the breast (18 percent). The latter tumor frequently involved several noncontiguous vertebrae (50 percent). This information underscores the difficulty of confidently predicting the level of epidural tumor using plain films alone when a tumor commonly spreads to several noncontiguous vertebrae, as in the case of breast cancer, or when the plain films are negative in the setting of epidural disease, as in the case of lung cancer. The finding of tumor involvement at multiple vertebral levels with breast cancer has been confirmed recently. In a series of 42 patients with myelographically documented ESCC, at least two vertebral metastases were seen on plain films in 90 percent of cases, and three or more lesions were present in nearly 75 percent.[74] Other studies have demonstrated that prostatic cancer also has a very high incidence of spreading to multiple vertebral levels, as demonstrated radiologically and at autopsy.[58, 156]

In another series,[164] 88 percent of patients with spine metastases were found to have abnormal plain films. The series from MSKCC[63, 144] found that when epidural tumor was present on myelography, vertebral involvement was seen on plain films in approximately 85 percent of patients, closely correlating with the overall frequency noted in the other studies.

Plain films may be misleadingly normal in some cases of spinal metastases. For example, although intramedullary spinal cord metastases account for only approximately 5 percent of spinal metastases,[144] they need to be considered in cancer pa-

tients with back pain and myelopathy; yet intramedullary metastases are associated with normal plain radiographs of the spine in 75 percent of cases.[68] Similarly, normal plain radiographs of the spine are seen in approximately two thirds of patients with ESCC secondary to lymphoma.[71] Thus, whereas plain films of the spine are frequently abnormal in patients with epidural spinal metastases, they cannot be relied upon confidently to rule in or rule out the presence of epidural tumor or to design the radiation treatment port.

Radionuclide Bone Scanning

Radionuclide bone scanning is more sensitive than plain radiography for visualizing skeletal metastases.[59] This additional sensitivity is gained at the expense of specificity because other skeletal conditions such as degenerative joint disease may also cause abnormal scans. In patients with metastatic disease, this results in a false-positive rate of spine metastasis that has been reported to range from 20 to 74 percent;[99] plain films, CT, or other techniques often are necessary to differentiate among these diagnoses. Occasionally, false-negative radionuclide scans also occur.[187]

In a series of patients with suspected vertebral column metastases,[153] an abnormal myelogram was found in 65 percent of those with abnormal bone scans, while an abnormal myelogram was found in 32 percent of those with normal bone scans. This study concluded that radionuclide bone scanning does not improve the accuracy of predicting the presence or absence of epidural tumor over that obtained by plain films alone.

In a study[74] of patients with suspected spinal cord compression from breast cancer, radionuclide bone scans were positive in 100 percent of patients with myelographically proven epidural metastases; but in 90 percent of these cases, there were multiple levels of involvement. Among patients with negative myelograms, positive radionuclide bone scans were found in 47 percent. These studies indicate that radionuclide bone scanning, although more sensitive than plain films of the spine, is inadequate to confirm or exclude the presence and level(s) of epidural spinal cord metastases and thus plan therapy.

Myelography

The importance of myelography in evaluating and managing patients with suspected metastatic spinal cord compression already has been noted.[7, 29, 35, 63, 147, 173] The arguments for myelography as outlined by Barron and colleagues[7] were as follows: (1) Plain roentgenograms may be normal in the presence of epidural tumor; (2) Abnormalities on plain films may be confused with osteoporosis or Paget's disease; and (3) Other sites of epidural involvement may be present aside from that shown on plain films.

These arguments in favor of myelography have been supported by more recent clinical studies. In the MSKCC study[63] of 130 cases of ESCC from metastatic cancer, myelography identified a complete block or high-grade partial block in the absence of bony involvement on routine studies in 15 percent of cases. Although myelography was performed in only 52 percent of cases reported from London Hospital,[173] it showed multiple levels of epidural involvement in 10 percent of all cases and 29 percent of cases secondary to breast cancer. Another study[113] showed that myelography may reveal the presence of spinal cord compression in the face of a normal neurological examination. Of 59 patients with radicular pain but no neurological deficit, 15 (25 percent) were found to have a complete spinal subarachnoid block on myelography.

Recently, other studies[25, 152, 153] quantified the value of myelography in patients with suspected metastatic spinal cord compression. In a study by Rodichok et al,[152] plain radiography correctly identified the level of spinal cord compression in only 13 of 18 (72 percent) patients presenting with myelopathy.[152] In a follow-up study, it was found that those patients diagnosed at an early stage of epidural disease were much more likely to remain ambulatory until death compared with those diagnosed later in their course. These findings resulted in a subsequent detailed study of the role of myelography in cancer patients at risk for ESCC.[153] Patients were divided into five groups: group 1—myelopathy; group 2—radiculopathy; group 3—plexopathy; group 4—back pain with normal neurological examination and abnormal plain spine film or bone scan; group 5—back pain with normal neurological examination and normal radiological studies.

Of 26 patients in group 1, with myelopathy, 20 (77 percent) had abnormal myelograms. Of these 20, 19 had abnormal plain films at the site of epidural tumor. Of the remaining six patients with negative myelograms, abnormal plain films were found in two that could have resulted in radiation therapy of asymptomatic sites. The authors believed this to be potentially important because three of the six were thought to have radiation myelopathy that could have been exacerbated by further irradiation.

Of 43 patients with radiculopathy but no signs of cord involvement (group 2), 27 (63 percent) had positive myelograms. When the plain films were positive for metastatic disease at the clinical level of radiculopathy, the chance of epidural disease was 91 percent. When the plain films were negative at the level of radiculopathy, 33 percent had evidence of epidural neoplasm on myelography. Of seven myelograms performed in Group 3, one had an epidural defect.

Among 43 patients in group 4 (back pain with normal neurological examination and abnormal plain film or bone scan), 63 percent had epidural tumor on myelogram. Of patients in group 5 (back pain, normal neurological examination and normal plain films/bone scan), none showed evidence of epidural tumor. Combining groups 4 and 5 yields a cohort of cancer patients presenting to their physician with nonradicular back pain and normal neurological examinations; based on the above data, of this large cohort, 44 percent can be expected to have epidural tumor. Similarly, prior to radiological studies, the overall risk of epidural disease in those complaining of radicular pain with a normal neurological examination is 63 percent.

This detailed analysis underscores the importance of early diagnostic evaluation of cancer patients complaining of back pain and radicular pain. Given the above findings, the authors of the study[153] concluded that most cancer patients with back pain require myelography; prompt myelography is particularly needed in patients with myelopathy and radiculopathy associated with normal plain films or diffuse spinal metastases.

The above conclusions have been supported by another study of the impact of myelography on radiotherapy of malignant spinal cord compression.[25] Patients with neurological deficits due to spinal cord compression were seen in consultation by a neurosurgeon and underwent plain radiographs of the spine. A mock radiation therapy port was then designed using the clinical and plain radiography information. The additional information obtained by myelography was then used to evaluate the adequacy of the mock radiation therapy ports. The mock radiation therapy ports were found inadequate in 69 percent of cases.

When myelography is performed in patients suspected of ESCC, the entire spinal axis should be examined unless there is a contraindication.[144, 145, 154] This approach permits the rostral and caudal extent of the block to be visualized and establishes whether multiple levels of metastatic involvement are present. This information is of value in determining radiation therapy ports and surgery if planned.

Case Illustration

A 64-year-old man presented with a 6-week history of progressive left shoulder pain; more recently, his pain radiated into the ulnar aspect of his arm and his chest in a radicular distribution. He was seen in an emergency room for this complaint. He had a 40 pack year smoking history and had an unexplained 20-pound weight loss in the previous 3 months. General physical examination was unremarkable except for expiratory wheezes. A detailed neurologic examination was entirely within normal limits. A plain radiograph of the cervical and thoracic spine was normal; however, a chest radiograph demonstrated a left apical pulmonary mass and hilar adenopathy. The patient underwent a needle biopsy and an adenocarcinoma was found. Due to the history of axial and radicular pain, he underwent a myelogram by lumbar approach. A complete block secondary to an epidural mass was found at the T3 level. Intrathecal contrast was administered via a C1–2 approach and the upper border of the block was found to be at T1. A postmyelographic CT scan through the area demonstrated a paravertebral mass, not seen on the plain films, which had invaded the epidural space through the intervertebral foramina.

Comment. Although epidural invasion through the intervertebral foramina often occurs with lymphoma (due to the paravertebral location of lymph nodes), it also may occur with other forms of malignancy. Superior sulcus tumors[138] frequently invade the brachial plexus and extend into the epidural space through foramina.[28, 98] In such cases, the vertebrae are not invaded and plain radiographs and radionuclide bone scans may be unrevealing.

Computerized Tomography

CT scanning has been demonstrated to be more sensitive and specific for identifying neoplasms of the vertebral column and paravertebral structures than bone scanning and plain films.[19, 79, 130, 145, 195] When used following myelography with water-soluble contrast material, CT has helped to locate an extension of tumor from vertebrae and paravertebral structures to the epidural space. For example, using spinal CT myelograms in 30 patients harboring epidural metastases at 106 vertebral levels, Weissman and associates[195] have demonstrated that epidural tumor extension occurs via three mechanisms: (1) direct extension from metastasis to the adjacent vertebra (81 percent); (2) craniocaudal extension from tumor arising in vertebrae at rostral or caudal levels (17 percent); and (3) epidural extension from paravertebral tissues through intervertebral foramina (2 percent).

Conversely, 85 of 109 (78 percent) vertebrae with cortical disruption from tumor invasion demonstrated epidural extension as well.[195] However, the absence of cortical disruption at a single vertebral level could not exclude the presence of epidural disease at that level, since epidural tumor was seen in 21 of 183 vertebral levels at which no cortical disruption was present. In all but one of these cases, the epidural tumor was due to extension from craniocaudal levels or paravertebral tissues. The risk of craniocaudal extension in the epidural space was significant, with 20 percent of patients studied showing this phenomenon; 10 percent of patients with epidural tumor demonstrated craniocaudal extension of more than two vertebral levels. This is important therapeutically because standard radiotherapy ports using plain films include two vertebral levels above and below the spinal metastasis. In this 10 percent of patients, however, the radiotherapy port would have been inadequate to encompass the entire epidural tumor. The authors state, "This, coupled with our findings of a 38 percent incidence of synchronous noncontiguous epidural deposits, emphasizes the need for careful myelographic documentation of the extent of the tumor before instituting therapy."[195]

Despite the excellent bony detail afforded by spinal CT, the same authors found limitations in identifying the presence or absence of vertebral cortical disruption from tumor invasion, especially in cases of severe osteoporosis, which may make cortical margins indistinct, and in cases of osteoblastic metastases arising from carcinoma of the prostate. They concluded that in cases of suspected epidural tumor, patients with back pain, normal neurological examination, and evidence of metastases on plain films should undergo myelography. In similar cases with normal or equivocal plain films, they recommended spinal CT scanning. If evidence of vertebral cortical disruption is found on the CT scan, then the patient is referred for myelography. Due to its sensitivity in demonstrating paravertebral soft tissues, spinal CT may be the initial diagnostic study of choice in patients suspected of harboring paravertebral metastases with epidural extension.

In a later study, O'Rourke and colleagues[130] studied the value of spinal CT and spinal CT metrizamide myelography in detecting spinal metastases in cancer patients with new spinal lesions on radionuclide bone scanning. Patients with an abnormality on bone scanning underwent plain radiographs of the spine. Group 1 consisted of patients with normal plain films. Group 2 consisted of those with compression fracture on plain radiograph. Group 3 consisted of those with evidence of metastasis on plain films.

Patients in group 1 underwent spinal CT. CT myelography was performed in all patients in groups 2 and 3 and those in group 1 with cortical bone discontinuity. Using this algorithm, it was found that CT scanning of the spine could differentiate benign from malignant disease in most cases and that the presence of cortical bone discontinuity was associated with epidural tumor in 20 of 31 (64 percent) of cases. Unlike the previous study noted,[195] no mention was made of epidural tumor at levels other than those with cortical bone destruction.

O'Rourke and colleagues[130] recommended the following algorithm for the evaluation of spinal metastasis: Patients with abnormal bone scan or back pain and no neurological findings would undergo plain spine films and then spinal CT. If no metastases are found, no further workup is needed at that time; if spinal metastases are found but the cortical bone is intact, then a follow-up CT scan would be performed in 1 month or as clinically indicated. If spinal metastasis with cortical bone discontinuity or soft tissue mass was seen, then CT myelography is recommended to rule out cord compression. The authors indicate that cases of benign and malignant disease would be differentiated using this protocol. The authors did not address the issue of therapy in this study,[130] but validated the usefulness of their clinical approach in a follow-up study.[149]

Magnetic Resonance Imaging

MRI is a sensitive, noninvasive imaging modality for a variety of different spinal disorders.[105, 124, 202] MRI is acquiring a major role in the evaluation of patients with metastatic ESCC.[33, 117, 159, 181, 201] In recent studies, it has been found to rival the sensitivity and specificity of both myelography[118, 171] and CT.[10] With the advent of contrast-enhanced MRI with gadolinium, its role and value in the evaluation and management of these patients is further increased.[180, 181] Figures 5–7 and 5–8 demonstrate examples of the excellent imaging potential of MRI for ESCC.

In an early study of noncontrast MRI of the spine, MRI appeared more sensitive than radionuclide bone scanning in the detection of vertebral metastases.[159] In another study[10] of tumors involving the osseous spine, MRI was compared with CT scanning for defining the anatomic relationships of the tumor, vertebral column, spinal canal, paravertebral tissues, and vascular involvement; MRI was found superior to CT without intrathecal contrast injection and equal to CT with contrast. CT scanning without contrast was found superior to MRI in detecting cortical bone destruction, due to the poor signal intensity of cortical bone with MRI.[191]

In a recent study comparing spinal MRI (0.5 Tesla) with myelography in 31 patients with cancer, Hagenau and colleagues[72] evaluated these two modalities in detecting epidural metastases in patients with myelopathy (n = 10) and those with pain but no myelopathy (n = 21). MRI was found comparable to myelography in detecting large epidural tumor masses that compressed the cord. Small epidural masses and those causing root compression were better identified using myelography in nine cases; MRI was superior in only one case. These authors concluded that myelography continued to be the preferred imaging technology.

In another recent study, spinal MRI was performed in 58 patients with epidural metastases and compared with myelography in 22 of these patients.[171] In 60 of 64 studies performed in 58 patients, MRI was found to be diagnostic. In the 22 patients undergoing both procedures, myelography was diagnostic in 20 studies and MRI yielded the same diagnosis in 19 of 22 cases. The authors concluded that when a technically satisfactory MRI study could be obtained, it was equivalent to myelography or CT myelography in detecting clinically significant epidural disease. In the same

study, the authors found T1-weighted images optimal for demonstrating spinal cord compression, whereas T2-weighted images were best for identifying subarachnoid space compression without cord impingement. Furthermore, paravertebral masses that would have been missed on myelography were recognized with MRI. Finally, because a spinal MRI required 60 to 90 minutes, compared with the 2 hours required for myelography or CT myelography, patients seemed to tolerate the MRI better. It should be recognized, however, that movement artifact degrades the quality of MRI images; because patients with spinal metastases are often in pain, especially when lying supine, pain control as well as claustrophobia remains problematic with MRI. Finally, the authors note that the cost of a spinal MR examination in most institutions is equal to or less than a myelogram followed by CT.

With the advent of contrast-enhanced MRI with gadolinium-DTPA, the value of MRI is further increased.[180, 181] Preliminary studies have reported that some regions of epidural tumor demonstrate marked enhancement while other areas show minimal or no enhancement.[181] In some cases, lesions that were hypointense on noncontrast MRI became isointense with surrounding bone following the administration of gadolinium-DTPA, decreasing the ability to detect these epidural metastases (see Fig. 5–8). Sze and colleagues[181] concluded that contrast-enhanced MRI was helpful in delineating and characterizing some epidural neoplasms when compared with precontrast MRI scans.

Although the detection of vertebral and epidural neoplasms is sometimes obscured by contrast administration, enhanced MRI scans may be very useful in the evaluation of patients with suspected epidural tumor. Gadolinium administration may help differentiate epidural tumor from disc herniation because herniated disc material should not enhance immediately following contrast administration, unlike tumor.[180] Furthermore, contrast-enhanced scans may demonstrate areas of active tumor involvement more readily than noncontrast studies. In patients with diffuse metastases on nonenhanced scans, biopsy of

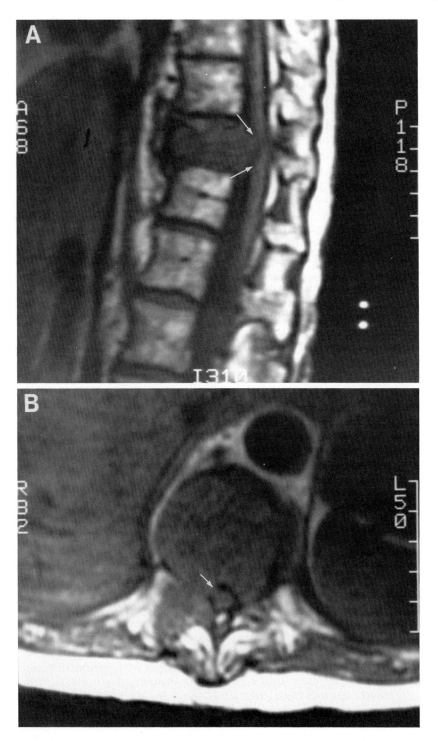

Figure 5–7. Noncontrast MRI of spine showing epidural metastasis at the T9 level due to breast cancer. (A) Saggital view showing destruction of the vertebral body with extension into the spinal canal resulting in cord compression (arrows). (B) Axial view showing tumor extending into the pedicle and compromising the spinal canal (arrow).

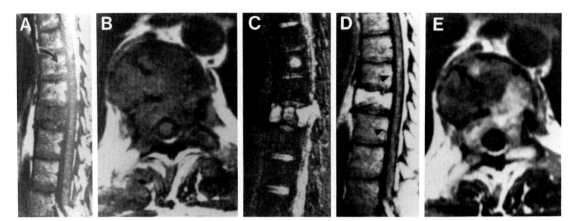

Figure 5–8. Gadolinium-enhanced MRI of the spine of a 36-year-old patient with a plasmacytoma. (A) and (B) Sagittal (A) and axial (B) images showing partial collapse of the T10 vertebral body and replacement of normal high signal of bone marrow with low-intensity tumor. In addition, a poorly defined hypointense focus is seen in the T8 vertebral body (arrow, A). (C) T2-weighted images show both lesions. (D) and (E) After the administration of gadolinium-DTPA, the T1-weighted sagittal (D) and axial (E) images show enhancement of the T10 vertebral body. The previously well seen hypointense region of tumor in T8 is not easily seen due to the fact that it is isointense with the remainder of the vertebral body on this enhanced study. The axial scan (E) shows greater enhancement on the left than the right side of the vertebral body. Although tumor may permeate the entire vertebral body, results of multiple biopsy attempts on the right side were negative, whereas results of biopsy on the left revealed tumor. (From Sze, G et al, [181] with permission.)

enhancing areas of vertebral involvement has resulted in a greater yield than biopsy of nonenhancing abnormal regions.[180] Gadolinium also may reveal specific areas of spinal cord compression more readily than noncontrast studies alone.[180, 181] In addition, contrast administration may have a role in evaluating response to therapy. Preliminary studies suggest that successfully treated bone metastases do not enhance with gadolinium, whereas unresponsive metastases continue to enhance.[180, 181]

Clinical Approach to the Patient Suspected of Spinal Metastasis

Cancer patients with clinical evidence of spinal metastases fall into three groups: (1) patients with back or neck pain with or without referred or radicular pain; (2) those with mild, stable, or equivocal evidence of spinal cord compression; and (3) patients with new or rapidly progressive symptoms and/or signs of spinal cord compression. (As elsewhere in this chapter, the terms myelopathy and spinal cord compression include cauda equina dysfunc-

tion and compression.) The goal of diagnosis is to recognize those patients with spinal metastases before neurological abnormalities arise because the outcome of therapy is so much more favorable in the first two groups.[63, 182] No single approach or algorithm can apply to all patients or supersede clinical judgment;[17] because circumstances often require that the approach be modified for individual cases, the following is only a guide to the workup.

In cancer patients with back or neck pain and normal neurologic examinations who are not suspected of harboring ESCC, many physicians initially obtain a radionuclide bone scan and plain spine radiograph. If these studies reveal findings that explain the patient's symptoms (e.g., vertebral metastasis at the level of pain), many medical oncologists and radiotherapists treat with systemic agents and/or radiotherapy without further diagnostic studies. In such cases, it must be recognized that clinically unsuspected epidural metastases may be present at the level of the known vertebral metastasis, adjacent to it, or at a distant vertebral level. Therefore, it is important to follow the patient's clinical course carefully and proceed with MRI or myelography if neurological signs consistent with spinal cord compression develop.

Alternatively, because many cancer patients with back and/or projected pain and normal neurological examinations harbor clinically unsuspected ESCC, many physicians recommend spinal MRI or myelography in planning therapy.[145] If MRI is unavailable or cannot be performed, then a plain radiograph of the spine may identify vertebral metastases. According to a recent study, if the plain film shows greater than 50 percent collapse of the vertebra due to metastasis, there is a nearly 90 percent risk of epidural tumor; if there is pedicle erosion, epidural tumor may be found in approximately 30 percent; only 7 percent had epidural tumor if the metastasis was restricted to the vertebral body without collapse.[20] Thus, myelography or MRI may be selected in those patients with a positive plain radiograph or those who have a significant risk of epidural extension. If the radiograph is negative for metastases or shows limited involvement, spinal CT scanning of the symptomatic areas may be performed next. Those with CT scans that are negative for metastases *and* in whom there is a low clinical suspicion for epidural tumor are next considered for lumbar puncture to evaluate for leptomeningeal metastases. Alternatively, myelography or MRI is still recommended in cancer patients with a negative CT scan for metastasis but in whom there is a high clinical suspicion for epidural tumor, or for those with CT scans that are positive for vertebral metastases with cortical disruption bordering the vertebral canal, or paraspinal mass.[149] All patients with spine metastases should undergo careful follow-up to identify neurological deterioration that might lead to consideration of other options for treatment.

For cancer patients with mild, stable, or equivocal symptoms and/or signs of spinal cord compression, a total spine MRI (if available) is performed by the next day. If MRI is unavailable, then an immediate radiograph of the spine is performed, followed by total spine myelography by the next day. Total spine studies are performed because some patients will have unsuspected metastases at multiple levels. During their evaluation, patients in this group should be closely observed to identify progressive myelopathy. Cancer patients with new or rapidly progressive signs of spinal cord compression should be given high-dose intravenous dexamethasone[194] (Posner recommends 100 mg[145]) to reduce spinal cord edema[188] and reduce the risk of spinal coning.[81] Then an immediate total spine MRI or myelogram is performed.

Because spinal MRI and myelography occasionally yield false-negative results in cases of spinal cord compression, the physician often must consider other diagnostic studies following a negative MRI or myelogram in the cancer patient with a myelopathy. For example, if the noncontrast spinal MRI is negative, the physician should consider a contrast-enhanced spinal MRI and CSF analysis to identify leptomeningeal metastases (see Chapter 7). Myelography should still be considered when clinical suspicion of a compressive lesion remains but none is identified on the spinal MRI; in such cases, CSF may be obtained for analysis at the time of myelography. Because neurologic deterioration may occur following myelography, neurosurgical consultation should be available.[81] Finally, contrast-enhanced MRI may demonstrate intramedullary metastases not seen on either myelography or plain MRI (see Chapter 6).

Therapy

Metastatic epidural spinal cord compression is most commonly treated with corticosteroids and radiation therapy; selected patients undergo surgical decompression.[145] Corticosteroids have been found to reduce vasogenic spinal cord edema[188] and usually help control pain and improve neurological function. The dosage and form of corticosteroid vary.[190a] We often use doses of 10−100 mg of dexamethasone intravenously stat, followed by 4−24 mg qid; the lower doses are used for patients with mild pain and no, or equivocal, signs of myelopathy; the highest doses are used in patients with prominent, or rapidly progressive, myelopathy. Occasional patients will report pain or burning in the perineal region when high-dose corticosteroids are administered intravenously. Tapering of high-dose steroids is begun within 48 to 72 hours and patients are followed closely for signs of steroid-induced complications such as glucose intolerance and infection. As the steroids are tapered, patients are observed for deterioration in neurological function and the dose is increased if this occurs. Many patients can be tapered off steroids within 2–3 weeks.[194]

Radiation therapy has become the primary mode of treatment of metastatic ESCC because such patients often harbor widespread metastatic disease and are poor surgical candidates. When radiotherapy is selected for treatment, it should commence once the diagnosis of metastatic ESCC is established. The upper and lower extent of the epidural neoplasm should be defined by imaging studies so that the entire area of cord compression and epidural tumor is treated. Because epidural metastases may occur at multiple levels, we routinely image the entire rostrocaudal spinal axis with MRI (or myelography) in patients with clinical manifestations of ESCC. In addition to identifying all levels of ESCC, this strategy allows the design of radiotherapy ports that include adjacent asymptomatic metastatic epidural deposits. If these adjacent epidural metastases are not included in the original treatment field and later require radiotherapy, the amount of radiation tolerated may be limited by overlapping spinal radiotherapy ports.

The prognosis for patients undergoing radiotherapy for metastatic ESCC depends upon their neurological function at the time treatment begins. Patients who are ambulatory at the time of diagnosis usually retain this ability following radiotherapy, but only about half of patients who are paraparetic at presentation regain ambulation, and paraplegic patients rarely are restored to ambulation with radiotherapy.[63]

Surgical decompression of metastatic ESCC has, until recently, consisted of laminectomy. However, several retrospective studies and one prospective study have shown that laminectomy followed by radiation therapy is not superior to radiation therapy alone.[56, 63, 199] Alternatively, because the metastatic tumor is usually anterior to the cord in the vertebral body, a surgical approach consisting of vertebral body resection followed by stabilization has been recently reported with promising results. Carefully selected paraparetic and paraplegic patients have been reported to ambulate following this surgical approach.[73, 168] There have been no randomized controlled studies to compare anterior vertebral body resection with radiotherapy alone.

The indications for surgical decompression of metastatic ESCC are evolving. We believe that surgical decompression should be considered in: (1) patients without a diagnosis; (2) patients who are neurologically deteriorating due to spinal cord compression, who have been previously irradiated at the site of spinal cord compression, and whose medical condition permits surgery; and (3) those with progressive neurological deterioration during radiation therapy. Intractable pain and radioresistant tumors are considered indications for surgical decompression in selected cases.

PRIMARY SPINAL NEOPLASMS

As indicated earlier, primary epidural spinal tumors arise from cellular elements that form the vertebral column and supporting structures. Their frequency is estimated to be approximately three times less than that of spinal metastases.[137] Their neurological presentation is similar to that of metastatic neoplasms, pain being the prominent first complaint, followed by symptoms and signs of neural compression. We briefly review the more common primary epidural spinal tumors (Table 5–5).

Multiple Myeloma

Multiple myeloma, a plasma cell neoplasm that proliferates in bone marrow, is the most common primary tumor of bone.[57] The neoplastic cells usually secrete

Osteogenic Sarcoma

Osteogenic sarcoma is the second most common primary bone tumor. It usually occurs in childhood and adolescence, but has a second peak of incidence in later life, often occurring in association with Paget's disease, previously irradiated bone, or other predisposing factor.[44, 116, 166, 170, 178] It may arise from transformation of an osteoblastoma or osteochondroma.[43, 57]

The spine is a rare site of primary involvement but is a frequent site of metastatic spread from a primary osteogenic sarcoma elsewhere.[55, 57, 132, 139, 166] Pain is the most common initial complaint; in the Mayo Clinic series,[32] pain was usually present for several months, but ranged from 2 1/2 weeks to 2 years. Neurological signs of spinal cord compression were often found. Serum alkaline phophatase is elevated in approximately one half of patients.[116] Among other abnormalities, radiographic studies often demonstrate both lytic and blastic changes of bone.[57, 116] The histological appearance can be variable and correlation of the clinical history, physical examination, and radiographic features can be very helpful in diagnosis and treatment planning.[32, 57]

The treatment of osteogenic sarcoma has undergone major advances in recent years. In addition to surgery, developments in radiation therapy and chemotherapy have altered the management of this disease. There are several chemotherapy protocols that have been used for primary and metastatic disease.[116]

an immunoglobulin protein and the disease is often associated with skeletal destruction, hypercalcemia, immunodeficiency, and impaired renal function. It generally affects older individuals, with a median age in the seventh decade, but may affect those much younger.[11] Osteosclerotic myeloma, a rare variant, may be associated with polyneuropathy, organomegaly, endocrinopathy, M protein and skin changes (POEMS syndrome).[94, 150]

Epidural spinal cord compression is the most common neurological complication of multiple myeloma, occurring in approximately 10 to 15 percent of cases.[7, 26] The clinical presentation is similar to that of metastatic deposits.[7] In addition to ESCC, neurological involvement[26] includes a variety of different forms of peripheral neuropathy[94, 95] that may, at times, be difficult to differentiate from spinal root involvement.

The myeloma cell causes bone resorption through an osteoclast-activating factor.[126] Vertebral bodies often demonstrate osteolytic defects without reactive bone formation.[57, 69] Vertebral body involvement typically occurs before the pedicles are invaded because there is normally less red marrow in the pedicles.[85, 101] Radiographs may show a solitary sclerotic vertebra (ivory vertebra). Radionuclide bone scans are often unremarkable; conventional radiographs have been found to be more sensitive.[69, 114] CT scanning, myelography, and MRI may show the spinal and epidural involvement by tumor.

Multiple myeloma is usually radiosensitive and most patients with ESCC can be treated with corticosteroids and radiotherapy, as in the therapy of metastatic epidural tumors.

Chordoma

Chordoma is a rare neoplasm that arises from notochordal remnants and shows a predilection for the sacrococcygeal area (50 percent) and base of the skull (35 percent); the remaining cases are found elsewhere in the vertebral column.[51, 83, 116] Patients are usually over the age of 30 years. Although chordomas may metastasize, the high morbidity and mortality of this neoplasm is due to frequent local recurrence, the most common cause of death.[123, 151] One review of the literature[67] found only 1 percent of 222 patients disease-free at 10 years.

The most common early symptom is pain. As the tumor grows, neural structures are involved; when it occurs in the sacrococcygeal region, bowel and bladder symptoms and saddle anesthesia may occur. The duration of symptoms varies between 2 weeks and 9 years, usually more than a year.[175] With sacrococcygeal chordomas, a presacral mass may be palpable on rectal examination. When the tumor occurs at other levels of the spine, it causes radicular and spinal cord symptoms and signs similar to those of other epidural tumors. Radiographically, there are a variety of different appearances.[102] The lesion may be osteolytic, osteoblastic, or contain both elements, or, at times, plain films may show no abnormalities.[32] Diagnosis is established by biopsy.

Surgery is the primary therapy of chordomas, with many patients benefiting from repeated surgical resections for tumor recurrence. In addition, radiation therapy may cause tumor regression that lasts for many years.[100] Proton beam radiation therapy may be especially effective in controlling local disease.[116] Postoperative radiation therapy has been recommended in many cases of incomplete surgical resection.[100]

Chondrosarcoma

Chondrosarcomas are cartilaginous neoplasms without direct osteoid formation that arise in bone.[116] Chondrosarcomas may arise de novo in bone, follow irradiation of bone, or may develop in preexisting Paget's disease or benign cartilage tumors such as osteochondroma or endochondromas.[4, 57] They generally occur in individuals over 30 years of age; fewer than 5 percent occur in patients under 20.[32, 39, 80, 83]

Chondrosarcomas typically occur in long bones or pelvis but may occur in the vertebral column. Initially, they tend to involve the vertebral bodies more frequently than the vertebral arch.[57] The initial symptom of spinal chondrosarcoma is usually pain; in the Mayo Clinic series, the period of pain ranged from 2 weeks to 11 years, but symptoms often persisted for 4–5 years prior to diagnosis.[32] As the epidural tumor grows, neural compression develops and symptoms and signs of radiculopathy and myelopathy referable to the level occur. Although they have a highly unpredictable biological behavior, chondrosarcomas may grow quite extensively locally before metastases appear. Radiographically, the lesions may appear as lytic lesions associated with lobular calcifications, but other appearances have been described.[57, 116]

Surgical resection is the treatment of choice of chondrosarcoma, with repeated surgical resections often helpful for recurrent disease.[57] These tumors are relatively radioresistant but radiotherapy may delay progression of the disease.[116]

Ewing's Sarcoma

Ewing's sarcoma is a rare, primitive round-cell tumor of bone usually occurring in childhood, adolescence, or early adult life.[141] This tumor usually arises in long bones but may rarely originate in the vertebral column. Since it frequently metastasizes to bone, spinal involvement more often is due to a metastasis from a primary site elsewhere than to a primary Ewing's sarcoma of the spine.[39, 177] When the tumor arises in the axial skeleton, the sacrum is the most common site of origin.[196]

Pain is the most frequent initial complaint and often may be present for a few months, although much shorter courses have also been noted.[32, 57] Neurological abnormalities referable to radicular and spinal cord dysfunction usually follow. Radiological studies may reveal a variety of different appearances.[32, 102, 189] On histological study, a variety of patterns may be seen.[32, 112] The use of radiation therapy and chemotherapy has dramatically improved the prognosis for patients with Ewing's sarcoma.[141]

Benign Tumors and Tumor-like Conditions

Symptomatic primary benign bone tumors of the spine are unusual and are rare causes of spinal cord compression. For example, vertebral hemangiomas have been found in approximately 10 percent of routine autopsies,[32, 57, 62, 161] but they are rarely symptomatic. However, when benign vertebral tumors do become symptomatic, they often present with pain and thus must be considered in the differential diagnosis of patients with axial and radicular pain. The more common neoplasms and tumor-like conditions include osteochondroma or exostosis,[23, 27, 52, 91] osteoid osteoma,[86, 97, 179] osteoblastoma,[86, 97, 133] giant cell tumors,[38, 42, 163] aneurysmal bone cysts,[165, 176] fibrous dysplasia,[60] eosinophilic granuloma,[158] and hemangioma. In addition, spinal cord compression secondary to extramedullary hematopoiesis[77, 108, 135, 172] has been described in cases of myelofibrosis, sideroblastic anemia, sickle cell anemia, thalassemia, and other myeloproliferative disorders. Furthermore, epidural lipomatosis in the setting of Cushing's disease or corticosteroid administration also may cause spinal cord compression.[5, 89, 109]

The radiographic appearance may suggest the diagnosis, as in the case of osteochondroma[169] or hemangioma;[57, 104] tissue confirmation may be necessary in some cases. When neural compression occurs secondary to an expanding mass or collapse of the vertebral body, the symptoms and signs are similar to those of other epidural tumors.

LIPOMA

Spinal lipomas are primary tumors of the spinal canal that may be part of the dysraphic state (developmental) or, less commonly, exist as an isolated neoplasm. The former, part of multiple congenital anomalies, may be associated with a subcutaneous palpable soft-tissue mass and abnormal fusion of the vertebrae, and are discussed elsewhere.[30, 50, 186] Alternatively, lipomas that occur as isolated tumors may be either intradural or extradural and are discussed in more detail in Chapter 6. Such "isolated" intradural and extradural lipomas account for approximately 1 percent of all primary spinal neoplasms.[64] One study[47] found that of nondevelopmen-

tal spinal lipomas, two fifths were epidural and three fifths were intradural.

Extradural lipomas affect both sexes equally and may present at any age.[64] Unlike intradural lipomas, which typically have a prolonged history of symptoms prior to diagnosis, extradural lipomas usually have a duration of symptoms lasting less than one year.[64] Although any segmental level may be involved, the thoracic spine appears to be the most common site.[64] There is no characteristic constellation of clinical symptoms or signs distinguishing epidural spinal lipomas from many other epidural tumors. In one review,[64] no bony changes were seen on plain films in two thirds of cases. Surgery is the treatment of choice.[64, 186] Epidural lipomas must be differentiated from steroid-induced lipomatosis, which may cause spinal cord compression.[5, 61, 89]

REFERENCES

1. Abrams, HL, Spiro, R, and Goldstein, N: Metastases in carcinoma. Analysis of 1000 autopsied cases. Cancer 3:74–85, 1950.
2. Al-Mefty, O, Harkey, LH, Middleton, TH, Smith, RR, and Fox, JL: Myelopathic cervical spondylotic lesions demonstrated by magnetic resonance imaging. J Neurosurg 68:217–222, 1988.
3. Alter, M: Statistical aspects of spinal cord tumors. In Vinken, PJ and Bruyn, GW (eds): Handbook of Clinical Neurology, Vol 19. North-Holland Publishing, Amsterdam, 1975, pp 1–22.
4. Aprin, H, Riseborough, EJ, and Hall, JE: Chondrosarcoma in children and adolescents. Clin Orthop 166:226–232, 1982.
5. Arroyo, IL, Barron, KS, and Brewer, EJ: Spinal cord compression by epidural lipomatosis in juvenile rheumatoid arthritis. Arthritis Rheum 31:447–451, 1988.
6. Arseni, CN, Simionescu, MD, and Horwath, L: Tumors of the spine: A follow-up study of 350 patients with neurosurgical considerations. Acta Psychiat Scand 34:398–410, 1959.
7. Barron, KD, Hirano, A, Araki, S, et al: Experiences with metastatic neoplasms involving the spinal cord. Neurology 9:91–106, 1959.
8. Batson, OV: The function of the vertebral veins and their role in the spread of metastases. Ann Surg 112:138–148, 1940.
9. Batson, OV: The vertebral vein system. Caldwell Lecture, 1956. American Journal Roentgenology, Radium Therapy and Nuclear Medicine 78:195–212, 1957.

10. Beltran, J, Noto, AM, Chakeres, DW, et al: Tumors of the osseous spine: Staging with MR imaging versus CT. Radiology 162:565–569, 1987.

11. Bergsagel, DE and Rider, WD: Plasma cell neoplasms. In DeVita, VT, Hellman, S and Rosenberg, SA (eds): Cancer: Principles and Practice of Oncology. JB Lippincott, Philadelphia, 1985, pp 1753–1795.

12. Bernat, JL, Greenberg, ER, and Barrett, J: Suspected epidural compression of the spinal cord and cauda equina by metastatic carcinoma. Cancer 51:1953–1957, 1983.

13. Berretoni, BA and Carter, JR: Mechanisms of cancer metastasis to bone. J Bone Joint Surg 68A:308–312, 1986.

14. Blight, A: Cellular morphology of chronic spinal cord injury in the cat: Analysis of myelinated axons by live sampling. Neuroscience 10:521–543, 1983.

15. Blight, A: Delayed myelination and macrophage invasion: A candidate for secondary damage in spinal cord injury. Central Nervous System Trauma 2:299–315, 1985.

16. Blight, A: Morphometric analysis of experimental spinal cord injury in the cat: Relation of injury intensity to survival of myelinated axons. Neuroscience 19:321–341, 1986.

17. Blois, MS: Medicine and the nature of vertical reasoning. N Engl J Med 318:847–851, 1988.

18. Boland, PJ, Lane, JM, and Sundarasen, N: Metastatic disease of the spine. Clin Orthop 169:95–102, 1982.

19. Braunstein, EM and Kuhns, LR: Computed tomographic demonstration of spinal metastases. Spine 8:912–915, 1983.

20. Browne, TR, Adams, RD, and Robertson, GH: Hemangioblastoma of the spinal cord. Arch Neurol 33:435–441, 1976.

21. Bumpus, HC: Carcinoma of the prostate. Surg Gynecol Obstet 43:150–155, 1926.

22. Bunn, PA, Schein, PS, Banks, PM, and DeVita, VT: Central nervous system complications in patients with diffuse histiocytic and undifferentiated lymphoma: Leukemia revisited. Blood 47:3–10, 1976.

23. Burr, T and Morch, MM: Hereditary multiple exostoses with spinal cord compression. J Neurol Neurosurg Psychiat 46:96–97, 1983.

24. Cairncross, JG and Posner, JB: Neurological complications of malignant lymphoma. In Vinken, PJ and Bruyn, GW (eds): Handbook of Clinical Neurology, Vol 39. North-Holland Publishing, Amsterdam, 1980, pp. 27–62.

25. Calkins, AR, Olson, MA, and Ellis, JH: Impact of myelography on the radiotherapeutic management of malignant spinal cord compression. Neurosurgery 19:614–616, 1986.

26. Camacho, J, Arnalich, F, Anciones, B, Pena, JM, Gil, A, Barbado, FJ, Puig, JG, and Vazquez, JJ: The spectrum of neurologic manifestations in myeloma. Journal of Medicine 16:597–611, 1985.

27. Carmel, PW and Cramer, FJ: Cervical cord compression due to exostosis in a patient with hereditary multiple exostoses. J Neurosurg 28:500–503, 1968.

28. Cascino, TL, Kori, S, Krol, G, and Foley, KM: CT of the brachial plexus in patients with cancer. Neurology 33:1553–1557, 1983.

29. Chade, HO: Metastatic tumours of the spine and spinal cord. In Vinken, PJ and Bruyn, GW (eds): Handbook of Clinical Neurology, Vol 20. North-Holland Publishing, Amsterdam, 1976, pp 415–433.

30. Chapman, PH: Congenital intraspinal lipomas: Anatomical considerations and surgical treatment. Childs Brain 9:37–47, 1982.

31. Citrin, DL, Bessent, RG, and Greig, WR: A comparison of the sensitivity and accuracy of Tc-99 phosphate bone scan and skeletal radiograph in the diagnosis of bone metastases. Clin Radiol 28:107–117, 1977.

32. Cohen, DM, Dahlin, DC, and MacCarty, CS: Apparently solitary tumors of the vertebral column. Mayo Clin Proc 39: 509–528, 1964.

33. Cohen, MD, Klatte, EC, Baehner, R, et al: Magnetic resonance imaging of bone marrow disease in children. Radiology 151:715–718, 1984.

34. Coman, DR and DeLong, RP: The role of the vertebral venous system in the metastasis of cancer to the spinal column. Cancer 4:610–618, 1951.

35. Constans, JP, De Divitiis, E, Donzelli, R, et al: Spinal metastases with neurological manifestations: Review of 600 cases. J Neurosurg 59:111–118, 1983.

36. Covelli, HD, Zaloznik, AJ, and Shekitka, KM: Evaluation of bone pain in carcinoma of the lung: Role of the localized false-negative scan. JAMA 244:2625–2627, 1980.

37. Cushing, H: Some experimental and clinical observations concerning states of increased intracranial tension. Am J Med Sci 124:375–400, 1902.

38. Dahlin, DC: Giant cell tumor of the vertebrae above the sacrum: A review of 31 cases. Cancer 39:1350–1356, 1977.

39. Dahlin, DC: Bone Tumors: General Aspects and Data on 6,221 Cases, ed 3. Charles C Thomas, Springfield, Ill, 1978.

40. del Regato, JA: Pathways of metastatic spread of malignant tumors. Seminars in Oncology 4:33–38, 1977.

41. Destouet, JM, Kyriakos, M, and Gilula, LA: Fibrous histiocytoma (fibroxanthoma) of a cervical vertebra. Skeletal Radiol 5:241–246, 1980.

42. DiLorenzo, N, Spallone, A, Nolletti, A, et al; Giant cell tumors of the spine: A clinical study of six cases with emphasis on the radiological features. Neurosurgery 6:29–34, 1980.

43. Doron, Y, Gruszkiewicz, J, Gelli, B, and Peyser, E: Benign osteoblastoma of the vertebral column and skull. Surg Neurol 7:86–90, 1977.

44. Dowdle, JA, Winter, RB, and Dehner, LP: Post-

radiation osteosarcoma of the cervical spine in childhood. A case report. J Bone Joint Surg 59A:969–971, 1977.

45. Eaton, LM and Craig, WM: Tumor of the spinal cord: Sudden paralysis following lumbar puncture. Proceedings of the Staff Meetings of the Mayo Clinic 15:170–172, 1940.

46. Edelstyn, GA, Gillespie, PJ, and Grebbell, FS: The radiological demonstration of skeletal metastases. Clin Radiol 18:158–162, 1967.

47. Ehni, G and Love, JG: Intraspinal lipomas. Report of cases; review of the literature, and clinical and pathologic study. Acta Neurol Psychiat 53:1–28, 1945.

48. Elsberg, CA: Extradural spinal tumors: Primary, secondary, metastatic. Surg Gynecol Obstet 46:1–20, 1928.

49. Elsberg, CA: Surgical Diseases of the Spinal Cord, Membranes and Nerve Root. Paul B. Hoeber, New York, 1941.

50. Emery, JL and Lendon, RG: Lipomas of the cauda equina and other fatty tumors related to neurospinal dysraphism. Dev Med Child Neurol (Suppl 20)2:62–70, 1969.

51. Eriksson, B, Gunterberg, B, and Kindblom, L-G: Chordoma: A clinicopathologic review of 48 cases of chordoma. Cancer 56:182–187, 1985.

52. Esposito, PW, Crawford, AH, and Vogler, C; Solitary osteochondroma occurring on the transverse process of the lumbar spine: A case report. Spine 10:398–400, 1985.

53. Ewing, J: Neoplastic Diseases, ed 3. WB Saunders, Philadelphia, 1928.

54. Fidler, IJ and Hart, IR: Principles of cancer biology: Cancer metastasis. In DeVita, VT, Hellman, S, and Rosenberg, SA (eds): Cancer: Principles and Practice of Oncology. JB Lippincott, Philadelphia, 1985, pp 113–124.

55. Fielding, JW, Fietti, VG, Hughes, JE, and Gabrielian, JC: Primary osteogenic sarcoma of the cervical spine. J Bone Joint Surg 58A:892–894, 1976.

56. Findlay, GFG: Averse effects of the management of malignant spinal cord compression. J Neurol Neurosurg Psychiatry 47:761–768, 1984.

57. Friedlander, GE and Southwick, WO: Tumors of the spine. In Rothman, RH and Simeone, FA (eds): The Spine. WB Saunders, Philadelphia, 1982, pp 1022–1040.

58. Galasko, CSB: The anatomy and pathways of skeletal metastases. In Weiss, L and Gilbert, HA (eds): Bone Metastasis. GK Hall, Boston, 1981, pp. 49–63.

59. Galasko, CSB: The development of skeletal metastases. In Weiss, L and Gilbert, HA (eds): Bone Metastasis. GK Hall, Boston, 1981, pp 83–113.

60. Garfin, SR and Rothman, RH: Fibrous dysplasia (polyostotic): Case report. Skeletal Radiol 15:72–76, 1986.

61. George, WE Jr, Wilmot, M, Greenhouse, A, et al: Medical management of steroid induced epidural lipomatosis. N Engl J Med 308:316–319, 1983.

62. Ghormley, RK and Adson, AW: Hemangioma of

vertebrae. J Bone Joint Surg 39:887–895, 1941.

63. Gilbert, RW, Kim, JH, and Posner, JB: Epidural spinal cord compression from metastatic tumor: Diagnosis and treatment. Ann Neurol 3:40–51, 1978.

64. Giuffre, R: Spinal lipomas. In Vinken, PJ and Bruyn, GW (eds): Handbook of Clinical Neurology, Vol 20. North-Holland Publishing, Amsterdam, 1976, pp 389–414.

65. Gledhill, RF and McDonald, WI: Morphological characteristics of central demyelination and remyelination: A single-fiber study. Ann Neurol 1:552–560, 1977.

66. Graif, M and Steiner, RE: Contrast-enhanced magnetic resonance imaging of tumours of the central nervous system: A clinical review. Br J Radiol 59:865–873, 1986.

67. Gray, SW, Singhabhandu, B, Smith, RA, et al: Sacrococcygeal chordoma: Report of a case and review of the literature. Surgery 78:573–582, 1975.

68. Grem, JL, Burgess, J, and Trump, DL: Clinical features and natural history of intramedullary spinal cord metastasis. Cancer 56:2305–2314, 1985.

69. Grossman, CB and Post, MJD: The adult spine. In Gonzalez, CF, Grossman, CB and Masdeau, JC (eds): Head and Spine Imaging. John Wiley & Sons, New York, 1985, pp 781–858.

70. Gudesblatt, M, Cohen, JA, Gerber, O, and Sacher, M: Truncal ataxia presumably due to malignant spinal cord compression (letter). Ann Neurol 21:511–512, 1987.

71. Haddad, P, Thaell, JF, Kiely, JM, and others: Lymphoma of the spinal extradural space. Cancer 38:1862–1866, 1976.

72. Hagenau, C, Grosh, W, Currie, M, and Wiley, RG: Comparison of spinal magnetic resonance imaging and myelography in cancer patients. J Clin Oncol 5:1663–1669, 1987.

73. Harrington, KD: Anterior cord decompression and spinal stabilization for patients with metastatic lesions of the spine. J Neurosurg 61:107–117, 1984.

74. Harrison, KM, Muss, HB, Ball, M, et al: Spinal cord compression in breast cancer. Cancer 55:2839–2844, 1985.

75. Hashimoto, M: Pathology of bone marrow. Acta Haematol 27:193–216, 1962.

76. Hashizume, Y, Iljima, S, Kishimoto, H, and Hirano, A: Pencil-shaped softening of the spinal cord: Pathologic study in 12 cases. Acta Neuropathol (Berl) 61:219–224, 1983.

77. Heffez, DS, Sawaya, R, Udvarhelyi, GB, and Mann, R: Spinal epidural extramedullary hematopoiesis with cord compression in a patient with refractory sideroblastic anemia. J Neurosurg 57:399–406, 1982.

78. Henson, RA and Parsons, M: Ischaemic lesions of the spinal cord: An illustrated review. Q J Med 36:205–222, 1967.

79. Hermann, G and Hermann, P: Computerized tomography of the spine in metastatic disease. Mt Sinai J Med (NY) 49:400–405, 1982.

80. Hirsch, LF, Thanki, A, and Spector, HB: Primary spinal chondrosarcoma with eighteen-year follow up: Case report. Neurosurgery 14:747–749, 1984.

81. Hollis, PH, Malis, LI, and Zappulla, RA: Neurological deterioration after lumbar puncture below complete spinal subarachnoid block. J Neurosurg 24:253–256, 1986.

82. Hughes, JT: Venous infarction of the spinal cord. Neurology 21:794–800, 1971.

83. Huvos, AG: Bone Tumors: Diagnosis, Treatment, and Prognosis. WB Saunders, Philadelphia, 1979.

84. Ikeda, H, Ushio, Y, Hayakawa, T, et al: Edema and circulatory disturbance in the spinal cord compressed by epidural neoplasms in rabbits. J Neurosurg 52:203–209, 1980.

85. Jacobson, G, Poppel, MH, Shapiro, JH, et al: The vertebral pedicle sign. A roentgen finding to differentiate metastatic carcinoma from multiple myeloma. AJR 80:817–821, 1958.

86. Janin, Y, Epstein, JA, Carras, R, et al: Osteoid osteomas and osteoblastomas of the spine. Neurosurgery 8:31–38, 1981.

87. Johnson, M, Carey, F, and McMillan, RM: Alternative pathways of arachidonate metabolism: Prostaglandins, thromboxane and leukotrienes. Essays Biochem 19:41–141, 1983.

88. Jooma, R and Hayward, RD: Upward spinal coning: Impaction of occult spinal tumors following relief of hydrocephalus. J Neurol Neurosurg Psychiatry 47:386–390, 1984.

89. Jungreis, CA and Cohen, WA: Spinal cord compression induced by steroid therapy: CT findings. J Comput Assist Tomogr 11:245–247, 1987.

90. Kahn, E: The role of the dentate ligaments in spinal cord compression and the syndrome of lateral sclerosis. J Neurosurg 4:191–199, 1947.

91. Karian, JM, DeFillip, G, Buchheit, WA, et al: Vertebral osteochondroma causing spinal cord compression: Case report. Neurosurgery 14:483–484, 1984.

92. Karp, SJ and Ho, RTK: Gait ataxia as a presenting symptom of malignant epidural spinal cord compression. Postgrad Med J 62:745–747, 1986.

93. Kato, A, Ushio, Y, Hayakawa, T, et al: Circulatory disturbance of the spinal cord with epidural neoplasm in rats. J Neurosurg 63:260–265, 1985.

94. Kelly, JJ, Kyle, RA, Miles, JM, and Dyck, PJ: Osteosclerotic myeloma and peripheral neuropathy. Neurology 33:202–210, 1983.

95. Kelly, JJ, Kyle, RA, Miles, JM, O'Brien, PC, and Dyck, PJ: The spectrum of peripheral neuropathy in myeloma. Neurology 31:24–31, 1981.

96. Kikaldy-Willis, WH, Paine, KWE, Cauchoix, J, et al: Lumbar spinal stenosis. Clin Orthop 99:30–50, 1974.

97. Kirwan, EO'G, Hutton, PAN, Pozo, JL, et al: Osteoid osteoma and benign osteoblastoma of the spine. J Bone Joint Surg 66B:21–26, 1984.

98. Kori, SH, Foley, KM, and Posner, JB: Brachial plexus lesions in patients with cancer: 100 cases. Neurology 31:45–50, 1981.

99. Kori, SH, Krol, G, and Foley, KM: Computed tomographic evaluation of bone and soft tissue metastases. In Weiss, L and Gilbert, HA (eds): Bone Metastasis. GK Hall, Boston, 1983, pp 245–257.

100. Kornblith, PL, Walker, MD, and Cassady, JR: Neurologic Oncology. JB Lippincott, Philadelphia, 1987.

101. Kricun, ME: Red-yellow marrow conversion: Its effects on the location of some solitary bone lesions. Skeletal Radiol 14:10–19, 1985.

102. Kricun, ME: Conventional radiography. In Kricun, ME (ed): Imaging Modalities of Spinal Disorders. WB Saunders, Philadelphia, 1988, pp 59–288.

103. Kuban, DA, El-Mahdi, AM, Sigfred, SV, et al: Characteristics of spinal cord compression in adenocarcinoma of prostate. Urology 28:364–369, 1986.

104. Laredo, J-D, Reizine, D, Bard, M, and Merland, J-J: Vertebral hemangiomas: Radiological evaluation. Radiology 161:183–189, 1986.

105. Lee, SH, Coleman, PE, and Hahn, FJ: Magnetic resonance imaging of degenerative disk disease of the spine. Radiol Clin North Am 26:949–964, 1988.

106. Levitt, P, Ransohoff, J, and Spielholz, N: The differential diagnosis of tumors of the conus medullaris and cauda equina. In Vinken, PJ and Bruyn, GW (eds): Handbook of Clinical Neurology, Vol 19. North-Holland Publishing, Amsterdam, 1975, pp 77–90.

107. Lewis, DW, Packer, RJ, Raney, B, et al: Incidence, presentation, and outcome of spinal cord disease in children with systemic cancer. Pediatrics 78:438–442, 1986.

108. Lewkow, LM and Shah, I: Sickle cell anemia and epidural extramedullary hematopoiesis. Am J Med 76:748–751, 1984.

109. Lipson, SJ, Naheedy, MH, and Kaplan, MH: Spinal stenosis caused by epidural lipomatosis in Cushing's syndrome. N Engl J Med 302:36, 1980.

110. Liskow, A, Chang, CH, DeSanctis, P, et al: Epidural cord compression in association with genitourinary neoplasms. Cancer 58:949–954, 1986.

111. Liu, CN and Chambers, WW: An experimental study of the corticospinal system in the monkey (Macaca mulatta). The spinal pathways and preterminal distribution of degenerating fibers following discrete lesions of the pre- and postcentral gyri and bulbar pyramid. J Comp Neurol 123:257–284, 1964.

112. Llombart-Bosch, A, Blache, R, and Peydro-Olaya, A: Ultrastructural study of 28 cases of Ewing's sarcoma: Typical and atypical forms. Cancer 41:1362–1373, 1978.

113. Longeval, E, Holdebrand, J, and Vollont, GH: Early diagnosis of metastases in the epidu-

ral space. Acta Neurochir 31:177–184, 1975.

114. Ludwig, H, Kumpan, W, and Sinzinger, H: Radiography and bone scintigraphy in multiple myeloma: A comparative analysis. Br J Radiol 55:173–181, 1982.

115. MacGregor, RJ, Sharpless, SK, and Luttges, M: A pressure vessel model of nerve compression. J Neurol Sci 24:295–304, 1975.

116. Malawer, MM, Abelson, HT, and Suit, HD: Sarcomas of bone. In DeVita, VT, Hellman, S, and Rosenberg, SA (eds): Cancer: Principles and Practice of Oncology. JB Lippincott, Philadelphia, 1985, pp 1293–1342.

117. Maravilla, KR, Lesh, P, Weinreb, JC, et al: Magnetic resonance imaging of the lumbar spine with CT correlation. AJNR 6:381–385, 1985.

118. Masaryk, TJ, Modic, MT, Geisinger, MA, et al: Cervical myelopathy: A comparison of magnetic resonance and myelography. J Comput Tomogr 10:184–194, 1986.

119. McAlhany, HJ and Netsky, MG: Compression of the spinal cord by extramedullary neoplasms: A clinical and pathological study. J Neuropath Exp Neurol 14:276–287, 1955.

120. McNeil, BJ: Value of bone scanning in neoplastic disease. Semin Nucl Med 14:277–286, 1984.

121. Meyer, A: Herniation of the brain. Arch Neurol Psychiat 4:387–400, 1920.

122. Miller, F and Whitehall, R: Carcinoma of the breast metastatic to skeleton. Clin Orthop 184:121–127, 1984.

123. Mindell, ER: Current concept review: Chordoma. J Bone Joint Surg 63:501–505, 1981.

124. Modic, MT, Masaryk, T, and Paushter, D: Magnetic resonance imaging of the spine. Radiol Clin North Am 24:229–245, 1986.

125. Moore, EW, Freireich, EJ, Shaw, RK, and Thomas, LB: The central nervous system in acute leukemia. Arch Intern Med 105:451–467, 1960.

126. Mundy, GR, Raisz, LG, Cooper, RA, et al: Evidence for the secretion of an osteoclast stimulating factor in myeloma. N Engl J Med 291:1041–1046, 1974.

127. Nakashima, K and Shimamine, T: Anatomopathologic study of pencil-shaped softening of the spinal cord. Advances in Neurological Science (Tokyo) 18:153–166, 1974.

128. Neustaedter, M: Incidence of metastases to the nervous system. AMA Archives of Neurology and Psychiatry 51:423–425, 1944.

129. Norstrom, CW, Kernohan, JW, and Love, JG: One hundred primary caudal tumors. JAMA 178:1071–1077, 1961.

130. O'Rourke, T, George, CB, Redmond, J, et al: Spinal computed tomography and computed tomographic metrizamide myelography in the early diagnosis of metastatic disease. J Clin Oncol 4:576–583, 1986.

131. Ochoa, J, Fowler, TJ, and Gilliatt, RW: Anatomical changes in peripheral nerves com-

132. Ogihara, Y, Sekiguchi, K, and Tsuruta, T: Osteogenic sarcoma of the fourth thoracic vertebra: Long-term survival by chemotherapy only. Cancer 53:2615–2618, 1984.

133. Omojola, MF, Fox, AJ, and Vinuela, FV: Computed tomographic metrizamide myelography in the evaluation of thoracic spinal osteoblastoma. AJNR 3:670–673, 1982.

134. Onuigbo, WIB: Historical concepts of cancer metastasis with special reference to bone. In Weiss, L and Gilbert, HA (eds): Bone Metastasis. GK Hall, Boston, 1981, pp 1–10.

135. Oustwani, MB, Kurtides, ES, Christ, M, and Ciric, I: Spinal cord compression with paraplegia in myelofibrosis. Arch Neurol 37:389–390, 1980.

136. Paget, S: The distribution of secondary growths in cancer of the breast. Lancet 1:571–573, 1889.

137. Paillas, J-E, Alliez, B, and Pellet, W: Primary and secondary tumours of the spine. In Vinken, PJ and Bruyn, GW (eds): Handbook of Clinical Neurology, Vol 20. North-Holland Publishing, Amsterdam, 1976, pp 19–54.

138. Pancoast, HK: Superior pulmonary sulcus tumor: Tumor characterized by pain, Horner's syndrome, destruction of bone and atrophy of hand muscles. JAMA 99:1391–1396, 1932.

139. Patel, DV, Hammer, RA, Levin, B, et al: Primary osteogenic sarcoma of the spine. Skeletal Radiol 12:276–279, 1984.

140. Pedersen, AG, Bach, F, and Melgaard, B: Frequency, diagnosis, and prognosis of spinal cord compression in small cell bronchogenic carcinoma. Cancer 55:1818–1822, 1985.

141. Pizzo, PA, Miser, JS, Cassady, JR, and Filler, RM: Solid tumors of childhood. In DeVita, VT, Hellman, S, and Rosenberg, SA (eds): Cancer: Principles and Practice of Oncology. JB Lippincott, Philadelphia, 1985, pp 1511–1589.

142. Portenoy, R, Lipton, RB, and Foley, KM: Back pain in the cancer patient: An algorithm for the evaluation and management. Neurology 37:134–137, 1987.

143. Posner, JB: Neurologic complications of systemic cancer. DM 25:1–60, 1978.

144. Posner, JB: Spinal metastases: diagnosis and treatment. In Posner, JB (ed): Neuro-Oncology Course at Memorial Sloan-Kettering Cancer Center, New York, 1981, pp 42–54.

145. Posner, JB: Back pain and epidural spinal cord compression. Med Clin North Am 71:185–204, 1987.

146. Price, RA and Johnson, WW: The central nervous system in childhood leukemia: I. The arachnoid. Cancer 31:520–533, 1973.

147. Rasmussen, TB, Kernohan, JW, and Adson, AW: Pathologic classification, with surgical consideration, of intraspinal tumors. Ann Surg 111:513–530, 1940.

148. Rechtine, GR, Hassan, MO, and Bohlman, HH: Malignant fibrous histiocytoma of the cervi-

cal spine: Report of an unusual case and description of light and electron microscopy. Spine 9:824–830, 1984.

149. Redmond, J, Freidl, KE, Cornett, P, Stone, M, O'Rourke, T, and George, CB: Clinical usefulness of an algorithm for the early diagnosis of spinal metastatic disease. J Clin Oncol 6:154–157, 1988.

150. Resnick, D, Greenway, GD, Bardwick, PA, et al: Plasma-cell dyscrasia with polyneuropathy, organomegaly, endocrinopathy, M-protein and skin changes: The POEMS syndrome. Radiology 140:7–22, 1981.

151. Rich, TA, Schiller, A, Suit, HD, et al: Clinical and pathologic review of 48 cases of chordoma. Cancer 56:182–187, 1985.

152. Rodichok, LD, Harper, GR, Ruckdeschel, JC, et al: Early diagnosis of spinal epidural metastases. Am J Med 70: 1181–1188, 1981.

153. Rodichok, LD, Ruckdeschel, JC, Harper, GR, et al: Early detection and treatment of spinal epidural metastases: The role of myelography. Ann Neurol 20:696–702, 1986.

154. Rodriguez, M and Dinapoli, RP: Spinal cord compression: With special reference to metastatic epidural tumors. Mayo Clin Proc 55:442–448, 1980.

155. Rogalsky, RJ, Black, B, and Reed, MH: Orthopedic manifestations of leukemia in children. J Bone Joint Surg 68A:494–501, 1986.

156. Rubin, J, Lome, LG, and Presman, D: Neurological manifestation of metastatic prostatic carcinoma. J Urol 111:799–802, 1974.

157. Rudge, P, Ochoa, J, and Gilliatt, RW: Acute peripheral nerve compression in the baboon. J Neurol Sci 23:403–420, 1974.

158. Sanchez, RL, Llovet, J, Moreno, A, et al: Symptomatic eosinophilic granuloma of the spine: Report of two cases and review of the literature. Spine 7:1721–1726, 1984.

159. Sarpel, S, Sarpel, G, Yu, E, et al: Early diagnosis of spinal-epidural metastasis by magnetic resonance imaging. Cancer 59:1112–1116, 1987.

160. Schliack, H and Stille, D: Clinical symptomatology of intraspinal tumors. In Vinken, PJ and Bruyn, GW (eds): Handbook of Clinical Neurology, Vol 19. North-Holland Publishing, Amsterdam, 1975, pp 23–49.

161. Schnyder, P, Fankhauser, H, and Mansouri, B: Computed tomography in spinal hemangioma with cord compression: Report of two cases. Skeletal Radiol 15:372–375, 1986.

162. Schramm, J, Shigeno, T, and Brock, M: Clinical signs and evoked response alterations associated with chronic experimental cord compression. J Neurosurg 58:734–741, 1983.

163. Schwimer, DC, Bassett, LW, Mancuso, AA, et al: Giant-cell tumor of the cervicothoracic spine. AJR 136:63–67, 1981.

164. Selwood, RB: The radiologic approach to metastatic cancer of the brain and spine. Br J Radiol 45:647–651, 1972.

165. Shacked, I, Tadmor, R, Wolpin, G, et al: Aneurysmal bone cyst of a vertebral body with acute paraplegia. Paraplegia 19:294–298, 1981.

166. Shives, TC, Dahlin, DC, Sim, FH, et al: Osteosarcoma of the spine. Skeletal Radiol 68A:660–668, 1986.

167. Siegal, T, Siegal, TZ, Sandbank, U, et al: Experimental neoplastic spinal cord compression: Evoked potentials, edema, prostaglandins, and light and electron microscopy. Spine 12:440–448, 1987.

168. Siegal, T, Tiqva, P, and Siegal, T: Vertebral body resection for epidural compression by malignant tumors. J Bone Joint Surg 67A: 375–382, 1985.

169. Sinclair, DC, Fedindel, WH, and Falconer, MA: The intervertebral ligaments as a source of segmental pain. J Bone Joint Surg 30B: 515–521, 1948.

170. Smith, J: Radiation-induced sarcoma of bone: Clinical and radiographic findings in 43 patients irradiated for soft tissue neoplasms. Clin Radiol 33:205–221, 1982.

171. Smoker, WRK, Godersky, JC, Knutzon, RK, Keyes, WD, Norman, D, and Bergman, W: The role of MR imaging in evaluating metastatic spinal disease. AJR 149:1241–1248, 1987.

172. Stahl, SM, Ellinger, C, and Baringer, JR: Progressive myelopathy due to extramedullary hematopoiesis: Case report and review of the literature. Ann Neurol 5:485–489, 1979.

173. Stark, RJ, Henson, RA, and Evans, SJW: Spinal metastases: A retrospective survey from a general hospital. Brain 105:189–213, 1982.

174. Stein, RJ: "Silent" skeletal metastases in cancer. Am J Clin Path 13:34–41, 1943.

175. Stillwell, DL: The nerve supply of the vertebral column and its associated structures in the monkey. Anat Rec 125:139–169, 1956.

176. Stillwell, WT and Fielding, JW: Aneurysmal bone cyst of the cervicodorsal spine. Clin Orthop 187:144–146, 1984.

177. Subbaro, K and Jacobson, HG: Primary malignant neoplasms. Semin Roentgenol 14:44–57, 1979.

178. Sundarasen, N, Huvos, AG, Rosen, G, et al: Postradiation osteosarcoma of the spine following treatment of Hodgkin's disease. Spine 11:90–92, 1986.

179. Swee, RG, McLeod, RA, and Beabout, JW: Osteoid osteoma. Detection, diagnosis, and localization. Radiology 130:117–123, 1979.

180. Sze, G: Gadolinium-DTPA in spinal disease. Radiol Clin North Am 26:1009–1024, 1988.

181. Sze, G, Krol, G, Zimmerman, RD, and Deck, MDF: Gadolinium-DTPA: Malignant extradural spinal tumors. Radiology 167:217–223, 1988.

182. Tang, SG, Byfield, JE, Sharp, TR, Utley, JF, Quinol, L, and Seagren, SL: Prognostic factors in the management of metastatic

epidural spinal cord compression. J Neuro-Oncology 1:21–28, 1983.

183. Tarlov, IM: Spinal cord compression studies. III. Time limits for recovery after gradual compression in dogs. Arch Neurol 71:588–597, 1953.

184. Tarlov, IM and Klinger, H: Spinal cord compression studies. II. Time limits for recovery after acute compression in dogs. AMA Archives of Neurology and Psychiatry 71:271–290, 1954.

185. Tarlov, IM, Klinger, H, and Vitale, S: Spinal cord compression studies. I. Experimental techniques to produce acute and gradual compression. AMA Archives of Neurology and Psychiatry 70:813–819, 1953.

186. Thomas, JE and Miller, RH: Lipomatous tumors of the spinal canal. Mayo Clin Proc 48:393–400, 1973.

187. Thrupkaew, A, Henken, R, and Quinn, JL: False negative bone scans in disseminated metastatic diseases. Radiology 113:383–386, 1975.

188. Ushio, Y, Posner, R, Posner, JB, et al: Experimental spinal cord compression by epidural neoplasms. Neurology 27:422–429, 1977.

189. Vanel, D, Contesso, G, Couanet, D, et al: Computed tomography in the evaluation of 41 cases of Ewing's sarcoma. Skeletal Radiol 9:8–13, 1982.

190. Vanel, D, Hagey, C, Rebibo, G, et al: Study of three radio-induced malignant fibrohistiocytomas of bone. Skeletal Radiol 9:174–178, 1983.

190a. Vecht, CJ, Haaxma-Reichett, H, Van Putten, WLJ, et al: Initial bolus of conventional versus high-dose dexamethasone in metastative spinal cord compression. Neurology 39: 1255–1257, 1989.

191. von Einsiedel, HG and Stepan, R: Magnetic resonance imaging of spinal cord syndromes. Eur J Radiol 5:127–132, 1985.

192. Wasserstrom, WR, Glass, JP, and Posner, JB: Diagnosis and treatment of leptomeningeal

metastases from solid tumors: Experience with 90 patients. Cancer 49:759–772, 1982.

193. Waxman, SG: Demyelination in spinal cord injury. J Neurol Sci 91:1–14, 1989.

194. Weissman, DE: Glucocorticoid treatment for brain metastases and epidural spinal cord compression: A review. J Clin Oncol 6:543–551, 1988.

195. Weissman, DE, Gilberg, M, Wang, H, et al: The use of computed tomography of the spine to identify patients at high risk for epidural metastases. J Clin Oncol 3:1541–1544, 1985.

196. Whitehouse, GH and Griffiths, GJ: Roentgenologic aspects of spinal involvement by primary and metastatic Ewing's tumor. J Can Assoc Radiol 27:290–297, 1976.

197. Young, JM and Funk, FJ: Incidence of tumor metastasis to the lumbar spine: A comparative study of roentgenographic changes and gross lesions. J Bone Joint Surg 35A:55–64, 1953.

198. Young, RC, Howser, DM, Anderson, T, et al: Central nervous system complications of non-Hodgkin's lymphoma. Am J Med 66:435–443, 1979.

199. Young, RF, Post, EM, and King, GA: Treatment of spinal epidural metastases: Randomized prospective comparison of laminectomy and radiotherapy. J Neurosurg 53:741–748, 1980.

200. Yuill, GM: Leukemia: Neurological involvement. In Vinken, PJ and Bruyn, GW (eds): Handbook of Clinical Neurology, Vol 39. North-Holland Publishing, Amsterdam, 1980, pp 1–25.

201. Zimmer, WD, Bergquist, TH, McLeod, RA, et al: Bone tumors: Magnetic resonance imaging versus computed tomography. Radiology 155:709–718, 1985.

202. Zimmerman, RA and Bilaniuk, LT: Imaging of tumors of the spinal canal and cord. Radiol Clin North Am 26:965–1007, 1988.

Chapter 6

NEOPLASTIC CAUSES OF SPINAL CORD COMPRESSION: INTRADURAL-EXTRAMEDULLARY AND INTRAMEDULLARY TUMORS

Neoplastic disease involving the spine may be classified according to the location of the tumor: epidural, intradural-extramedullary, and intramedullary (Fig. 6–1). As reviewed in Chapter 5, the majority of epidural neoplasms are metastatic in nature. Intradural-extramedullary tumors and intramedullary neoplasms, on the other hand, are often primary tumors of the spine. Their clinical importance is demonstrated by the fact that among neurosurgical series, which tend to exclude cases of metastatic disease, intradural-extramedullary and intramedullary tumors comprise the majority of spinal tumors.[1, 134]

In some cases, a definite distinction cannot be made between an intramedullary and intradural-extramedullary location because the tumor may extend into both locations. In the present chapter, we group tumors according to their more frequent site.

INTRADURAL-EXTRAMEDULLARY TUMORS

Many intradural-extramedullary neoplasms are histologically benign tumors. If the condition is diagnosed and treated early in its course, neurological function will be preserved and the tumor usually cured. However, if not recognized and surgically resected, these benign neoplasms will generally cause progressive neurological dysfunction and ultimately loss of spinal cord and cauda equina function. (As in other chapters, the term spinal cord compression includes cauda equina compression unless otherwise indicated.) As reported in 1888, the first successful surgical removal of a spinal neoplasm was that of an intradural-extramedullary tumor.[57] Thus it has been recognized for more than a century that there is a great premium on the early diagnosis and treatment of these benign neoplasms.

In most neurosurgical series, intradural-extramedullary neoplasms are primarily represented by the histologically benign meningioma and nerve sheath tumor.[1, 78, 112, 117, 134] For example, in one review,[1] nerve sheath tumor and meningioma were responsible for 52 to 72 percent of all spinal tumors among the four neurosurgical series cited. However, as discussed in Chapter 5, these series are biased in that patients selected for inclusion in neurosurgical series are more apt to have benign localized growths than metastatic disease. In addition to meningiomas and nerve sheath tumors, vascular neoplasms and

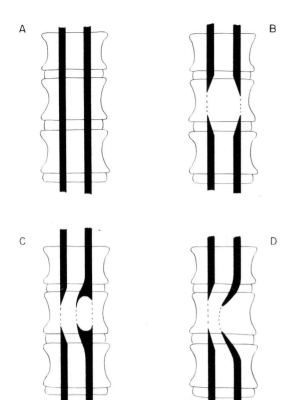

Figure 6–1. Masses within the spinal canal may be classified according to location relative to the spinal cord and dura mater. (A) Normal. (B) Intradural-intramedullary. (C) Intradural-extramedullary. (D) Epidural. (From Leeds, NE et al, [96] p 350, with permission.)

malformations, epidermoids, and lipomas also are found in this location.

Leptomeningeal metastases from systemic cancer or central nervous system malignancies also may present as intradural-extramedullary neoplasms. Among the cancer population, this complication is frequent. For example, it has been estimated that approximately 5 percent of patients dying of systemic cancer develop leptomeningeal metastases.[56, 119] Furthermore, in some forms of non-Hodgkin's lymphoma, the prevalence of leptomeningeal metastases may range from 5 to 29 percent.[17, 71, 97, 101, 109, 120] The clinical manifestations of leptomeningeal metastases are protean and the diagnostic evaluation is often different from that of other intradural-extramedullary tumors. For these reasons, leptomeningeal metastases are reviewed separately in Chapter 7.

Meningioma

Among primary neoplasms of the spine, meningiomas vie with nerve sheath tumors as the most common.[1, 117] For example, meningiomas were found to comprise approximately 25 percent of 1,322 primary spinal tumors in a large Mayo Clinic series.[134] In other series,[115, 122] meningiomas were responsible for 33 percent and 47 percent of primary spinal tumors.

Meningiomas may arise from any of the cell elements that form the meninges, but the majority stem from arachnoid cells.[129] Although over 90 percent of cases are purely intradural in location,[16, 99] the remaining 7 to 10 percent may be extradural.[16, 99, 112] In many of the latter cases, the tumor may extend from an intradural to an extradural location.[99] Extradural meningiomas are considered more biologically aggressive than those in the intradural location and have been associated with a shorter clinical history.[16, 99]

LOCATION

Meningiomas may occur at any level along the spinal axis, but the cervical and thoracic regions are more commonly involved than the lumbar region. In a review of the literature,[112] among a total of 705 reported spinal meningiomas, 17 percent of cases were in the cervical spine, 81 percent in the thoracic spine, and 2 percent in the lumbar region. In a more recent series from the Cleveland Clinic[99] consisting of 97 spinal meningiomas, the cervical spine was the site of involvement in 17 percent, the thoracic spine in 75 percent, and the lumbar spine in only 7 percent of cases.

Of further clinical importance, the Cleveland Clinic study examined the relationship between sex and location.[99] Among women, 83 percent of the meningiomas were found in the thoracic region. Men had a nearly equal frequency of cervical (41 percent) and thoracic (47 percent) lesions. The reason for this predilection to the thoracic spine in women is unknown.

The location of meningiomas in the transverse plane of the vertebral canal also has been studied. Most meningiomas at-

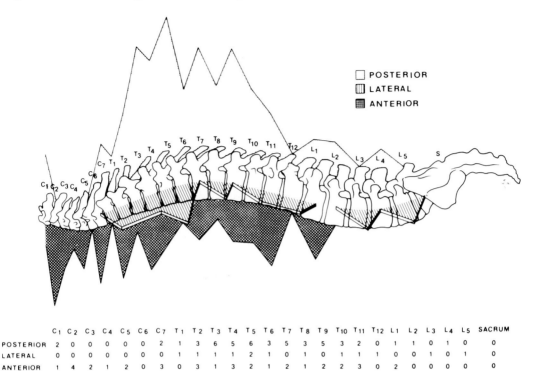

	C1	C2	C3	C4	C5	C6	C7	T1	T2	T3	T4	T5	T6	T7	T8	T9	T10	T11	T12	L1	L2	L3	L4	L5	SACRUM
POSTERIOR	2	0	0	0	0	0	2	1	3	6	5	6	3	5	3	5	3	2	0	1	1	0	1	0	0
LATERAL	0	0	0	0	0	0	0	1	1	1	1	2	1	0	1	0	1	1	1	0	0	1	0	1	0
ANTERIOR	1	4	2	1	2	0	3	0	3	1	3	2	1	2	1	2	2	3	0	2	0	0	0	0	0

Figure 6−2. The distribution of the location of meningiomas relative to the spinal cord along the spinal axis in a series of 97 cases. (From Levy, WJ et al, [99] with permission.)

tach to the insertion of the dentate ligament and may extend anteriorly or posteriorly.[112] Thus they may be classified as anterior or posterior to the dentate ligament or may be lateral. Among 179 cases from the literature,[112] 61 percent were posterior to the dentate ligament, 28 percent were anterior, and the remaining 11 percent extended too far to classify. The anterior-posterior location of meningiomas was analyzed with respect to their vertebral level of involvement in the Cleveland Clinic series[99] (Fig. 6−2). Eleven of 13 meningiomas above C7 were in the anterior location. Alternatively, at and below the level of C7, there were 22 anterior and 45 posterior meningiomas.

PATHOLOGY

In the Cleveland Clinic series,[99] 59 percent of meningiomas of the spinal canal were meningothelial and 21 percent were psammomatous. Another study[33] found psammomatous tumors to be the most frequent histology, followed by meningothelial tumors. Fibroblastic, angioblastic,

and transitional tumors were less frequent in both series.[33, 99] Although invasive tumors are occasionally seen, malignant meningiomas appear rare. Calcium may be seen histologically and occasionally radiographically as well.[16]

Occasionally multiple meningiomas are encountered. Multiple spinal meningiomas may occur in von Recklinghausen's disease, associated with other forms of neoplasia, or as an isolated event. Multiple spinal meningiomas rarely occur in isolation.[112] In one series,[33] multiple meningiomas occurred in 7 percent of 45 patients, but they were found in only 2 percent of the Cleveland Clinic series of 97 patients.[99]

CLINICAL FEATURES

Sex and Age

Spinal meningiomas are much more frequently encountered in women than in men. In many series, approximately 80 percent of cases occur in women.[33, 78, 99, 112] In Rand's series,[122] 95 percent of patients were women. As mentioned previously, in women the thoracic spine is disproportionately more frequently involved than the cervical spine, whereas in men, meningiomas are more evenly distributed in the cervical and thoracic region.[99, 112]

Spinal meningiomas have a peak incidence between the ages of 40 and 70 years. Symptoms develop under 30 years of age in only 10 percent of cases, and the tumor infrequently occurs under the age of 15.[78, 112] The average age of males (51 years) and females (54 years) was not significantly different in the series from the Cleveland Clinic.[99]

Duration of Symptoms. The duration of symptoms referable to spinal meningiomas is quite variable. Occasional patients have abrupt onset of symptoms, often precipitated by trauma.[99] More frequently, symptoms begin insidiously and progress over several months. In one series,[33] 75 percent of patients had symptoms greater than 6 months, whereas in the Cleveland Clinic series[99] the average duration was 23 months prior to diagnosis; in one case, the symptoms were present for 20 years. Occasionally the symptoms may appear to have remissions and exacerbations and thus suggest demyelinating disease.[78]

Symptoms and Signs

Spinal meningiomas may represent a difficult diagnostic problem; in a recent series,[99] one third of patients had been previously misdiagnosed. As in most other types of spinal tumor, pain is the most common presenting complaint.[99] Oddsson[115] reported the occurrence of pain in 85 percent of cases; in the Cleveland Clinic series,[99] it was a presenting complaint in 72 percent. Pain may be axial or radicular in nature; Nittner[112] reported radicular pain as a major complaint in 50 percent of cases.

Sensory disturbances in the form of paresthesias, cold and hot sensations, and numbness have been reported in approximately one third of cases at the time of diagnosis.[99, 112] Sensory disturbances may be of a radicular nature or may be due to ascending tract dysfunction. The sensory disturbances may ascend as the more peripheral spinothalamic fibers are compressed before central fibers.

Dissociated sensory disturbances and the Brown-Séquard syndrome are infrequent.[78, 99, 112] Sensory disturbances including a sensory level were found in over three quarters of patients in a recent series.[99]

Subjective motor weakness is frequently seen in patients with spinal meningiomas and is usually bilateral. Hemiparesis is uncommon but may occur with meningiomas in the region of the craniocervical junction.[112] Usually motor symptoms begin ipsilateral to the side of the tumor but occasionally they may begin contralaterally, with progression to include both sides;[78] this clinical presentation may be due to contrecoup compression.[108] Although weakness was a subjective complaint in 66 percent of cases in the Cleveland Clinic series,[99] objective signs of paresis and reflex changes were present in approximately 80 percent of patients at diagnosis.

Sphincter dysfunction is a less frequent, albeit important, presenting complaint.[33, 99] No patient in one series[33] presented with sphincter disturbance; 40 percent of the patients in the Cleveland Clinic series complained of bowel or bladder disturbance, while only 15 percent had objective evidence of sphincter dysfunction.

LABORATORY AND DIAGNOSTIC IMAGING STUDIES

Diagnostic Imaging Studies

Abnormalities on plain spine radiographs suggesting tumor occur in only approximately 10 percent of patients with spinal meningiomas.[5, 16, 112] These abnormalities include widening of the interpedicular distance at the level of the tumor, bony erosion, and calcification. Enlargement of an intervertebral foramen may occur if the tumor grows in an hourglass shape, although this finding is more frequently seen with nerve sheath tumors.[112] Plain films are not usually helpful in distinguishing intradural meningiomas from extradural meningiomas because both infrequently may cause bony erosion.[16, 112] An increase in the interpedicular distance is not specific for meningiomas because nerve sheath tumors, intramedullary tumors, and other intraspinal masses may similarly widen the spinal canal. The relatively nonspecific findings of kyphosis and scoliosis may be seen in up to one third of patients.[112]

Although calcification of spinal meningiomas is not often seen on plain films, CT scanning occasionally will show calcification of the tumor and hyperostosis of adjacent bones.[94] CT scanning following intravenous contrast administration may demonstrate dense enhancement of the tumor.[62] Extradural extension of meningiomas also may be seen on CT scanning.

Intradural-extramedullary neoplasms have a rather characteristic pattern on

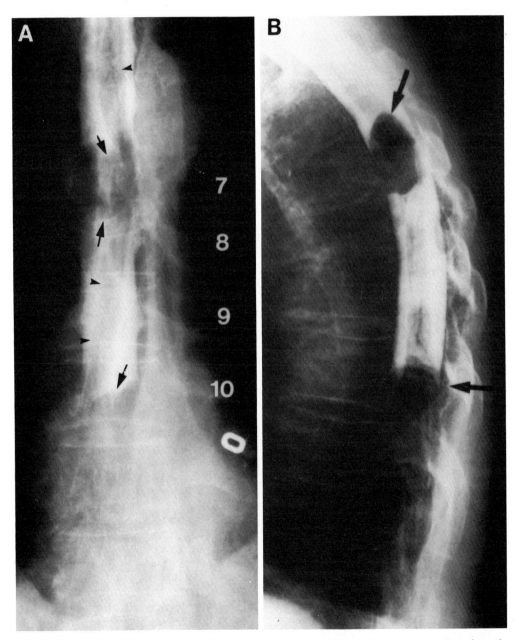

Figure 6—3. The myelographic appearance of two meningiomas. (A) The meningioma (arrows) on the right side of the vertebral canal at T7 displaces the spinal cord (arrowhead) to the left. The meningioma (arrow) on the left at T10 displaces the cord (arrowheads) to the right. (B) This lateral view shows the two meningiomas (arrows) at T7 and T10. (Courtesy of Dr. Helmuth Gehbauer.)

myelography (Fig. 6–3). The spinal cord is displaced away from the mass and the subarachnoid space above and below the tumor is enlarged. In epidural and intramedullary neoplasms, the subarachnoid space is narrowed adjacent to the tumor. Differentiation of an intradural nerve sheath tumor from a meningioma based on myelography alone may be difficult.[5] Postmyelographic CT scanning may better define the anatomical relationship between the spinal cord and the meningioma.

Although noncontrast MRI has been found less sensitive in the diagnosis of intradural-extramedullary tumors than of epidural tumors, it has been used in the localization of spinal meningiomas.[90, 106] The spinal cord may appear displaced with enlargement of the subarachnoid space, as seen by myelography. The transverse anatomical relationship of the meningioma to the spinal cord also may be demonstrated (Fig. 6–4). The administration of contrast agents with MRI has been shown to improve its sensitivity for intradural-extramedullary spinal tumors.[58, 137, 138] The full role of MRI in evaluating patients with spinal meningiomas is yet to be determined.

Cerebrospinal Fluid. The CSF usually shows the nonspecific findings of elevated protein. Nittner's review[112] reported that the lumbar CSF protein was elevated in 76 to 90 percent of cases. There may be a slight degree of pleocytosis but there is albumino-cytologic dissociation in 85 percent of cases.[112]

THERAPY

Surgery is the treatment of choice for spinal cord compression from meningioma. Complete removal with the attached dura usually leads to no recurrence, but incomplete removal of spinal meningiomas may have an excellent prognosis with no recurrence or recurrence delayed by several years.[99] Epidural meningiomas and calcified meningiomas, however, often do not have such an excellent prognosis.[99]

As with other slow growing mass lesions, an excellent recovery often occurs following surgery even if there is a severe neurological deficit at the time of diagnosis. In the Cleveland Clinic series,[99] 85 percent of patients had a favorable result with surgical removal. Thus patients with spinal meningioma are usually restored to ambulation unless they are paraplegic preoperatively; even some paraplegic patients become ambulatory in long-term follow-up.

Nerve Sheath Tumors

Nerve sheath tumors arise from cells that ensheathe the axons of the peripheral nervous system. Such tumors may occur on spinal nerve roots and thereby cause spinal cord compression. The cells surrounding axons include Schwann cells, fibroblasts, and perineurial fibroblasts.[129] There has been considerable debate among pathologists as to the cell of origin of nerve sheath tumors, which has resulted in the use of several terms to describe such tumors, including schwannoma, neurofibroma, neurinoma, perineurofibroblastoma, and neurilemoma.[129]

Rubinstein[129] has classified nerve sheath tumors as schwannomas and neurofibromas. Schwannomas are typically solitary tumors composed of Schwann cells, and are far more frequently found on sensory nerve roots than on motor roots. When a manifestation of von Recklinghausen's neurofibromatosis, schwannomas may be multiple and associated with gliomas, meningiomas, and other neoplasms. Alternatively, neurofibromas arise from both Schwann cells and fibroblasts. In the setting of von Recklinghausen's neurofibromatosis, they are often multiple and may undergo malignant change, developing into a neurofibrosarcoma.[129] Despite these pathological and biological differences, clinical series of spinal tumors[1, 16, 52, 112, 117, 122] often do not distinguish between schwannomas and neurofibromas when discussing nerve sheath tumors. Therefore, in this text, "nerve sheath tumor" refers to both schwannomas and neurofibromas unless otherwise stated. It is to be recognized, however, that a neurofibroma (or, less commonly, a schwannoma) in the setting of von Recklinghausen's disease has very different implications for clinical evaluation and management than does a solitary schwannoma.

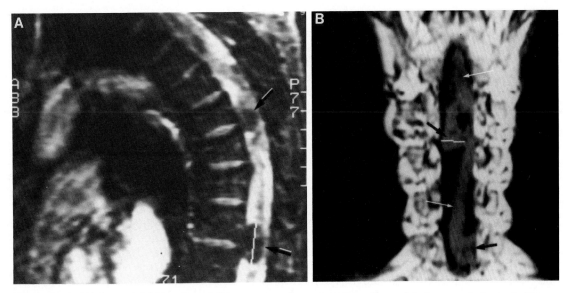

Figure 6—4. (A) A sagittal MR image of the same two thoracic meningiomas (black arrows) shown in Figure 6—3. (B) A coronal MR image of the meningiomas (black arrows) displacing cord (white arrows). (Courtesy of Dr. Helmuth Gehbauer.)

FREQUENCY AND LOCATION

Nerve sheath tumors have been considered to be among the most common primary spinal tumors. In one extensive series of spinal tumors,[134] they were the most common, constituting 29 percent of all cases. In a review of 4,885 histologically proven spinal tumors culled from the literature,[112] nerve sheath tumors accounted for 23 percent and meningiomas for 22 percent.

Nerve sheath tumors are more evenly distributed along the spinal axis than meningiomas. Among three series[12, 52, 124] with a total of 322 cases, 26 percent were cervical, 41 percent were thoracic, 31 percent were lumbar, and 2 percent were sacral. In the setting of von Recklinghausen's disease, multiple spinal nerve sheath tumors, which may be associated with other neoplasms and pigmented skin lesions, may be frequently encountered.[112]

In relation to the meninges, nerve sheath tumors may be totally intradural, completely extradural or extend both intradurally and extradurally. Among 163 cases,[124] 67 percent were intradural, 16.5 percent were intradural and extradural, and 16.5 percent were extradural. Intradural tumors are nearly always juxtamedullary; rarely, they may be intramedullary.[112, 134]

Many nerve sheath tumors form dumbbell-shaped masses that extend through the intervertebral foramen. In one series,[52] 19 percent of nerve sheath tumors were dumbbell shaped. The extraspinal extension of such tumors can be massive and may, at times, be seen on chest radiograph or palpated on physical examination of the neck or abdomen. Although in the transverse plane they may occur in any anatomical position in relation to the spinal cord, more tumors are located in the posterior and lateral locations than anteriorly.[52]

CLINICAL FEATURES

Sex and Age. Nerve sheath tumors affect both sexes equally.[12, 52, 112] They may occur in individuals ranging from childhood to the very elderly, but most are found in the middle-age years. Although one author reported that significant numbers were found between ages 11 and 70, more than 60 percent of cases were encountered from age 31 through 60.[52] In his series, the average age was 43.5 years (compared with 53 years as the average age of patients with spinal meningiomas[99]).

Symptoms and Signs

In an extensive literature review,[112] pain was the initial symptom in 74 percent of cases. The pain may be axial, radicular, and/or remote (referred lower in the spine or legs in cases of cervical or thoracic neoplasms). It is often exacerbated by Valsalva maneuvers, coughing, sneezing, and recumbency.[41, 124] When symptoms and signs were analyzed according to level of spinal involvement, pain was a presenting complaint in 49 percent of cervical, 68 percent of thoracic, and 91 percent of lumbosacral tumors.[52]

Motor and sensory symptoms and signs are occasional presenting complaints but are frequently found at the time of diagnosis. These neurological disturbances may be of radicular and/or funicular origin. In one series,[112] the presenting complaint was motility disturbance in 15 percent and sensory abnormalities in 9 percent of cases. However, by the time of diagnosis, motor disturbances were present in 85 percent of cases and sensory abnormalities in 70 percent. A similarly high incidence of motor and sensory symptoms and signs has been found at the time of diagnosis in other series.[52]

Sphincter disturbance and sexual dysfunction form the fourth principal symptom. Such disturbances were found to be the presenting complaint in only 2.5 percent of Nittner's published experience,[112] but at the time of diagnosis, approximately 54 percent of patients had such vegetative disturbances.

Out of the four principal clinical features (pain, motor disorder, sensory abnormalities, and sphincter dysfunction) most patients are found to have a combination of at least two of them at diagnosis. For example, more than 97 percent of cases cited by Nittner[112] had two abnormalities and 93 percent had three such clinical abnormalities at diagnosis; 65 percent had all four. A similar experience was reported by another author.[52]

The duration of symptoms prior to diagnosis of a spinal nerve sheath tumor averages 1 to 4 years. The shortest average course or symptoms is seen in cervical lesions, and the longest among lumbar neoplasms.[52] Occasionally, the duration of symptoms may be only weeks in length, and in exceptional cases, it may persist for decades. The longest reported course was over 28 years.[112]

LABORATORY AND DIAGNOSTIC IMAGING STUDIES

Diagnostic Imaging Studies

As in many clinical series, neurofibromas and schwannomas are often grouped together as nerve sheath tumors in the radiological literature.[94, 106] Abnormalities on plain radiographs are often encountered in contradistinction to the experience with spinal meningiomas. In three series, the incidence of abnormalities on plain film in cases of spinal nerve sheath tumors ranged from 43 percent to 52 percent.[12, 16, 52] Those most commonly encountered include widening of the intervertebral foramen, erosion of the pedicle or vertebral body, and widening of the interpedicular distance. In the case of large extradural thoracic tumors, the mass may be evident on chest radiograph. Spinal nerve sheath tumors associated with normal plain films were more likely to be complete intradural, whereas those with extension into the extradural space are characteristically associated with plain film abnormalities and are often of the dumbbell variety.[16]

Prior to the advent of CT and MRI, myelography was essential for the diagnosis of most cases of spinal nerve sheath tumor. In cases of intradural tumor, a mass is usually seen displacing the cord with widened subarachnoid space just above and below the lesion. Although such neoplasms arise from nerve sheath elements, they occasionally demonstrate no anatomical contact with a nerve root on myelography.[12] Although criteria have been proposed to distinguish nerve sheath tumors from meningiomas on myelography, they may be difficult to differentiate.[16, 52, 112] As in the case of any intraspinal neoplasm, occasionally lumbar puncture below a compressing lesion may be associated with neurological deterioration, and appropriate treatment must be undertaken emergently to prevent permanent neurological damage.[74]

CT scanning is a sensitive technique for evaluating nerve sheath tumors if the spinal segment affected by the tumor is imaged.[118] The noncontrast CT scan often shows a mass slightly more dense than spinal cord.[26] With intravenous contrast, uniform tumor enhancement is typical.[25, 26, 68] The relationship of the tumor to the spinal cord may be identified by CT scanning following the intrathecal administration of contrast material.[140]

MRI has recently been shown to demonstrate spinal nerve sheath tumors.[5, 106] Its full utility has yet to be elucidated, but it is likely to become an important technique.[137, 138] The value of paramagnetic contrast agents also has been reported.[131]

Cerebrospinal Fluid

The cerebrospinal fluid in cases of spinal nerve sheath tumor usually shows no signs of pleocytosis but typically reveals an increase in protein. Of 98 CSF analyses,[52] only 12 patients had an elevated CSF white cell count. Some of the CSF analyses were blood-stained. In patients with CSF pleocytosis, the tumors were intradural.

The CSF protein content was elevated in 82 percent (82/98) of cases and was higher in cases of intradural tumor than when the tumor was totally extradural. As expected, it appeared also to be higher in those with higher grade blocks than in those with smaller lesions.

THERAPY

Surgery is the optimal therapy of spinal cord compression resulting from nerve sheath tumors. Resection often leads to an excellent recovery of neurological function even if the patient has signs of severe neurological dysfunction at the time of diagnosis, apparently due to the ability of the spinal cord to adapt to compression from these slow-growing lesions.

With total removal of these lesions, recurrence is rare. However, because these tumors are often intimately attached to nerve roots, complete resection may not be possible without sacrificing the root.[93] In the setting of neurofibromatosis, multiple nerve sheath tumors may be present that may not be surgically resectable.

Case Illustration

A 30-year-old businessman presented with right-sided weakness and gait difficulty. He had noted progressive weakness of the right arm over a period of 18 months. In addition, he observed weakness and stiffness of the right and, more recently, the left lower extremities. His disability, however, did not prevent him from engaging in athletics. One week before neurological evaluation, he developed transient right hemiplegia after being struck on the head with a soccer ball. On neurological examination, there were no café au lait spots. Cranial nerves and funduscopic examinations were normal. He had disuse atrophy of the right upper extremity associated with spastic weakness. There was spastic weakness of both lower extremities, with the right more affected than the left. The left upper extremity motor examination was normal. Sensory examination was unremarkable. Jaw jerk was normal, deep tendon reflexes were increased throughout, and plantar responses were flexor bilaterally. Gait was slightly ataxic.

The clinical impression was a high cervical or foramen magnum neoplasm. An MRI was performed (Fig. 6–5). Severe spinal cord compression from an extra-axial mass was seen to the left of and anterior to the spinal cord. The patient underwent complete resection of the C1–2 mass, which was found to be a neurofibroma. He had a complete return of neurological function several months after the operation.

Comment. This case illustrates several important clinical points. This benign tumor in the region of the foramen magnum caused weakness to progress from the ipsilateral upper extremity to the ipsilateral leg and then to the contralateral leg, as often seen in foramen magnum mass lesions (See Chapter 2). The symptoms were slowly progressive but the patient markedly deteriorated following incidental trauma, as is sometimes seen with spinal cord compression. Furthermore, despite severe spinal cord compression as seen on the MRI, the patient had a paucity of neurological signs consistent with the long evolution of spinal cord compression. Finally, the patient had an excellent outcome following surgical removal at a time when he still had good neurological function.

Vascular Malformations and Tumors

The classification and nomenclature of vascular tumors and malformations have

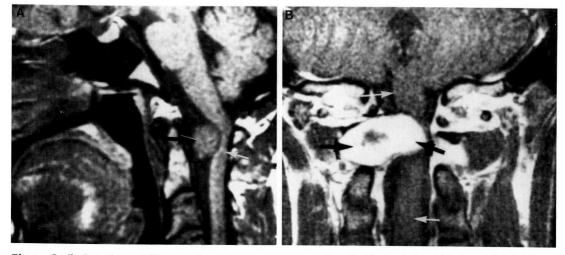

Figure 6−5. Spinal neurofibroma at C1−2 level. (A) This nonenhanced sagittal MRI demonstrates the neurofibroma (black arrow) anterior and compressing the spinal cord (white arrow). (B) This gadolinium-enhanced coronal MRI demonstrates the tumor (black arrow) lateral to the spinal cord (white arrows). (Courtesy of Dr. Joseph Piepmeier.)

represented a great problem for the pathologist and clinician from the time these lesions were first described.[18] Several pathological classifications have been proposed for vascular malformations and vascular tumors (Table 6−1). Although vascular malformations are hamartomas, where as the vascular tumors (hemangioblastomas and hemangiopericytomas) are true neoplasms, all are capable of growth and compression of neighboring tissue (Fig. 6−6). They may be very difficult to differentiate clinically because both may present as enlarging mass lesions,

may hemorrhage, or may cause ischemic neurological symptoms. Finally, they may be difficult to separate clinically because in 48 percent of spinal hemangioblastomas,[14, 80] an associated meningeal varicosity or arteriovenous malformation (AVM) is found.

FREQUENCY

The frequency of vascular malformations and neoplasms of the spine is difficult to ascertain with certainty because the malformations may be clinically silent. Collectively, vascular malformations and neoplasms have been estimated to account for approximately 5 to 10 percent of space-occupying lesions of the spine.[80, 121] Vascular malformations are much more frequent than vascular tumors of the spine.[80] Arteriovenous malformation is the most common histological type represented.[80]

A review of spinal hemangioblastomas[14, 42, 134] reported that they represent approximately 2 percent of all spinal tumors, 3 percent of intramedullary neoplasms, 2 percent of extramedullary-intradural tumors, and 4 percent of extradural tumors. It should be recognized that these surgical series tend to exclude metastatic neoplasms.

Table 6−1 CLASSIFICATION OF SPINAL VASCULAR MALFORMATIONS AND VASCULAR TUMORS*

Vascular malformations
    Capillary telangiectasia
    Cavernous angioma
    Arteriovenous malformation
        Dural
        Intradural
    Venous malformation
Vascular tumors
    Capillary hemangioblastoma
Vascular tumors of the meninges
    Hemangioblastoma
    Hemangiopericytoma

*Adapted from classification proposed by Rubinstein.[129]

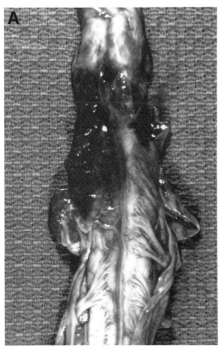

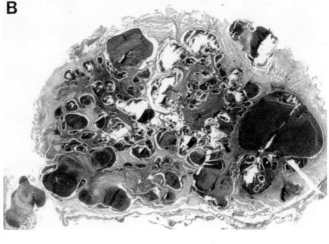

Figure 6-6. A cavernous angioma involving the spinal cord. (A) Surface of the cord. (B) Axial section of the cord. (Courtesy of Dr. L. Forno.)

VASCULAR MALFORMATIONS

Spinal AVMs have been classified arteriographically as dural and intradural.[88] Dural AV fistulas are defined as a vascular nidus in the dura that is supplied by a dural branch of an intercostal artery or lumbar artery and that drains into spinal veins via an AV shunt. Intradural AVMs are defined as lesions in which the vascular nidus is in the spinal cord or pia and which are supplied by medullary arteries. Intradural AVMs may be further classified as intramedullary AVMs (juvenile and glomus types) and direct AV fistulas, which may be extramedullary or intramedullary. Dural AV fistulas are considered more common than intradural AVMs.[128]

The etiology of AVMs is controversial. It has been suggested that dural AVMs may be acquired and intramedullary AVMs congenital in origin.[128]

The pathogenetic explanations for neurological dysfunction in spinal AVMs include venous hypertension, arterial steal, and subarachnoid hemorrhage. In the case of dural AVMs, it is suggested that the valveless venous system allows high venous pressure from the AV fistula to be transmitted to the spinal veins, causing congestive myelopathy. Arterial steal and subarachnoid hemorrhage are not considered likely explanations for the pathogenesis of neurological dysfunction in dural AVMs. However, with indradural AVMs, all three mechanisms are considered likely explanations.[128]

Location. Although spinal vascular malformations may be found at any level of the spinal axis, they are more frequently encountered in the caudal spine than at rostral levels. One pathological review[80] reported the following frequencies: cervical, 10 to 15 percent; cervicothoracic and upper thoracic, 20 to 30 percent; lower thoracic, lumbar, and lumbosacral, 50 to 70 percent. Alternatively, the thoracic spine is the most frequently involved level for hemangioblastomas. Intradural AVMs have been found to be more uniformly distributed along the spinal axis than dural AVMs, which show a predilection for the low thoracic and lumbar areas.[128] Another review[14] of 85 hemangioblastomas found the following levels of involve-

Table 6−2 HISTOLOGICALLY DEMONSTRATED CASES OF SPINAL CORD HEMANGIOBLASTOMA*

	No. (%) of Patients	
Sex		
Male	42	(52.5)
Female	38	(47.5)
No. of Hemangioblastomas		
Single	59	(78.7)
Multiple	16	(21.3)
Position of Hemangioblastoma		
Intramedullary	45	(60.0)
Extramedullary-intradural	16	(21.3)
Intramedullary and extramedullary	8	(10.7)
Extradural	6	(8.0)
Level of Hemangioblastomas		
Cervical	30	(37.5)
Cervicothoracic	3	(3.7)
Thoracic	38	(47.5)
Lumbar	13	(16.2)
Lumbosacral	3	(3.7)
Sacral	2	(2.5)
Cauda eqina	7	(8.7)
Syringomyelia		
Present	34	(43.0)
Absent	45	(57.0)
Meningeal Varices		
Present	34	(47.9)
Absent	37	(52.1)
Lindau disease	26	(32.5)
Coincident Hemangioblastomas		
Any location	26	(32.5)
Medulla	18	(22.5)
Cerebellum	15	(18.7)
Retina	14	(17.5)
Supratentorial area	3	(3.7)
Visceral Lesions of Lindau Disease	18	(22.5)
Family History of Hemangio-blastoma		
Present	11	(23.9)
Absent	35	(76.1)

*From Browne, TR, et al, [14] p 439, with permission.

ment: cervical, 38 percent; thoracic, 48 percent; and lumbar, 16 percent (Table 6−2).

Clinical Features

Spinal vascular malformations occur more commonly in men than in women. Over two thirds of patients in most series are men.[36, 121, 128] Vascular malformations may present at any age but the average age of onset of symptoms and diagnosis is 30 to 40 years.[36, 121] The average age of patients presenting with dural AVMs is greater than that of patients with intradural AVMs. In one series,[128] the average age of patients with dural AV fistulas was 49 years (range: 22 to 72); whereas the average age of those with intradural AVMs was 27 (range: 4 to 58), with 65 percent of patients under 25 years of age.

The symptoms caused by vascular malformations are similar to those of other space-occupying lesions of the spine— pain, motor deficit, sensory loss, and sphincter disturbance (Table 6−3). Pain may be local, funicular, and/or radicular in nature. When due to hematomyelia or subarachnoid hemorrhage, it is meningeal, radicular, or funicular in origin.

As shown in Table 6−3, paresis was the most common presenting symptom in dural AVMs, whereas hemorrhage, common in intradural AVMs, was not seen in dural fistulas. Weakness is usually manifested as spastic paraparesis; loss of pain and temperature is the most common sensory complaint. When a sensory level is present, it often corresponds to the level of the vascular nidus. Spinal bruits usually indicate high-flow intradural lesions. Some authors have found that intermittent neurogenic claudication may be the presenting complaint of spinal arteriovenous malformations.[82, 144, 149] Madsen and Heros[102] review the pathogenesis of neuro-

Table 6−3 INITIAL SYMPTOMS AND SYMPTOMS AT DIAGNOSIS OF SPINAL AVM*†

Symptom	Initial Symptoms		Symptoms at Diagnosis‡	
	Dural AVMs	Intradural AVMs	Dural AVMs	Intradural AVMs
Back pain	2	8	11	10
Root pain	4	2	7	20
Paresis	12	16	21	50
Sensory change	5	5	18	40
Impotence	1	2	14	23
Hemorrhage	0	17	0	28
Bowel disturbance	1	1	17	24
Bladder dysfunction	2	3	22	40
Total cases	27	54	27	54

*From Rosenblum, B, et al, [128] p 798, with permission.

†AVM = arteriovenous malformation.

‡The values listed indicate the number of patients with those symptoms when the diagnosis of spinal AVM was established. Most patients had several of the symptoms.

genic claudication and postulate a mechanism that could explain some of the neurological manifestations of spinal AVMs.

The temporal profile of clinical presentation of vascular malformations varies widely, with the onset of symptoms classified as apoplectiform (due to thrombosis or hemorrhage), remitting, or progressive. When remitting or progressive, the duration of symptoms may date back over several years or even decades.[121] Although some authors have found an apoplectiform onset unusual,[15, 36] one report[121] listed the frequency of the temporal course of symptoms and signs as follows: apoplectiform, 30 to 50 percent; remittent, 20 to 40 percent; and progressive, 30 percent. When the symptoms and signs are fluctuating, an erroneous diagnosis of multiple sclerosis may be considered. Precipitating factors found to play a role in the onset of spinal AVMs in occasional patients include physical exertion, trauma, and pregnancy.[36, 121, 128]

Spinal vascular malformations may be associated with AVMs elsewhere and with other physical findings. In the Klippel-Trenaunay-Weber syndrome, an accompanying cutaneous angioma is associated with a spinal vascular malformation. Other dysplasias associated with spinal angiomas have been reported.[80] Cerebral and spinal aneurysms may also be seen.[128] Furthermore, a vertebral angioma may be seen on radiological study of the spine.[121]

The Foix-Alajouanine syndrome[48, 59] has been considered an example of progressive myelopathy secondary to an intradural vascular malformation. This syndrome is characterized by a subacute or chronic progressive course leading over a period of months to paraplegia. Spasticity is said to occur early, but evolves into a flaccid, areflexic paraplegia, associated with sensory loss and impairment of sphincter function. Pathologically, in most cases there is evidence for a diffuse AVM of the spinal cord, with multiple small infarcts and occasional hemorrhagic lesions. The end stage is marked by severe necrosis of gray and white matter, most marked in lumbosacral segments but extending upwards in some cases to thoracic levels. Blood vessels show thickened, cellular, and fibrotic walls. The pathogenesis of the disorder is uncertain but a spinal phlebothrombosis has been suggested as an etiologic possibility.[15, 75, 103]

Laboratory and Diagnostic Imaging Studies. The CSF may show elevated protein and evidence of recent bleeding, but a normal CSF profile does not exclude a spinal angioma.[36, 121] Myelography is reported to be abnormal in over 90 percent of cases of spinal vascular malformations and is specific for the diagnosis in nearly two thirds.[36] Spinal angiography has also been found to be specific and critical for identifying the feeding vessels and draining veins as well as the vascular nidus.[22, 36] CT scanning is often abnormal but the enhancement seen may be difficult to differentiate from neoplasms. Dynamic CT imaging, in which CT images are obtained successively every few seconds, may help distinguish between a neoplasm and a vascular malformation.[68] MRI is likely to be helpful in the evaluation of these lesions.[35, 107]

Therapy. The management of spinal AVMs is controversial and difficult. With the advent of microsurgical techniques and spinal angiography, the surgical treatment has improved. Thus a dural AVM with a single feeding vessel may respond to ligation.[110] For intradural AVMs, endovascular embolization has become an alternative to surgery or has been performed preoperatively.[22] However, both surgery and embolization carry the significant risk of worsening the neurological deficit. Thus in some cases, no intervention is recommended. Patients should be managed by physicians with a large experience with these rare and often devastating lesions.[22, 110, 128]

SPINAL VASCULAR NEOPLASMS

Clinical Features of Spinal Hemangioblastomas

Some of the clinical features of spinal cord hemangioblastomas, which affect both sexes equally, are shown in Table 6–2.[14] The average age of patients with spinal hemangioblastomas is approximately 30 years. In the spinal cord, the lesions are single in nearly 80 percent of cases. Lindau disease, comprised of hemangioblastomas occurring at multiple sites throughout the central nervous system, was found in nearly one third of the patients in one review.[14] The associated hemangioblastomas were most common in the medulla, cerebellum, and retina. Of clinical importance is the observation that when cerebellar or retinal hemangioblastomas coexisted with spinal lesions, the former usually became clinically symptomatic before those in the spine.

As most hemangioblastomas are situated in the posterior aspect of the cord, sensory loss and radicular pain are common early symptoms. As the other spinal tracts become involved, symptoms and signs extend to include motor findings. Spinal hemangioblastomas may remain clinically silent throughout life and be found incidentally at autopsy.[91, 127]

Laboratory and Diagnostic Imaging Studies

The CSF in cases of spinal hemangioblastoma is often xanthochromic and has an elevated protein.[63] Plain film abnormalities were found in 37 percent of the cases shown in Table 6–2.[14] The most commonly encountered findings were widening of the interpedicular distance and the anteroposterior diameter of the vertebral canal. Several contiguous vertebrae are often found to have erosion of vertebral bodies and pedicles due to the expanding intraspinal mass.[87]

When performed, myelography is abnormal in over 90 percent of cases.[14] Depending upon the location of the tumor, both intramedullary and extramedullary masses may be found. When an associated syringomyelia has developed, the cord may be widened. When dilated serpiginous vessels are encountered, the diagnosis should be considered. Spinal angiography has been useful in the evaluation of these lesions.[70, 86, 150] CT scanning often reveals a soft-tissue mass with dramatic contrast enhancement,[68] and a cyst or syringomyelic cavity may be demonstrated. Several abnormalities may be seen using MRI, including diffuse enlargement of the cord, cystic areas, and edema extending several segments beyond the limits of the tumor.[135] Following the administration of paramagnetic contrast agents, enhance-

ment has been reported in spinal hemangioblastomas.[106] The nidus of tumor may enhance, distinguishing it from an adjacent cyst.[137, 139]

Therapy. The definitive treatment of spinal hemangioblastomas is surgery.[14] Although microsurgical techniques have been a major advance, larger lesions or strategically placed tumors may make complete removal impossible without unacceptable neurological injury. For this reason, radiation therapy has been used following incomplete resection of the hemangioblastoma, or occasionally as primary therapy.[14] When the hemangioblastoma nodule cannot be completely resected, it usually recurs. Infantile spinal hemangiomas may respond to steroid therapy.[93]

Epidermoid and Dermoid Cysts and Teratomas

Epidermoid and dermoid cysts and teratomas comprise approximately 1 to 2 percent of primary spinal tumors. In the Mayo Clinic analysis of 1,322 tumors of the spine, 18 (1.4 percent) were one of these histological types. Of this group, 10 were intramedullary tumors, but these neoplasms also may reside in the extramedullary-intradural space. Among children, these tumors account for nearly 5 percent of primary spinal tumors.[123]

The wall of an epidermoid cyst is composed of connective tissue lined by stratified squamous epithelium.[2, 30, 31, 142] The central cavity of the cyst contains fat-laden keratinized debris produced by the epithelium.[105] The wall of a dermoid cyst has a similar composition but also contains such dermal appendages as hair follicles, sebaceous glands, and occasional sweat glands.[10] The central cavity of a dermoid cyst may contain hair and glandular secretions. When either cyst is present in the subarachnoid space, it may be surrounded by signs of chronic inflammation because these cysts may release their contents, resulting in arachnoiditis.[19, 34]

Epidermoid and dermoid cysts may arise either as a result of an error in development in which cutaneous ectoderm is enclosed within the neural tube[8] or, possibly, as a result of introduction of skin at the time of lumbar puncture.[11, 23, 53] Evidence suggests that epidermoid tumors may develop years following lumbar punctures.[145] When the tumors occur in the setting of a developmental error, other anomalies may be found, such as spina bifida occulta, posterior dermal sinuses, syringomyelia, and diastematomyelia.[8, 145] Dermal sinus tracts, beginning in the skin, may extend into the spinal canal and terminate intradurally in a dermoid cyst.[100, 145, 148]

Other related tumors and cysts may be more complex, exhibiting elements of mesodermal tissue, and thus are classified as teratomas.[51, 146] Teratomas in the spinal canal are rare, with the majority appearing in childhood.[77] Other developmental abnormalities, such as spina bifida, are often found in association with such teratomas.[76]

CLINICAL FEATURES

Epidermoid and dermoid cysts are slow-growing mass lesions. They may occur at any level of the spinal axis[76] but more often are found in the lumbar region and therefore cause symptoms referable to the cauda equina and conus medullaris. When they arise higher in the spinal canal, symptoms and signs referable to these levels develop.

In cases associated with developmental anomalies, cutaneous stigmata consisting of hypertrichosis, pigmented skin, and cutaneous angiomas may be found. Repeated bouts of sterile meningitis due to rupture of the cysts may herald their presence. Examination of the CSF under polarized light may demonstrate the presence of keratin released by an epidermoid cyst. In cases of developmental origin, vertebral defects may be noted on plain films of the spine. Myelography and CT myelography[68] may demonstrate dermoids and epidermoids. MRI is expected to be useful in their evaluation.[106]

Lipoma

Spinal lipomas are rare primary tumors of the spinal canal composed of lobules of adult adipose tissue.[40, 42, 129] Many intraspinal lipomas are associated with other developmental defects of the vertebral arches, dura, and subcutaneous tissue. These lesions thus may be considered as part of a myelovertebral malformation rather than as an isolated spinal neoplasm. Such developmental lipomas are often transdural when seen in association with meningocele or myelomeningocele. A tethered conus medullaris may also be seen in such cases. The developmental lipomas associated with spinal dysraphism commonly occur in the caudal spinal canal and present in the early decades of life;[20, 43, 55] they are excluded from the present discussion.

Intradural spinal lipomas constitute approximately 1 percent of primary spinal tumors. In the large Mayo Clinic series,[134] there were 6 (0.5 percent) lipomas among 1,322 primary spinal neoplasms. Another study[55] found 6 (1.6 percent) intradural spinal lipomas among 378 primary spinal tumors. The tumors most frequently are located on the posterior surface of the spinal cord in the midline; this observation has led to the suggestion that they arise from embryologically misplaced cells.[18]

The lipoma is often covered on its posterior surface by pia mater.[55] The neoplasm is usually adherent to the underlying spinal cord and may often extend into the substance of the cord itself. Lipomas are thus often both intramedullary and intradural-extramedullary in location. Any segmental level of the spinal axis may be the site of an intraspinal lipoma,[38] but the cervicothoracic region has been found to be a favored location.[55]

Although Giuffre[55] excluded spinal lipomatous malformations from his review, he still found that one third of intradural lipomas were associated with other lesions, predominantly malformations, including spina bifida occulta, cranial osteomas, craniopharyngioma, subcutaneous lipoma at the same level, hydrocephalus, extradural lipoma, and intracranial lipoma. Thus, as with teratomas and epidermoid and dermoid cysts, the distinction between developmental anomalies and true neoplasms may be difficult.[76, 146]

CLINICAL FEATURES

Intradural lipomas appear to show no predilection for either sex.[55] Although they may present at any age, approximately two thirds of patients report that symptoms began before age 30.[55] Symptoms often are present for long periods of time prior to diagnosis. In the Mayo Clinic series,[134] the average duration of symptoms prior to surgery was 11 years, 8 months; the longest duration was 31 years. In the more recent review by Giuffre,[55] 56 percent of patients had symptoms exceeding 3 years; in 10 percent, the symptoms were present for over 20 years. The tumor may come to clinical attention after trauma, Valsalva maneuver (such as a sneeze), or pregnancy.[54, 55]

Although pain was the first symptom in four of six patients in the Mayo Clinic series,[134] Giuffre[55] has commented on the infrequency of radicular pain in patients with intradural lipomas. In his review, numbness and ataxia were the most common presenting complaints. Despite the intramedullary location of some of these tumors, a suspended segmental sensory loss has been infrequently found.[55] As spinal cord compression or cauda equina compression ensues, the symptoms and signs are those of other space-occupying lesions of the spine. As with other spinal tumors, remissions and exacerbations have been reported in a minority of patients. The long duration of symptoms appears to be the most characteristic feature of intradural lipomas.

DIAGNOSTIC IMAGING STUDIES

Plain film abnormalities of the vertebral column are seen in approximately one half of cases of intradural lipoma.[55] Widening of the spinal canal, abnormal curvature, and congenital abnormalities are the most frequently encountered. Myelography usually shows a mass lesion.[55] On CT scanning, the tumor is usually seen as a noncontrast-enhancing, homogenous mass of low attenuation.[37, 68, 94] MRI is a sensitive technique for imaging lipomas and will probably play a dominant role in their diagnosis and management.[106] When the intraspinal lipoma is associated with

spinal dysraphism, many other abnormalities are seen.[5, 47]

THERAPY

Surgery is the treatment of choice of spinal cord compression due to lipoma.[55] Recovery or improvement in function typically follows. If feasible, complete resection is preferred, but laminectomy alone may lead to a long period of clinical stabilization.[141]

INTRAMEDULLARY TUMORS

Gliomas are among the most common intramedullary spinal neoplasms, found in 0.01 to 0.06 percent of routine autopsies.[130] In the Mayo Clinic series of primary tumors of the spinal canal,[134] gliomas were the third most common tumor (after nerve sheath tumor and meningioma), accounting for 22 percent of all neoplasms encountered. Gliomas arise from neuroglia and may be classified in the spinal cord as astrocytomas, ependymomas, oligodendrogliomas, spongioblastomas, and subependymal gliomas.[134]

Over 60 percent of spinal gliomas are ependymomas, with astrocytoma claiming 25 percent, and glioblastoma and oligodendroglioma comprising 7.5 percent and 3 percent, respectively.[130] Among children alone, however, spinal astrocytoma is more common than ependymoma. Approximately 50 percent of all spinal gliomas are located in the caudal segments and filum terminale.[130] Oligodendrogliomas of the spinal cord are extremely rare, with only 38 cases reported prior to a review published in 1980.[49] Subependymal gliomas are similarly rare.[134] Spongioblastomas have been classified as astrocytomas.[129] Although primary intramedullary spinal lymphoma[69] has been rarely reported, its frequency may increase as the incidence of primary CNS lymphoma rises.[73]

Ependymoma

Spinal ependymomas arise from ependymal cells and may occur as intramedullary growths throughout the length of the spinal cord or in the region of the cauda equina. Ependymal cells are those which line the central cavities of the central nervous system. In addition, ependymal cells have been found in abundance in the region of the filum terminale. Detailed histological studies of this structure found that the filum terminale is not merely a fibrous band but contains multiple islands of ependymal cells.[66] These observations may explain the high frequency of ependymomas in the caudal spine.[113]

When they occur within the spinal parenchyma, ependymomas characteristically form a cylindrical mass surrounded by normal spinal tissue. The spinal cord may enlarge to cause a complete subarachnoid block. The tumor may extend from the intramedullary region of the spinal cord to breach the pia mater into the subarachnoid space.[134] When the tumor develops in the filum terminale, it forms a nodular or fusiform swelling in the caudal spinal canal. The tumor often grows between and invades the cauda equina.

The majority of ependymomas are histologically benign, although remote metastases may occur.[130] The presence of ependymal rosettes is a characteristic and, essentially, a diagnostic feature.[129] According to the histological classification used by Sloof, Kernohan, and MacCarty, [134] ependymomas may be graded from 1 to 4, with grade 1 being the most benign form and grade 4, the most malignant. In their series of 169 cases, 108 were grade 1, 56 were grade 2, and 5 were grade 3 ependymomas; there were no grade 4 ependymomas. Furthermore, ependymomas may be classified as cellular, papillary, epithelial, myxopapillary, and mixed, according to their histological appearance. Although myxopapillary ependymomas are virtually restricted to the region of the conus medullaris and cauda equina, the other histological types also may occur in this region.[130]

FREQUENCY AND LOCATION

Ependymomas may arise at any level of the central nervous system. In a clinical survey of 74 ependymomas,[7] 64 percent were intracranial and 36 percent were spinal. Among primary spinal tumors, ependymomas were found in 13 percent (169) of the Mayo Clinic series of 1,322 primary spinal tumors.[134] Ependymomas constitute the most common histological type of intramedullary glioma in the spinal cord including the filum terminale. In the large Mayo Clinic series, 62 percent of intramedullary and filum terminale gliomas were ependymomas.

Within the spinal canal, ependymomas are classified as intramedullary tumors when at the level of the spinal cord, or as neoplasms of the cauda equina. Of the 169 cases in the Mayo Clinic series,[134] 57 percent were at the level of the cauda equina and 43 percent were intramedullary. In other series of ependymomas,[4, 7, 134] 49 percent occurred at the level of the cauda equina and 50 percent were intramedullary (20 percent cervical and 31 percent thoracic).[46]

When ependymomas arise within the substance of the spinal cord, they often extend over multiple segments. In one surgical series of intramedullary spinal cord tumors,[27] the mean length of solid tumor was 4.7 segments. Occasionally spinal ependymomas may metastasize throughout the neuraxis.[32]

Among primary caudal tumors, ependymoma has been reported as the most frequent histological type.[89] In a series of 100 primary caudal tumors,[113] ependymoma accounted for 88 percent of cases. The second most common tumor in this series was astrocytoma, responsible for 8 percent.

CLINICAL FEATURES

Sex and Age

Spinal ependymomas are more frequent in men than in women. Men accounted for 63 percent[7] and 59 percent[134] of cases in two series.

Spinal ependymomas may occur from childhood to late life but, unlike their intracranial counterparts, appear to be rare in infancy and early childhood.[46] The youngest patient among 169 cases in one series[134] was 6 years old; the youngest in another[7] was 14. The average age of patients with ependymomas of the filum terminale has been reported as 35 years, whereas the average age of those with intramedullary spinal cord ependymomas was 42 years.[134]

Duration of Symptoms

The interval of time between the onset of symptoms and diagnosis of spinal ependymoma ranges from days to years. In one series,[7] one patient presented after two days of leg weakness associated with coughing. At the other extreme, patient with a caudal tumor had a 20-year history of coccygeal pain. Trauma often appears to precipitate symptoms; in the same series,[7] 33 percent of patients with spinal ependymomas attributed their symptoms to trauma.

In the detailed analysis of the Mayo Clinic series,[134] the average duration of symptoms was 56 months for grade 1 ependymomas and 33 months for grade 2. The average duration was similar for grade 1 lesions in the spinal cord as compared with the filum terminale (52 vs. 58 months). For grade 2 tumors, however, the average preoperative duration was only 17 months for filum terminale lesions, compared with 49 months for intramedullary ones. Among the entire series for all sites, two thirds had symptoms for less than 4 years.[134]

Symptoms and Signs

The primary symptoms and signs in spinal ependymoma may be classified as pain, motor dysfunction, sensory disturbance, and sphincter disturbances. Pain, the most common initial symptom, may be due to vertebral compression (local), nerve root irritation (radicular), and/or ascending spinal tract involvement (funicular). Although these types of pain may occur separately, they more often occur in combination. As discussed in Chapter 2, the pain associated with intramedullary tumors is more often funicular than radicular.[133] Furthermore, funicular pain is usually bilateral, poorly localized, diffuse, and burning in nature. Alternatively, pain due to cauda equina compression is usually radicular in nature, although it may commonly be bilateral.

Among the 149 patients with spinal ependymomas, 117 experienced pain as the presenting symptom.[134] Back pain was the most common (60 patients), but back

and limb pain (9 patients), lower extremity pain alone (16 patients), neck/upper extremity pain (14), and truncal pain (6) also were reported. Coccygeal pain has also been seen as a presenting complaint.[7, 46] In the series cited above,[134] three patients initially reported rectal discomfort.

In the same series,[134] the second most common presenting complaint was sensory disturbance. Twenty-one of 149 patients initially had sensory symptoms, generally in the form of numbness, coldness, and hypesthesia. The sensory disturbances could involve any region of the body. Motor disturbance was the third most common presenting symptom, reported in 15 patients. As with sensory complaints, motor disturbances more frequently involved the legs than the arms but could occur at any location. Sphincter disturbance or impotence was the presenting complaint in 5 patients.

LABORATORY AND DIAGNOSTIC IMAGING STUDIES

The cerebrospinal fluid usually shows an elevated protein concentration, especially when the tumor causes a block of cerebrospinal pathways.[7, 134] Occasionally a dry tap is encountered, especially with tumors of the filum terminale. A CSF pleocytosis is occasionally encountered; the average number of cells in the cerebrospinal fluid in the Mayo Clinic series[134] was 5 to 6 per cubic millimeter.

Plain films of the spine have been reported as abnormal in a minority of patients with spinal ependymomas.[134] The abnormalities usually consist of widening of the interpedicular distance, erosion of the medial surface of the pedicle, and concavity of the posterior surface of the vertebral body. In one series,[7] these abnormalities were encountered in 38 percent of patients.

With myelography, intramedullary spinal tumors may show widening of the spinal cord. Alternatively, the width of the spinal cord may appear normal despite the presence of an intramedullary neoplasm. In the region of the filum terminale, an ependymoma may displace and compress the cauda equina. CT scanning is often complementary to myelography in cases of spinal ependymoma. A thin rim of intra-thecal contrast may be seen on CT that is not evident with plain myelography, thus demonstrating the intramedullary location of the tumor. Nonenhanced CT scanning of ependymomas frequently demonstrates a decreased attenuation or isodense tumor as compared with the cord.[68] Ependymo-mas may contrast-enhance following intra-venous contrast administration.[62, 68, 95] Contrast enhancement of ependymomas may be prominent and has been found to be similar to that of intramedullary astrocytomas.[95] MRI has been found use-ful in distinguishing syringomyelia from intramedullary tumors with or without associated tumor cavities.[29, 35, 106] With the use of paramagnetic contrast-en-hanced MRI, the spinal ependymomas may be readily seen. Thus MRI is the initial imaging modality of choice in evaluating intramedullary spinal cord neoplasms.[29] Patients with spinal ependymomas should be evaluated for an intracranial ependy-moma that is presenting with a drop metastasis.

THERAPY

The therapy of spinal ependymomas is controversial. While conservative surgery followed by radiotherapy has been recommended by some investigators,[132] the advent of improved surgical tech-niques has led to radical surgical resec-tion of these lesions without postopera-tive radiotherapy.[27] Clinical improvement or stabilization was reported in 21 of 29 patients (72 percent) undergoing radical resection of intramedullary tumors (14 of the 29 patients had ependymomas).[27] Postoperative radiotherapy has been rec-ommended in cases of incomplete resection,[93, 132, 136] although its value has been questioned.[111]

The prognosis for survival of patients with spinal ependymomas is relatively fa-vorable. Of 51 patients with spinal ependy-momas reported in one study,[111] 72 per-cent were alive at 10 years. Patients with cauda equina tumors have a better prog-nosis than those with intramedullary neo-plasms, and those with myxopapillary his-tology fare better than those with cellular pattern.[111]

Astrocytoma

Astrocytomas and ependymomas are the two most common intramedullary tumors of the spinal cord.[45] In the Mayo Clinic series,[134] 86 (7 percent) of the en-tire group of 1,322 primary spinal tumors were astrocytomas. Although ependymo-mas (13 percent) were the most com-monly encountered intramedullary tu-mor if the filum terminale is included in that designation, among tumors arising within the spinal cord *per se*, astrocytoma was the most common. Astrocytoma of the filum terminale is unusual, with only 7 percent of the cases of astrocytoma appearing in this region in the Mayo Clinic series.[134] In a surgical series of intramedullary tumors (excluding the filum terminale),[27] there were 14 ependymomas and 10 astrocytomas. Among purely intramedullary spinal tu-mors in children, astrocytomas are ap-proximately twice as frequent as ependymomas.[44, 126]

As in the brain, spinal astrocytomas are often histologically classified from grade 1 to 4. The less malignant grades 1 and 2 are much more frequently encountered in the spinal cord than are the higher grade lesions.[3] Among the Mayo Clinic series, 76 percent were either grade 1 or 2.[134] A much higher incidence of more malignant astrocytomas is encountered in the brain.[134] Cysts or syringomyelia may be associated with spinal cord astrocyto-mas.[85, 134]

LOCATION AND EXTENT

The thoracic spine is the most frequent location for spinal cord astrocytomas.[27, 134] In the Mayo Clinic series[134] 20 percent were in the cervical region, 13 percent in the cervicothoracic area, and 48 percent in the thoracic spine; only 5 percent were in the lumbar region alone. These observa-tions correspond to the expected frequency of spinal cord tumors based on the relative length and mass of the spinal cord.[3] Using microsurgical techniques, Cooper and Ep-stein[27] found that the mean length of solid tumor in patients with astrocytoma was 5.3 segments.

CLINICAL FEATURES

Sex and Age. Spinal cord astrocytomas are more frequently seen in men than in women.[3] Of 86 patients in the Mayo Clinic series,[134] 48 were males. These tumors may arise at any age, although the average patient is middle aged. Patients with lower-grade tumors tend to be slightly older than those with more malignant lesions; in one series,[92] the average age of patients with astrocytoma grade 1 or 2 was 40 years, whereas that of patients with astrocytoma grade 3 or 4 was 34. The Mayo Clinic series[134] found the average age of patients with astrocytoma grade 1 or 2 was 37 years, whereas that of patients with glioblastoma was 23.

Duration of Symptoms Although there is a considerable range, the mean duration of symptoms prior to diagnosis depends to some extent upon the grade of the astrocytoma. The average duration of symptoms in the Mayo Clinic series was reported to be 41 months for grade 1, 29 months for grade 2, 7 months for grade 3, and 4 months for grade 4 astrocytomas.[134] The range of duration of symptoms was very broad, especially for lower-grade tumors; the interval ranged from 1 month to 12 years for grade 1 astrocytomas.

Symptoms and Signs As in other spinal tumors, the most common presenting symptoms of patients with spinal astrocytomas are pain, motor disorders, sensory disturbances, and sphincter dysfunction. Pain is the most frequent presenting complaint,[134] and may be local, radicular, or funicular in nature, with the site of referral dependent upon the location of the tumor. Motor disturbances are the second most frequent presenting complaint and include weakness, spasticity, or atrophy. When the lesion is in the cervical spine, upper extremity atrophy may be accompanied by lower extremity spasticity. Sensory and sphincter disturbances are less frequent presenting complaints. Sensory abnormalities often occur in a suspended distribution (see Chapter 2). At the time of diagnosis, most patients have more than one symptom and usually demonstrate multiple abnormalities on their neurological examination.[134]

LABORATORY AND DIAGNOSTIC IMAGING STUDIES

The cerebrospinal fluid usually shows signs of elevated protein, varying according to the degree of spinal block. Pleocytosis is occasionally found; the average number of white cells in the Mayo Clinic series[134] was 7 per cubic millimeter. On rare occasions, malignant astrocytomas may spread via the subarachnoid pathways and seed the leptomeninges throughout the neuraxis.[83] In such cases, the CSF may show malignant cells.

Plain films of the spine are usually not helpful in evaluating patients with spinal astrocytomas. Among 74 patients undergoing such studies, only 5 demonstrated signs diagnostic of tumor.[134] Myelography is usually diagnostic of an intramedullary tumor but may occasionally be normal. CT scanning following the administration of intrathecal contrast is considered sensitive. A second series of CT scans obtained 12 to 24 hours following the intrathecal administration of contrast material may demonstrate the presence of an intramedullary cyst because the cystic cavities may be filled with dye on delayed studies.[27, 94] MRI may demonstrate the location and extent of these tumors, including the presence of an associated cyst or syringomyelia.[29, 35] Following the administration of paramagnetic contrast material, MRI has been found very useful in the characterization and delineation of intramedullary astrocytomas.[106, 139] Areas of contrast enhancement may identify regions of neoplastic tissue (Fig. 6–7).[139] MRI is the initial imaging procedure of choice for intramedullary spinal neoplasms.[29]

THERAPY

The therapy of intramedullary astrocytomas is controversial. While biopsy followed by radiotherapy has been recommended by many investigators,[132] recent advances in surgical techniques have led to reports of total or 99 percent removal of these tumors, followed by improvement or stabilization of the clinical status.[24, 27, 64, 93, 126] Postlaminectomy spinal deformities may be a significant postoperative complica

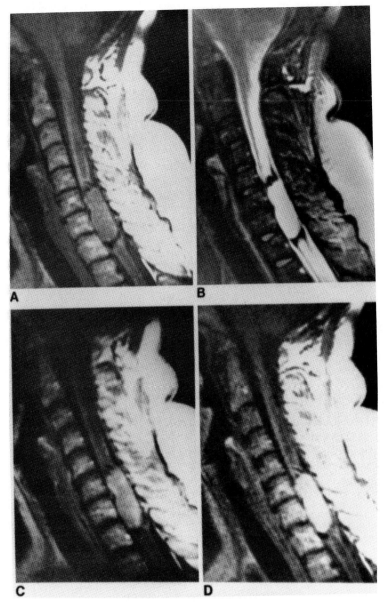

Figure 6–7. A 55-year-old woman with a spinal cord astrocytoma. (A) and (B) Noncontrast sagittal MR images demonstrate a central nidus with superior and inferior cysts. The markedly hypointense rim was shown pathologically to be hemosiderin deposition. (C) Gadolinium-enhanced MR sagittal image 30 minutes after administration of contrast material discloses peripheral enhancement of central lesion. (D)One-hour-delayed gadolinium-enhanced sagittal scan showing enhancement of the central focus. Associated syrinxes are not surrounded by enhancing cord parenchyma, suggesting they are probably benign reactive cysts (a finding confirmed at surgery) rather than tumor cysts. The necrotic nature of the tumor was shown pathologically and was probably responsible for delayed enhancement. (From Sze, G, et al,[139] with permission.)

tion, especially in children.[126] Although the benefits of postoperative radiotherapy are controversial, many authors recommend its use, especially in cases where there has been incomplete resection of the tumor.[93, 126]

Survival is related to the grade of the neoplasm. In children and adolescents, grade 1 and 2 astrocytomas have a 5-year and 10-year survival rate of approximately 80 percent and 55 percent, respectively,[126] while patients with grade 3 or 4 lesions have a median survival of less than 1 year.[24, 92, 126] Chemotherapy has been used in selected cases with malignant astrocytomas of the spinal cord.[24]

Intramedullary Metastasis

Intramedullary spinal cord metastases are rare and present difficult diagnostic and management problems. Approximately 100 cases had been reported as of a detailed review in 1985.[60] In a prospective autopsy study [21] of 1,066 patients with disseminated cancer, 200 had intraparenchymal central nervous system metastases; of this group, an intramedullary spinal cord metastasis was found in 10. Thus in a detailed autopsy series, less than 1 percent of patients dying of malignancy were found to have intramedullary spinal cord metastasis. Using the same data, however, it may be concluded that the spinal cord is more susceptible to metastasis than is the brain.[39] Although the weight of the spinal cord is only 2 percent that of the brain, the autopsies found that 5 percent of intraparenchymal CNS metastases were to the spinal cord.[21] In another study of patients with small-cell lung cancer,[114] which has a high incidence of CNS metastases, 49 percent of patients had CNS metastases but only 6 percent had intraspinal involvement. Among the patients with intraspinal invasion, all had leptomeningeal metastases as well.

SITE OF PRIMARY TUMORS

Carcinoma of the lung appears to be the most common primary tumor causing intramedullary spinal cord metastasis. In a review of 55 cases of spinal cord metastases in the literature,[60] 49 percent were due to lung cancer; breast cancer accounted for 15 percent, followed by lymphoma (9 percent), colorectal (7 percent), head and neck (6 percent), renal cell (6 percent), and miscellaneous other neoplasms. In a review of 13 autopsied cases,[28] lung cancer accounted for 85 percent, followed by breast cancer and melanoma, each responsible for 7.5 percent.

LOCATION AND PATHOLOGICAL FINDINGS

The spinal level of intramedullary spinal cord metastasis is roughly proportionate to the length of spinal cord. Thus among 55 cases,[60] the cervical region had 31 percent; the thoracic cord, 42 percent; and the lumber region, 15 percent. The cervicothoracic and thoracolumbar areas accounted for the remaining cases.

In gross pathological study, the spinal cord at the level of the tumor may or may not be enlarged.[28] Such absence of cord enlargement accounts for the lack of myelographic abnormalities in many cases. The metastasis may extend from one to several segments along the rostro-caudal axis.

The pathogenesis may be either direct metastasis to the cord, with occasional extension into the adjacent dorsal root or subarachnoid space, or, alternatively, leptomeningeal metastases with secondary extension into the spinal parenchyma. One pathological study [28] found 9 of 13 cases with direct metastasis to the spinal cord, and 4 cases representing extension from the subarachnoid space to the spinal parenchyma.

A pathological study [81] concluded that the majority of intramedullary metastases are the result of hematogenous dissemination to the cord directly rather than via transdural or perineural spread. It could not be determined whether the hematogenous spread occurred via venous or arterial routes, or both. In a case report in which an intramedullary metastasis was associated with a spinal infarct,[72] the authors suggested that the metastasis arose as a tumor embolus via the arterial system, which secondarily caused a spinal infarction.

CLINICAL FEATURES

As with epidural or leptomeningeal metastases from systemic cancer, intramedullary spinal cord metastases may herald the diagnosis of malignancy or develop years after the original diagnosis. In a review of 55 cases[60] (Table 6-4), the most frequent presenting complaints are pain and weakness. These symptoms usually occurred together in 33 percent of patients but a similar proportion of patients presented with either pain without weakness or weakness without pain. As presenting features, paresthesias and sphincter dysfunction were seen in 27 percent and 9 percent, respectively.

All 55 patients had weakness or paralysis on the initial examination. Weakness was found in the following patterns: paraparesis (23 patients), monoparesis (15 pa-

Table 6−4 NEUROLOGICAL SYMPTOMS AND SIGNS AT THE TIME OF INITIAL EVALUATION OF 55 PATIENTS WITH INTRAMEDULLARY SPINAL CORD METASTASIS*

Symptoms	No. of Patients (%)	
Pain	34	(62)
Nonradicular	16	(29)
Radicular	18	(33)
Motor deficit	35	(64)
Paresthesias	15	(27)
Bowel/Bladder dysfunction	5	(9)

Signs	No. of Patients (%)	
Motor deficit	55	(100)
Sensory level to pin, etc.	27	(49)
Dermatomal sensory loss	7	(13)
Paresthesias	15	(27)
Atrophy of musculature	3	(5)
Bowel/bladder dysfunction	39	(71)
Upgoing toes	17	(31)
Tenderness over spine	4	(7)
Pain on straight leg raising or neck flexion	6	(12)
Horner's syndrome	2	(4)
Completed neurological deficit		
Flaccid paralysis	25	(45)
Spastic paresis/plegia	5	(9)
Brown-Séquard syndrome	6	(11)

*From Grem, JL, et al, [60] p 2310, with permission.

tients), quadriparesis (9), and hemiparesis (8). An asymmetrical motor examination was found in 51 percent of cases. Atrophy was not common. Sensory deficits were seen in 64 percent, with a sensory level present in 49 percent. Despite a low incidence of bowel and bladder symptoms, signs of sphincter disturbance were seen in the majority (71 percent).

The time course between the onset of symptoms and the development of the full neurological deficit was less than 1 week in 22 percent, between 1 week and 1 month in 49 percent, and 5 weeks to 6 months in 24 percent. In 5 percent, neurological syndrome evolved for more than 6 months.[60]

LABORATORY AND DIAGNOSTIC IMAGING STUDIES

The cerebrospinal fluid in patients with intramedullary spinal cord metastasis is frequently abnormal but the abnormalities are usually nonspecific; the protein is often elevated and there may be pleocytosis. In the cases of leptomeningeal metastases with secondary invasion of the spinal cord, there may be cytological evidence of malignant cells.

Radiological studies are usually necessary to confirm the clinical impression. Plain films of the spine show evidence of vertebral metastases in 25 percent of cases;[60] the remainder are judged as normal.

Myelography was the most important diagnostic study prior to the advent of MRI. On myelography, the characteristic appearance of an intramedullary spinal cord metastasis is widening of the cord in two perpendicular views.[60] A lobulated mass or prominent pial vessels also may be seen on the surface of the cord.[39] In one study,[60] 48 percent of myelograms demonstrated evidence of widening (fusiform swelling) of the spinal cord on two views. A partial or complete block, lobular filling defect, or abnormal dilated blood vessels were also seen. In the remaining 42 percent of cases, however, the myelogram was normal.

CT scanning of the spine following the intrathecal administration of contrast may be very sensitive to recognizing slight enlargement of the spinal cord. High-resolution CT scanning of the spinal cord without intrathecal contrast may show the metastasis as an area of increased density in the spinal cord.[125]

MRI is expected to play a major role in the evaluation and management of these patients.[29, 139] Enhancement with gadolinium has been found to occur with intramedullary metastases.[50, 137]

Case Illustration

A 34-year-old woman was referred for increasing left upper extremity weakness and gait difficulty. She had a history of metastatic breast cancer to bone, lungs, liver, and brain. She had received whole brain irradiation 5 months earlier for a cerebellar metastasis. During the 2 weeks prior to referral, she noticed progressive left upper extremity weakness and occipital headache.

General physical examination showed an enlarged liver and ascites. On neurological examination, she had normal higher integrative functions and cranial nerves. There was no nystagmus. Funduscopic exam was benign.

There was weakness of the left arm (4 − /5) and left leg (4/5) but no weakness of the right side. No sensory deficit was found and there was no cerebellar disturbance. Gait was unsteady, with left lower extremity weakness. There were increased reflexes of the left side and sustained left ankle clonus. Both toes were downgoing on plantar stimulation. The differential diagnosis was considered to be recurrent brain or cervical spine metastasis (possibly leptomeningeal can-

cer) or, less likely, radiation-induced CNS dysfunction.

CT scan was performed to exclude recurrent cerebral metastases and showed no evidence of metastatic disease or hydrocephalus. A total spine MRI without and with gadolinium demonstrated an enhancing intramedullary metastasis in the cervical spine (Fig. 6−8) but no other evidence of metastases. The patient showed an excellent neurological response to

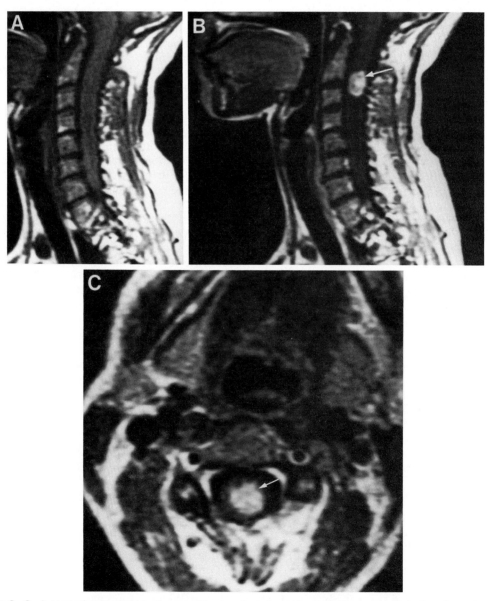

Figure 6−8. A cervical spine MRI is shown with an enhancing intramedullary metastasis from breast cancer. (A) Nonenhanced sagittal MRI shows a subtle cord abnormality. (B) Enhancement of an intramedullary mass is seen following the administration of gadolinium. (C) Axial section showing enhancing metastasis within the spinal cord.

corticosteroids and radiation therapy to the cervical spine.

DIFFERENTIAL DIAGNOSIS

Intramedullary spinal cord metastases cannot be clinically differentiated from epidural metastasis on the basis of symptoms or signs.[39] Pain, motor disturbances, sensory findings (dissociated or otherwise), and sphincter disturbances did not discriminate between these two locations.[39] In such cases, the clinician must resort to radiological procedures to discriminate between intramedullary and epidural metastasis. As discussed in Chapter 5, myelography and usually MRI will confidently demonstrate an epidural metastasis compressing the spinal cord.

When the cancer patient develops symptoms and signs of myelopathy and the radiological workup fails to reveal an epidural metastasis, the physician is confronted with a difficult diagnostic problem. The diagnostic possibilities include: metastatic disease (e.g., leptomeningeal metastases, intramedullary spinal cord metastasis); untoward effects of antineoplastic therapy (e.g., radiation myelopathy and myelopathy caused by intrathecal chemotherapy); remote effects of cancer (e.g., paraneoplastic necrotizing myelopathy); and a cause unrelated to the cancer or its treatment, such as multiple sclerosis, subacute combined degeneration, spondy-

losis, or trauma. The clinical differentiation of intramedullary spinal cord metastasis from radiation myelopathy, paraneoplastic necrotizing myelopathy and leptomeningeal metastases may present the clinician with a daunting task (Table 6–5).

The various clinical syndromes of radiation myelopathy are more fully discussed in Chapter 8. The most common syndrome is the early transient disorder consisting of Lhermitte's sign, which occurs within a few months of radiation therapy and is associated with a normal neurological examination. The second most common form of radiation myelopathy is the delayed chronic progressive myelopathy, which may more commonly be mistaken for intramedullary spinal cord metastasis. However, they usually can be differentiated by their tempo of evolution. The onset of symptoms of intramedullary spinal cord metastasis is usually abrupt, with a rapidly progressive course over days or weeks; infrequently it may progress over months or, rarely, years.[39] Chronic progressive radiation myelopathy, however, generally evolves over several months or years and may arrest at a stage of incomplete myelopathy.

The amount of radiation received also is important in the diagnosis of chronic progressive radiation myelopathy. Not only the total dose, but also the fractionation schedule and the length of the cord irradiated, are important parameters.[84] Factors

Table 6–5 NEUROLOGICAL FEATURES OF DIFFERENTIAL VALUE IN THE DIAGNOSIS OF A NONCOMPRESSIVE MYELOPATHY IN A PATIENT WITH CANCER*

| Myelopathy | Pain | Progression of Spinal Disease | | | Size of Affected Spinal Segments as Seen on Myelogram | | | Tumor Cells in CSF |
| | | Tempo | | Ascending or Descending | | | | |
		Subacute	Chronic		Normal	Enlarged	Small	
Intramedullary spinal cord metastasis	+	+	–	+	+	+	–	–
Leptomeningeal metastases	+	+	–	NA	+	–	–	+
Radiation myelopathy	–	–	+	–	+	+	+	–
Necrotizing myelopathy	–	+	–	+/–	+	+	–	–

*From Winkelman, MD, et al,[147] p 529, with permission. CSF indicates cerebrospinal fluid; NA, not applicable; +, present; –, absent; and +/–, may be present or absent.

such as hyperbaric oxygenation[143] and idiosyncratic sensitivity may allow radiation myelopathy to occur at levels otherwise considered safe.[13, 84] The primary tumor most frequently associated with radiation myelopathy has been head and neck cancer (82 percent of cases according to one report).[147] In this case, the cervical spinal cord is included in the radiation port due to its proximity to the primary tumor. On the other hand, the most common tumors associated with intramedullary spinal cord metastasis are lung and breast cancer (68 percent of cases according to one report).[147] In the irradiation of these primary malignancies, the spine usually does not receive radiation at doses sufficient to cause chronic progressive radiation myelopathy.

Occasionally intramedullary metastasis may be difficult to differentiate clinically from leptomeningeal metastases. Although leptomeningeal metastases usually cause symptoms and signs at multiple levels throughout the neuraxis, the cauda equina syndrome caused by metastases to this site alone may be identical to the clinical presentation of an intramedullary metastasis to the conus medullaris. As discussed in Chapter 2, often it is not possible on clinical grounds alone to discriminate between the conus medullaris and cauda equina syndromes.[98, 113]

In cases of leptomeningeal metastases, the CSF cytology and myelography, which may show thickening or nodularity of nerve roots and normal-size spinal cord, are helpful.[9, 61] Furthermore, head CT scanning may show evidence of leptomeningeal seeding or communicating hydrocephalus.[79] Although plain MRI has had limitations in the evaluation of leptomeningeal spread from tumor,[6] contrast-enhanced MRI may be more sensitive.[138, 139] It should be stressed that some patients develop intramedullary tumors secondary to leptomeningeal spread, so that the two may coexist.[28] Finally, clinical follow-up of the patient should differentiate between the two because their clinical courses are different.

Necrotizing myelopathy, discussed in Chapter 8, is a very rare remote effect of cancer that is in the differential diagnosis of myelopathy in the cancer patient with negative radiological studies; it thus must be differentiated from intramedullary spinal cord metastasis.[104] Patients with necrotizing carcinomatous myelopathy do not complain of local or radicular pain.[65, 116] Instead, they usually complain of vague, intermittent paresthesias in the lower extremities for weeks or months before an ascending transverse myelopathy develops. The necrotizing myelopathy usually begins in the thoracic spinal cord and then ascends and descends through the cord. Thus patients initially may have spastic paraplegia, followed by flaccid, areflexic paraplegia.[147] Radiological and CSF studies are nondiagnostic. As in cases of intramedullary metastasis, the course may be subacute. Because intramedullary metastases usually develop in the setting of widespread visceral and cerebral metastases, the law of parsimony would favor a diagnosis of intramedullary metastasis rather than a remote effect of cancer in such cases. Alternatively, visceral metastases occasionally may be found in patients with necrotizing carcinomatous myelopathy.

THERAPY

The management of intramedullary spinal metastasis is based on anecdotal reports because there are no large prospective series. Because many cases occur in the setting of widely disseminated disease, surgical therapy is infrequently undertaken. Furthermore, intramedullary metastases are often multiple or associated with intracerebral and/or leptomeningeal metastases; treatment therefore should consider the extent of CNS dissemination. Radiation therapy has been the primary treatment in most cases. The extent of the radiation port is determined by imaging studies, clinical involvement, and consideration of bone marrow tolerance (irradiation of the vertebral column may cause significant bone marrow suppression).[147] When leptomeningeal metastases are present, intrathecal chemotherapy may be used in addition to radiotherapy. The prognosis for patients with intramedullary spinal cord metastasis is poor, with over 80 percent dying within 3 months in one recent series.[60]

REFERENCES

1. Alter, M: Statistical aspects of spinal cord tumors. In Vinken, PJ and Bruyn, GW (eds): Handbook of Clinical Neurology, Vol 19. North-Holland Publishing, Amsterdam, 1975, pp 1–22.
2. Alves, AM and Norrell, H: Intramedullary epidermoid tumors of the spinal cord. Report of a case and review of the literature. Int Surg 54:239–243, 1970.
3. Arendt, A: Spinal gliomas. In Vinken, PJ and Bruyn, GW (eds): Handbook of Clinical Neurology, Vol 20. North-Holland Publishing, Amsterdam, 1976, pp 323–351.
4. Arseni, C and Ionesco, S: Les compressions médullaires dues a des tumeurs intra-rachidiennes. Étude clinico-statistique de 362 cas. J Chir (Paris) 75:582–595, 1958.
5. Banna, M: Clinical Radiology of the Spine and Spinal Cord. Aspen, Rockville, Md, 1985.
6. Barloon, TJ, Yuh, WTC, Yand, CJC, and Schultz, DH: Spinal subarachnoid tumor seeding from intracranial metastasis: MR findings. J Comp Assist Tomogr 11:242–244, 1987.
7. Barone, BM and Elvidge, AR: Ependymomas: A clinical survey. J Neurosurg 33:428–438, 1970.
8. Black, SPW and German, WJ: Four congenital tumors found at operation within the vertebral canal. With observations on their incidence. J Neurosurg 7:49–61, 1950.
9. Bleyer, WA and Byrne, TN: Leptomeningeal cancer in leukemia and solid tumors. Current Problems in Cancer 12:185–238, 1988.
10. Boldrey, EB and Elvidge, AR: Dermoid cysts of the vertebral canal. Ann Surg 110:273–284, 1939.
11. Boyd, HR: Iatrogenic intraspinal epidermoid. Report of a case. J Neurosurg 24:105–107, 1966.
12. Broager, B: Spinal neurinoma. Acta Psychiat Scand (Suppl)85:1–241, 1953.
13. Brown, WJ and Kagan, AR: Comparison of myelopathy associated with megavoltage irradiation and remote cancer. In Gilbert, HJ and Kagan, AR (eds): Radiation Damage to the Nervous System. Raven Press, New York, 1980, pp 191–206.
14. Browne, TR, Adams, RD, and Robertson, GH: Hemangioblastoma of the spinal cord. Arch Neurol 33:435–441, 1976.
15. Buchan, AM and Barnett, JM: Vascular malformations and hemorrhage of the spinal cord. In Barnett, HJM, Mohr, JP, Stein, BM, and Yatsu, FM (eds): Stroke: Pathophysiology,

16. Bull, JWD: Spinal meningiomas and neurofibromas. Acta Radiol 40:283–300, 1953.
17. Bunn, PA, Schein, PS, Banks, PM, and DeVita, VT: Central nervous system complications in patients with diffuse histiocytic and undifferentiated lymphoma: Leukemia revisited. Blood 47:3–10, 1976.
18. Burger, PC and Vogel, FS: Surgical Pathology of the Nervous System and Its Coverings. John Wiley & Sons, New York, 1976.
19. Cantu, RC and Wright, RL: Aseptic meningitic syndrome with cauda equina epidermoid tumor. J Pediatr 73:114–116, 1968.
20. Chapman, PH: Congenital intraspinal lipomas: Anatomical considerations and surgical treatment. Childs Brain 9:37–47, 1982.
21. Chason, JL, Walker, FB, and Landers, JW: Metastatic carcinoma in the central nervous system and dorsal root ganglia. Cancer 16:781–787, 1963.
22. Choi, IS and Berenstein, A: Surgical neuroangiography of the spine and spinal cord. Radiol Clin North Am 26:1131–1141, 1988.
23. Choremis, C, Oeconmos, D, Papadatos, C, and Gargoulas, A: Intraspinal epidermoid tumours (cholesteatomas) in patients treated for tuberculous meningitis. Lancet 32:437–439, 1956.
24. Cohen, AR, Wisoff, JH, Allen, JC, and Epstein, F: Malignant astrocytomas of the spinal cord. J Neurosurg 70:50–54, 1989.
25. Cohen, LM, Schwartz, AM, and Rockoff, SD: Benign schwannomas: Pathologic basis for CT inhomogeneities. AJR 147:141–143, 1986.
26. Coleman, BG, Arger, PH, Dalinka, MK, et al: CT of sarcomatous degeneration in neurofibromatosis. AJR 140:383–387, 1983.
27. Cooper, PR and Epstein, F: Radical resection of intramedullary spinal cord tumors in adults: Recent experience in 29 cases. J Neurosurg 63:492–499, 1985.
28. Costigan, DA and Winkelman, MD: Intramedullary spinal cord metastasis: A clinicopathological study of 13 cases. J Neurosurg 62:227–233, 1985.
29. Council, Scientific Affairs: Magnetic resonance imaging of the central nervous system. JAMA 259:1211–1222, 1988.
30. Craig, RL: A case of epidermoid tumor of the spinal cord. Review of the literature of spinal epidermoids and dermoids. Surgery 13:354–367, 1943.
31. Critchley, M and Ferguson, FR: The cerebrospinal epidermoids (cholesteatomata). Brain 51:334–384, 1928.
32. Davis, C and Barnard, RO: Malignant behavior of myxopapillary ependymoma: Report of three cases. J Neurosurg 62:925–929, 1985.
33. Davis, RA and Washburn, PL: Spinal cord meningiomas. Surg Gynecol Obstet 131:15–21, 1970.
34. Decker, RE and Gross, SW: Intraspinal dermoid

Diagnosis and Management. Churchill Livingstone, New York, 1986, pp 721–730.

tumor presenting as chemical meningitis. Report of a case without dermal sinus. J Neurosurg 27:60–62, 1967.

35. Di Chiro, G, Doppman, JL, Dwyer, AJ, Patronas, NJ, Knop, RH, Bairamian, D, Vermess, M, and Oldfield, EH: Tumors and arteriovenous malformations of the spinal cord: Assessment using MR. Radiology 156:689–697, 1985.

36. Djindjian, M: Clinical symptomatology and natural history of arteriovenous malformations of the spinal cord—a study of the clinical aspects and prognosis based on 150 cases. In Pia, HW and Djindjian, R (eds): Spinal Angiomas: Advances in Diagnosis and Therapy. Springer-Verlag, New York, 1978, pp 75–83.

37. Dosseter, RS, Kaiser, M, and Veiga-Pires, JA: CT scanning in two cases of lipoma of the spinal cord. Clin Radiol 30:227–231, 1979.

38. Drapkin, AJ: High cervical intradural lipoma. J Neurosurg 41: 699–704, 1974.

39. Edelson, RN, Deck, MDF, and Posner, JB: Intramedullary spinal cord metastases: Clinical and radiological findings in 9 cases. Neurology 22:1222–1231, 1972.

40. Ehni, G and Love, JG: Intraspinal lipomas. Report of cases; review of the literature, and clinical and pathologic study. Acta Neurol Psychiat 53:1–28, 1945.

41. Elsberg, CA: Tumors of the Spinal Cord and Membranes. Paul B Hoeber, New York, 1925.

42. Elsberg, CA: Surgical Diseases of the Spinal Cord, Membranes and Nerve Root. Paul B Hoeber, New York, 1941.

43. Emery, JL and Lendon, RG: Lipomas of the cauda equina and other fatty tumors related to neurospinal dysraphism. Dev Med Child Neurol (Suppl 20)2:62–70, 1969.

44. Epstein, F and Epstein, N: Intramedullary tumors of the spinal cord. In Shillito, J and Matson, DD (eds): Pediatric Neurosurgery: Surgery of the Developing Nervous System. Grune & Stratton, New York, 1982, pp 529–539.

45. Epstein, F and Epstein, N: Surgical treatment of spinal cord astrocytomas of childhood: A series of 19 patients. J Neurosurg 57:685–689, 1982.

46. Fischer, G and Tommasi, M: Spinal ependymomas. In Vinken, PJ and Bruyn, GW (eds): Handbook of Clinical Neurology, Vol 20. North-Holland Publishing, Amsterdam, 1976, pp 353–387.

47. Fitz, CR: The pediatric spine. In Gonzalez, CF, Grossman, CB, and Masdeu, JC (eds): Head and Spine Imaging. John Wiley & Sons, New York, 1985, pp 759–780.

48. Foix, C and Alajouanine, T: La myelite necrotique subaigue. Rev Neurol 2:1–42, 1926.

49. Fortuna, A, Celli, P, and Palma, L: Oligodendrogliomas of the spinal cord. Acta Neurochir 52:305–329, 1980.

50. Fredericks, RK, Elster, A, and Walker, FO: Gadolinium-enhanced MRI: A superior technique for the diagnosis of intraspinal metastases. Neurology 39:734–736, 1989.

51. Furtado, D and Marques, V: Spinal teratoma. J Neuropath Exp Neurol 10:384–393, 1951.

52. Gautier-Smith, PC: Clinical aspects of spinal neurofibromas. Brain 90:359–394, 1970.

53. Gibson, T and Norris, W: Skin fragments removed by injection needles. Lancet 2:983–985, 1958.

54. Giuffre, R: Intradural spinal lipomas. Review of the literature (99 cases) and report of an additional case. Acta Neurochir 14:69–95, 1966.

55. Giuffre, R: Spinal lipomas. In: Vinken, PJ and Bruyn, GW (eds): Handbook of Clinical Neurology, Vol 20. North-Holland Publishing, Amsterdam, 1976, pp 389–414.

56. Gonzalez-Vitale, JC and Garcia-Bunuel, R: Meningeal carcinomatosis. Cancer 37: 2906–2911, 1976.

57. Gowers, WR and Horsley, V: Case of tumour of spinal cord: Removal; recovery. Med Chir Tr, London 71:377–430, 1888.

58. Graif, M and Steiner, RE: Contrast-enhanced magnetic resonance imaging of tumours of the central nervous system: A clinical review. Br J Radiol 59:865–873, 1986.

59. Greenfield, JG and Turner, JWA: Acute and subacute necrotic myelitis. Brain 62:227–252, 1939.

60. Grem, JL, Burgess, J, and Trump, DL: Clinical features and natural history of intramedullary spinal cord metastasis. Cancer 56: 2305–2314, 1985.

61. Grogan, JP, Daniels, DL, Williams, AL, et al: The normal conus medullaris: CT criteria for recognition. Radiology 151:661–664, 1984.

62. Grossman, CB and Post, MJD: The adult spine. In Gonzalez, CF, Grossman, CB, and Masdeau, JC (eds): Head and Spine Imaging. John Wiley & Sons, New York, 1985, pp 781–858.

63. Guidetti, B and Fortuna, A: Surgical treatment of intramedullary hemangioblastoma of the spinal cord: Report of six cases. J Neurosurg 27:530–540, 1967.

64. Guidetti, B, Mercuri, S, and Vagnozzi, R: Long-term results of the surgical treatment of 129 intramedullary spinal gliomas. J Neurosurg 54:323–330, 1981.

65. Handforth, A, Nag, S, Sharp, D, et al: Paraneoplastic subacute necrotic myelopathy. Can J Neurol Sci 10:204–207, 1983.

66. Harmeier, JW: Normal histology of intradural filum terminale. AMA Archives of Neurology and Psychiatry 29:308–316, 1933.

67. Hashizume, Y, Iljima, S, Kishimoto, H, and Hirano, A: Pencil-shaped softening of the spinal cord: Pathologic study in 12 cases. Acta Neuropathol (Berl) 61:219–224, 1983.

68. Haughton, VM and Williams, AL: Computed Tomography of the Spine. CV Mosby, St Louis, 1982.

69. Hautzer, NW, Aiyesmoju, A, and Robitaille, Y: "Primary" spinal intramedullary lymphomas: A review. Ann Neurol 14:62–66, 1983.

70. Herdt, JR, Shimkin, PM, Ommaya, AK, et al:

Angiography of vascular intraspinal tumors. Journal Roentgenology Radium Therapy Nuclear Medicine 115:165–170, 1972.

71. Hermann, G and Hermann, P: Computerized tomography of the spine in metastatic disease. Mt Sinai J Med (NY) 49:400–405, 1982.

72. Hirose, G, Shimazaki, K, Takado, M, et al: Intramedullary spinal cord metastasis of the spinal cord associated with pencil-shaped softening of the spinal cord. J Neurosurg 52:718–721, 1980.

73. Hochberg, FH and Miller, DG: Primary central nervous system lymphoma (review article). J Neurosurg 68:835–853, 1988.

74. Hollis, PH, Malis, LI, and Zappulla, RA: Neurological deterioration after lumber puncture below complete spinal subarachnoid block. J Neurosurg 64:253–256, 1986.

75. Hughes, JT: Diseases of the spinal cord. In Blackwood, W and Corsellis, JAN (eds): Greenfield's Neuropathology. Year Book Medical Publishers, Chicago, 1976, pp 652–687.

76. Hughes, JT: Pathology of the Spinal Cord. WB Saunders, Philadelphia, 1978.

77. Ingraham, FD and Bailey, OT: Cystic teratomas and teratoid tumors of the central nervous system in infancy and childhood. J Neurosurg 3:511–532, 1946.

78. Iraci, G, Peserico, L, and Salar, G: Intraspinal neurinomas and meningiomas. A clinical survey of 172 cases. International Journal of Surgery 56:289–303, 1971.

79. Jaeckle, KA, Krol, G, and Posner, JB: Evolution of computed tomographic abnormalities in leptomeningeal metastases. Ann Neurol 17:85–89, 1985.

80. Jellinger, K: Pathology of spinal vascular malformations and vascular tumors. In Pia, HW and Djindjian, R (eds): Spinal Angiomas: Advances in Diagnosis and Therapy. Springer-Verlag, New York, 1978, pp 18–44.

81. Jellinger, K, Kothbauer, P, Sunder-Plassman, E, et al: Intramedullary spinal cord metastases. J Neurol 220:31–41, 1979.

82. Jellinger, K and Neumayer, E; Claudication of the spinal cord and cauda equina. In Vinken, PJ and Bruyn, GW (eds): Handbook of Clinical Neurology, Vol 12. North-Holland Publishing, Amsterdam, 1972, pp 507–547.

83. Johnson, DL and Schwarz, S; Intracranial metastases from malignant spinal-cord astrocytoma: Case report. J Neurosurg 66:621–625, 1987.

84. Kagan, AR, Wollin, M, Gilbert, HA, et al: Comparison of the tolerance of the brain and spinal cord to injury by radiations. In Gilberg, HA and Kagan, AR (eds): Radiation Damage to the Nervous System. Raven Press, New York, 1980, pp 183–190.

85. Kan, S, Fox, AJ, Vinuela, F, et al: Delayed CT metrizamide enhancement of syringomyelia secondary to tumor. Radiology 146:409–414, 1983.

86. Kendall, B: Application of angiography to tumors affecting the spinal cord. Proc R Soc Med 63:185–187, 1970.

87. Kendall, B and Russell, J: Hemangioblastoma of the spinal cord. Br J Radiol 39:817–823, 1966.

88. Kendall, BE and Logue, V: Spinal epidural angiomatous malformations draining into intrathecal veins. Neuroradiology 13:181–189, 1977.

89. Ker, NB and Jones, CB: Tumours of the cauda equina: The problem of differential diagnosis. J Bone Joint Surg 67B:358–361, 1985.

90. Kilgore, DP: Thoracic spine. In Daniels, DL, Haughton, VM, and Naidich, TP (eds): Cranial and Spinal Magnetic Resonance Imaging. An Atlas and Guide. Raven Press, New York, 1987, pp 263–284.

91. Kinney, TD and Fitzgerald, PJ: Lindau-von Hippel disease with hemangioblastoma of the spinal cord and syringomyelia. Arch Pathol 43:439–455, 1947.

92. Kopelson, G and Linggood, RM: Intramedullary spinal cord astrocytoma versus glioblastoma: The prognostic importance of histologic grade. J Neurosurg 50:732–735, 1982.

93. Kornblith, PL, Walker, MD, and Cassady, JR: Neurologic Oncology. JB Lippincott, Philadelphia, 1987.

94. Kricun, R and Kricun, ME: Computed Tomography. In Kricun, ME (ed): Imaging Modalities in Spinal Disorders. WB Saunders, Philadelphia, 1988, pp 376–467.

95. Lapointe, JS, Graeb, DA, Nugent, RA, and Robertson, WD: Value of intravenous contrast enhancement in the CT evaluation of intraspinal tumors. AJR 146:103–107, 1986.

96. Leeds, NE, Elkin, CM, Leon, E, et al: Myelography. In Kricun, ME (ed): Imaging Modalities in Spinal Disorders. WB Saunders, Philadelphia, 1988, pp 325–375.

97. Levitt, LJ, Dawson, DM, Rosenthal, DS, et al: CNS involvement in non-Hodgkin's lymphomas. Cancer 45:545–552, 1980.

98. Levitt, P, Ransohoff, J, and Spielholz, N: The differential diagnosis of tumors of the conus medullaris and cauda equina. In Vinken, PJ and Bruyn, GW (eds): Handbook of Clinical Neurology, Vol 19. North-Holland Publishing, Amsterdam, 1975, pp 77–90.

99. Levy, WJ, Bay, J, and Dohn, D: Spinal cord meningioma. J Neurosurg 57:804–812, 1982.

100. List, CF: Intraspinal epidermoids, dermoids, and dermal sinuses. Surg Gynecol Obstet 73:525–538, 1941.

101. Litam, JP, Cabanillas, F, Smith, TL, et al: Central nervous system relapse in malignant lymphomas: Risk factors and implications for prophylaxis. Blood 54:1249–1257, 1979.

102. Madsen, JR and Heros, RC: Spinal arteriovenous malformations and neurogenic claudication. Report of two cases. J Neurosurg 68:793–797, 1988.

103. Mair, WGP and Folkerts, JF: Necrosis of spinal cord due to thrombophlebitis (subacute necrotic myelitis). Brain 76:563–574, 1953.

104. Mancall, EL and Remedios, KR: Necrotizing myelopathy associated with visceral carcinoma. Brain 87:639–655, 1964.

105. Manno, NJ, Uihlein, A, and Kernohan, JW: Intraspinal epidermoids. J Neurosurg 19:754–765, 1962.

106. Masaryk, TJ: Spine tumors. In Modic, MT, Masaryk, TJ, and Ross, JS (eds): Magnetic Resonance Imaging of the Spine. Year Book Medical Publishers, Chicago, 1988, pp 183–213.

107. Masaryk, TJ, Ross, JS, Modic, MT, Ruff, RL, Selman, WR, and Ratcheson, RA: Radiculomeningeal vascular malformations of the spine: MR imaging. Radiology 164:845–849, 1987.

108. McAlhany, HJ and Netsky, MG: Compression of the spinal cord by extramedullary neoplasms: A clinical and pathological study. J Neuropath Exp Neurol 14:276–287, 1955.

109. Mead, GM, Kennedy, P, Smith, JL, Thompson, J, Macbeth, FRM, Ryall, RDH, Williams, CJ, and Whitehouse, JMA: Involvement of the central nervous system by non-Hodgkin's lymphoma in adults: A review of 36 cases. Q J Med 60:699–714, 1986.

110. Michelsen, WJ: Arteriovenous malformation of the brain and spinal cord. In Johnson, RT (ed): Current Therapy in Neurologic Disease—2. BC Decker, Toronto, 1987, pp 170–173.

111. Mork, SJ and Loken, AC: Ependymoma: A follow-up study of 101 cases. Cancer 40:907–915, 1977.

112. Nittner, K: Spinal meningiomas, neurinomas and neurofibromas and hourglass tumors. In Vinken, PJ and Bruyn, GW (eds): Handbook of Clinical Neurology, Vol 20. North-Holland Publishing, Amsterdam, 1976, pp 177–322.

113. Norstrom, CW, Kernohan, JW, and Love, JG: One hundred primary caudal tumors. JAMA 178:1071–1077, 1961.

114. Nugent, JL, Bunn, PA, Matthews, MJ, et al: CNS metastases in small cell bronchogenic carcinoma—increasing frequency and changing patterns with lengthening survival. Cancer 44:1885–1893, 1979.

115. Oddsson, B: Spinal Meningioma. HP Hansens, Kopenhagen, 1947.

116. Ojeda, VJ: Necrotising myelopathy associated with malignancy: A clinicopathological study of two cases and literature review. Cancer 53:1115–1123, 1984.

117. Onofrio, BM: Intradural extramedullary spinal cord tumors. Clin Neurosurg 25:540–555, 1978.

118. Osborn, RE and DeWitt, JD: Giant cauda equina schwannoma: CT appearance. AJNR 6:835–836, 1985.

119. Patchell, RA and Posner, JB: Neurologic complications of systemic cancer. Neurol Clin 3:729–750, 1985.

120. Perez-Soler, R, Smith, TL, and Cabanillas, F: Central nervous system prophylaxis with combined intravenous and intrathecal methotrexate in diffuse lymphoma of aggressive histologic type. Cancer 57:971–977, 1986.

121. Pia, HW: Symptomatology of spinal angiomas. In Pia, HW and Djindjian, R (eds): Spinal Angiomas: Advances in Diagnosis and Therapy. Springer-Verlag, New York, 1978, pp 48–74.

122. Rand, CW: Surgical experiences with spinal cord tumors. A survey over forty-year period. Bulletin of the Los Angeles Neurological Society 28:260–268, 1963.

123. Rand, RW and Rand, CW: Intraspinal Tumors of Childhood. Charles C Thomas, Springfield, Ill, 1960, pp 349–381.

124. Rasmussen, TB, Kernohan, JW, and Adson, AW: Pathologic classification, with surgical consideration, of intraspinal tumors. Ann Surg 111:513–530, 1940.

125. Reddy, SC, Vijayamohan, G, and Gao, GR: Delayed CT myelography in spinal intramedullary metastasis: Case report. J Comput Assist Tomogr 8:1182–1185, 1984.

126. Reimer, R and Onofrio, BM: Astrocytomas of the spinal cord in children and adolescents. J Neurosurg 63:669–675, 1985.

127. Rho, YM: Von Hippel-Lindau's disease: A report of five cases. Can Med Assoc J 101:135–142, 1969.

128. Rosenblum, B, Oldfield, EH, Doppman, JL, and DiChiro, G: Spinal arteriovenous malformations: A comparison of dural arteriovenous fistulas and intradural AVM's in 81 patients. J Neurosurg 67:795–802, 1987.

129. Rubinstein, LJ: Tumors of the Central Nervous System. AFIP, Washington, DC, 1972.

130. Russell, DS and Rubenstein, LJ: Pathology of Tumours of the Nervous System. Williams & Wilkins, Baltimore, 1989.

131. Schroth, G, Thron, A, Guhl, L, Voigt, K, Niendorf, H-P, and Garces, LR-N: Magnetic resonance imaging of spinal meningiomas and neurinomas. J Neurosurg 66:695–700, 1987.

132. Schwade, JG, Wara, WM, Sheline, GE, et al: Management of primary spinal cord tumors. Int J Radiat Oncol Biol Phys 4:389–393, 1978.

133. Schenkin, HA and Alpers, BJ: Clinical and pathological features of gliomas of the spinal cord. Arch Neurol Psychiatry 52:87–105, 1944.

134. Sloof, JL, Kernohan, JW, and MacCarty, CS: Primary Intramedullary Tumors of the Spinal Cord and Filum Terminale. WB Saunders, Philadelphia, 1964.

135. Solomon, RA and Stein, BM: Unusual spinal cord enlargement related to intramedullary hemangioblastoma. J Neurosurg 68:550–553, 1988.

136. Sonneland, PRL, Scheithauer, BW, and Onofrio, BM: Myxopapillary ependymoma: A clinicopathologic and immunocytochemical

study of 77 cases. Cancer 56:883–893, 1985.

137. Sze, G: Gadolinium-DTPA in spinal disease. Radiol Clin North Am 26:1009–1024, 1988.

138. Sze, G, Abramson, A, Krol, G, et al: Gadolinium-DTPA in the evaluation of intradural extramedullary spinal disease. AJNR 9:153–163, 1988.

139. Sze, G, Krol, G, Zimmerman, RD, and Deck, MDF: Intramedullary disease of the spine: Diagnosis using gadolinium-DTPA-enhanced MR imaging. AJNR 9:847–858, 1988.

140. Tadmor, R, Cacayorian, ED, and Kieffer, SA: Advantages of supplementary CT in myelography of intraspinal masses. AJNR 4:618–621, 1983.

141. Thomas, JE and Miller, RH: Lipomatous tumors of the spinal canal. Mayo Clin Proc 48:393–400, 1973.

142. Tytus, JS and Pennybacker, J: Pearly tumors in relation to the central nervous system. J Neurol Neurosurg Psychiatry 19:241–259, 1956.

143. Van den Brenk, HAS, Richter, W, and Hurley, RH: Radiosensitivity of the human oxygenated cervical spinal cord based on analysis of 357 cases receiving 4 MeV X rays in hyperbaric oxygenation. Br J Radiol 41:205–214, 1968.

144. Verbiest, H: Neurogenic intermittent claudication—lesions of the spinal canal and cauda equina, stenosis of the vertebral canal, narrowing of intervertebral foramina and entrapment of peripheral nerves. In Vinken, PJ and Bruyn, GW (eds): Handbook of Clinical Neurology, Vol 20. North-Holland Publishing, Amsterdam, 1976, pp 611–804.

145. Wilkins, RH and Odom, GL: Spinal intradural cysts. In Vinken, PJ and Bruyn, GW (eds): Handbook of Clinical Neurology, Vol 20. North-Holland Publishing, Amsterdam, 1976, pp 55–101.

146. Willis, RA: The Borderland of Embryology and Pathology. Butterworth, London, 1962.

147. Winkelman, MD, Adelstein, DJ, and Karlins, NL: Intramedullary spinal cord metastasis: Diagnostic and therapeutic considerations. Arch Neurol 44:526–531, 1987.

148. Wright, RL: Congenital dermal sinuses. Progress in Neurological Surgery 4:175–191, 1971.

149. Wyburn-Mason, R: Vascular Abnormalities and Tumors of the Spinal Cord and Its Membranes. Kimpton, London, 1943.

150. Yasargil, MG, Fiedeler, RW, and Rankin, ThP: Operative Treatment of Spinal Angioblastomas. In Pia, HW and Djindjian, R (eds): Spinal Angiomas: Advances in Diagnosis and Therapy. Springer-Verlag, Berlin, 1978, pp 171–188.

Chapter 7

NEOPLASTIC CAUSES OF SPINAL CORD COMPRESSION: LEPTOMENINGEAL METASTASES

Metastases to the leptomeninges from systemic malignancies or primary central nervous system neoplasms are a frequent cause of symptoms and signs of spinal cord and cauda equina dysfunction. Thus leptomeningeal cancer must be considered in the differential diagnosis of patients with these complaints and findings. This is especially true among patients with known malignancy because approximately 5 to 8 percent of patients dying of solid tumors develop leptomeningeal metastases.[30, 53]

CLINICAL ANATOMY

The spinal cord and spinal roots are surrounded by three meninges: the dura mater, arachnoid, and pia mater. The arachnoid and pia mater are collectively called the leptomeninges (Fig. 7–1; see Fig. 1–10).

The outermost covering, the dura mater, consists of a tough fibrous tissue that forms a barrier to prevent the invasion of neoplastic cells into the central nervous system. Despite the frequency of vertebral metastases with epidural extension, epidural neoplasms rarely breach the dura mater and enter the CNS. In cases of epidural tumors, therefore, the region of the nervous system jeopardized is that which is subject to compression, that is, the region adjacent to or underlying the tumor.

The leptomeninges are composed of the trabeculated arachnoid and pia mater. While the outer arachnoid membrane is apposed to the dura mater, the pia mater closely follows the contours of the cerebral cortex and spinal cord.[14] Within the brain and spinal cord, the pia mater merges with glial elements to form the pia-glial membrane.

The subarachnoid space is located between the outer arachnoid and the pia mater. In addition to containing cerebrospinal fluid (CSF), the subarachnoid space contains nerve roots, blood vessels, and connective tissue. As blood vessels penetrate the spinal cord, they are ensheathed by arachnoid and pia-glial tissues. A perivascular space, the Virchow-Robin space, is formed between the blood vessel and this adventitial sheath. This space has clinical significance because it is continuous with the subarachnoid space and, therefore, allows invasion of neoplastic cells deep into the substance of the spinal cord and brain.

The spinal roots are surrounded by sheaths of arachnoid and by extensions of the subarachnoid space that extend as far laterally as their exit from the vertebral canal. This also has clinical importance because leptomeningeal invasion can extend out in sheath-like fashion around the roots to this point.

Within the subarachnoid space, CSF flows freely from the ventricular system through the spinal axis to the region over the convexities of the cerebral hemi-

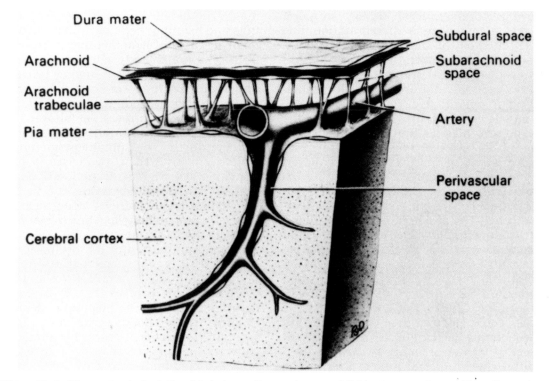

Figure 7—1. The anatomical relationship between the meninges and the brain parenchyma. (From Carpenter, MB, [14] with permission.)

spheres, where it is reabsorbed at the arachnoid villi of the dural sinuses. This unobstructed flow provides a pathway for the passage of neoplastic cells that have seeded any region of the subarachnoid space to spread throughout the neuraxis. With this spread, disturbances of cerebral, cranial nerve, and/or spinal functions are often encountered. Thus the clinical hallmark of leptomeningeal metastases is *multifocal neurological abnormalities* at different levels of the neuraxis.

PATHOGENESIS

The basic concepts underlying the metastatic process were discussed in Chapter 4. However, the specific mechanisms whereby malignant cells spread to the leptomeninges are important to review here because understanding them will aid the physician in the diagnosis and management of these patients.

Several mechanisms have been proposed to explain the pathogenesis of metastasis to the leptomeninges. The most frequent hypothesis suggests extension to the leptomeninges from a parameningeal site or via hematogenous routes. According to this hypothesis, neoplastic cells invade the leptomeninges from parameningeal foci such as brain or spinal cord parenchyma, the epidural space, choroid plexus, or bone marrow. In support of this explanation, it has been found that intraparenchymal CNS tumors such as malignant gliomas, ependymomas, medulloblastomas, and cerebral metastases may seed the leptomeninges.[23, 28, 37, 86] Leptomeningeal invasion also has been shown to occur via nerve roots from paravertebral locations and along vascular channels from bone marrow involvement.[33, 42] In cases of bone marrow involvement by lymphoma, epidemiological studies have demonstrated an increased risk of leptomeningeal metastases.[34, 40, 42] Metastatic involvement of the choroid plexus represents another access to seeding of the leptomeninges.[31]

Despite these reports, many patients with leptomeningeal metastases do not have a parameningeal tumor. In such cases, hematogenous dissemination has been cited as the most probable explanation.[77] There is strong experimental and clinicopathological support for this idea. In an experimental animal model, transvascular migration of leukemia cells has been shown to occur in arachnoidal veins in guinea pigs.[4] Clinicopathological reports have included a detailed histopathological study of the CNS of 126 children dying from leukemia.[59] Among the 70 cases with evidence of arachnoidal leukemia, the following pathogenesis was demonstrated: The arachnoidal veins bridging the subarachnoid space were the initial site of invasion by the leukemic cells; as the malignant cells invaded the supporting adventitia of the vessels, they extended into the CSF pathways of the subarachnoid space. Once in the CSF, the leukemic cells could follow the CSF pathways throughout the length of the neuraxis. Later, they were found to invade deep within the white and gray matter of the brain and spinal cord via the perivascular spaces. In the most advanced cases, direct invasion of the parenchyma of the brain and spinal cord was found when the pia-glial membrane was disrupted by the invading leukemic cells.

In addition to providing a route for CNS dissemination, the invasion of the blood vessels by malignant cells is significant in the pathogenesis of neurological symptoms and signs. Researchers found histopathological evidence of infarction and hemorrhage considered secondary to blood vessel invasion by leukemic cells.[59] A more recent report has shown that regional cerebral blood flow was diminished in nearly 90 percent of patients with leptomeningeal metastases.[67] Although the cause of reduced cerebral blood flow may be multifactorial, compression of blood vessels is one probable cause.

PATHOLOGICAL FINDINGS

The pathological findings of leptomeningeal metastases include diffuse and widespread multifocal infiltration of the leptomeninges. These findings are similar in cases of leptomeningeal metastases from solid tumors,[51] leukemia,[59] and lympho-

ma.[33] The detailed histopathological findings and extent of nervous system involvement in cases of leptomeningeal invasion from lymphoma and solid tumors have been reported in detail;[51] among 19 cases undergoing postmortem study, 15 demonstrated evidence of diffuse neoplastic involvement of the intracranial (supratentorial and infratentorial) and spinal leptomeninges. The spinal leptomeninges alone were involved in two cases, a phenomenon which has been described by others.[52] In two other cases, the basilar and spinal leptomeninges alone were involved. Intraparenchymal brain metastases were present in nearly half.

Gross examination of the brain, spinal cord, and roots often demonstrates tumor nodules studding these structures and the overlying leptomeninges (Fig. 7–2). Myelography is often very helpful in demonstrating these nodules in the cauda equina. In occasional cases, however, the leptomeninges may not reveal thickening on gross examination.[51]

Communicating hydrocephalus frequently has been found pathologically and clinically in cases of leptomeningeal metastases.[51] It is explained by the predilection of such metastases for the basilar meninges. The association between hydrocephalus and leptomeningeal metastases has been found for all types of cancer, but its pathogenesis was studied in a detailed report of patients (primarily children) with leukemia. In an autopsy study, Moore and colleagues[46] found that 75 percent of patients dying with leptomeningeal leukemia had communicating hydrocephalus at autopsy. The communicating hydrocephalus could not be explained on the basis of invasion of the pacchionian granulations in the dural sinuses or invasion of the choroid plexus; rather, it most closely correlated with the degree of arachnoidal and perivascular invasion of the basilar meninges. Thus the pathophysiology of communicating hydrocephalus may be explained by the obstruction of CSF flow caused by neoplastic infiltration of the basilar meninges. Clinically, communicating hydrocephalus may cause gait difficulties and sphincter disturbances that must be differentiated from spinal cord and cauda equina dysfunction.

The histopathological findings of lep-

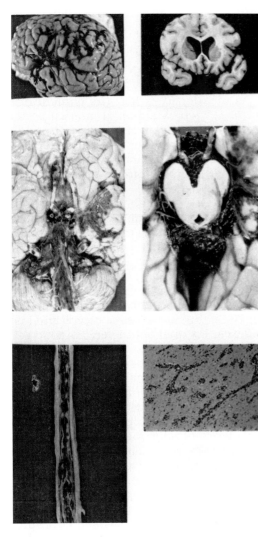

Figure 7–2. Leptomeningeal metastases due to melanoma. The pigmentation of the tumor identifies the regions where tumor is most heavily concentrated. (A) Lateral view of the cerebral hemisphere showing tumor concentrated in the Sylvian fissure and sulci. (B) Coronal section through the anterior portion of the Sylvian fissure demonstrates extension of leptomeningeal tumor into the brain parenchyma of both temporal cortices. The lateral ventricles are dilated secondary to communicating hydrocephalus. (C) The base of the brain is shown, with tumor involving several cranial nerves. (D) Transverse section through the midbrain showing tumor encircling brainstem at this level. (E) Anterior surface of the spinal cord demonstrates tumor on the surface of the cord and tumor nodules along nerve roots. (F) Microscopic section from a different patient with melanoma demonstrating tumor extending into the perivascular space deep within the basal ganglia. (From Olson, ME, Chernik, NL and Posner, JB,[51] with permission.)

tomeningeal metastases consist of sheets of tumor cells that are surrounded byfi-

brosis and generally a small amount of inflammation.[51] Tumor cells are often-found to congregate around spinal nerve roots. Although the cerebral convexities generally show less tumor involvement, the basilar meninges typically are heavily involved, as are the spinal cord and its nerve roots.

A histopathological study of leptomeningeal invasion by solid tumors[51] demonstrated (as in the case of leukemia[59]) that the brain and spinal cord parenchyma are invaded by tumor cells along the perivascular spaces. Invasion of the spinal parenchyma secondary to cancer in the leptomeninges was found in 4 of 40 cases of leptomeningeal metastases.[18] The intraparenchymal spinal cord extension occurred either secondary to invasion of the pia mater or from invasion along the perivascular spaces. Furthermore, along the spinal axis and basilar cisterns, tumor cells were found to encase and invade spinal roots and cranial nerve structures. Thus the histopathological findings in cases of leptomeningeal invasion from solid tumors and lymphoma are similar to those previously described in leptomeningeal leukemia.[46, 59]

PREVALENCE

The overall prevalence of leptomeningeal metastases among patients dying with systemic cancer appears to be approximately 5 to 8 percent.[53] The most common neoplasms that metastasize to the leptomeninges are breast and lung cancers, melanoma, non-Hodgkin's lymphoma, and leukemia.[42, 46, 51, 53, 77, 85] However, the prevalence of leptomeningeal metastases from individual neoplasms is difficult to ascertain because the evolution of therapy for primary tumors has been associated with a change in the frequency of metastases to the CNS.[57] For example, because the CNS represents a pharmacological sanctuary site,[12, 49, 63, 77, 83] the frequency of leptomeningeal leukemia dramatically increased as effective systemic treatments were developed for acute lymphoblastic leukemia.[85] Subsequently, with the advent of CNS prophylaxis for leptomeningeal leukemia, the frequency of this complication declined dramatically.[8, 12]

Although these evolving patterns must be considered, estimates of the risk for developing leptomeningeal metastases for individual tumors have emerged. Recent studies of small cell lung cancer have shown the risk to be approximately 9 to 18 percent.[3, 5, 63] Among patients receiving chemotherapy for breast cancer, approximately 5 percent developed leptomeningeal metastases.[83]

In cases of non-Hodgkin's lymphoma, the frequency of leptomeningeal metastases is quite variable; it has been reported to range from 5 to 29 percent[12, 34, 40, 41, 44, 56, 84] Several risk factors for involvement of the leptomeninges have been identified, including bone marrow and testicular involvement, extranodal disease, epidural invasion, diffuse histology, lymphoblastic lymphoma, and Burkitt's lymphoma.[13, 34, 40, 42, 56, 84]

The interval of time between the diagnosis of malignancy and the development of leptomeningeal metastases also is quite variable. Although leptomeningeal metastases usually occur in the setting of widespread systemic disease (as suggested by the risk factors identified above for non-Hodgkin's lymphoma), they may be present at the time of diagnosis of the primary tumor or even herald the presence of malignancy.[42, 63, 71, 77] Furthermore, because the CNS is a pharmacological sanctuary site, the leptomeninges may be the site of recurrence in the absence of other metastases, or may be affected while disease elsewhere is responding to chemotherapy.[5, 13, 42, 63, 71]

Leptomeningeal metastases may occur with or without coexisting intraparenchymal brain metastases or epidural spinal cord compression. The coexistence of these other metastases may make the clinical evaluation of these patients even more perplexing. For example, among a series of 90 patients with leptomeningeal metastases from solid tumors or lymphoma at Memorial Sloan-Kettering Cancer Center (MSKCC), one third had coexisting intraparenchymal brain metastases or epidural spinal cord compression;[77] one patient had all three conditions. The presence of intraparenchymal brain metastases may help support the clinical impression of leptomeningeal metastases or even an intramedullary spinal metastasis if cytologi-

cal and radiological confirmation is not forthcoming.[32, 79]

CLINICAL MANIFESTATIONS

As mentioned earlier, *the clinical hallmark of leptomeningeal metastases is multifocal involvement of the neuraxis at multiple levels.* Since conventional neurological teaching emphasizes the identification of a single anatomical lesion to explain the patient's entire neurological deficit, this may be a diagnostically challenging problem. For example, a patient with known malignancy may present with a chief complaint of back pain, gait difficulty, and burning dysesthesias of the lower extremities. Physical examination may reveal cognitive disturbances, facial asymmetry, asymmetric corneal responses, unilateral loss of biceps and knee reflexes, lax anal sphincter, apractic gait, and Babinski signs. In such a patient, although the history suggested spinal cord and/or cauda equina dysfunction alone, the physical examination may demonstrate evidence of dysfunction of the nervous system at multiple levels. Such multiple levels of neurological disturbance, in which more abnormal neurological signs than symptoms are found, are characteristic of leptomeningeal metastases.[77]

The symptoms and signs of patients with suspected leptomeningeal metastases may be classified as abnormalities of spinal and radicular function, meningeal inflammation and raised intracranial pressure, disturbances of cerebral function, and cranial nerve dysfunction.

Spinal/Radicular Symptoms and Signs

According to one detailed series from MSKCC, spinal and radicular symptoms and signs were present in 74 of 90 patients (82 percent) with leptomeningeal cancer[77] (Table 7–1). Lower extremity weakness was the most common symptom reported by patients. This weakness was of a lower motor neuron type and therefore was associated with depressed reflexes. The most common sign on physical examination (71 percent was reflex asymmetry.

Table 7–1 LEPTOMENINGEAL METASTASES FROM SOLID TUMORS IN 90 PATIENTS: SPINAL AND RADICULAR SYMPTOMS AND SIGNS*

Symptoms	Number of Patients (%)	
Lower motor neuron weakness	34	(38)
Paresthesias	31	(34)
Radicular pain	19	(21)
Back/neck pain	23	(25)
Bowel/bladder dysfunction	12	(13)
Signs	**Number of Patients (%)**	
Reflex asymmetry	64	(71)
Weakness	54	(60)
Sensory loss	24	(27)
Straight leg raising	11	(12)
Decreased rectal tone	10	(11)
Nuchal rigidity	7	(8)

*From Wasserstrom, WR, Glass, JP, and Posner, JB, [77] p 761, with permission.

Pain is a common presenting manifestation, reported in approximately one fourth of patients. The pain may be secondary to meningeal irritation or due to spinal/radicular compression. When the pain is radicular, it may mimic that of epidural metastasis or degenerative disc disease. As with other forms of neuropathic pain, it may be burning in character, or patients may describe the sensation of the extremity(ies) being wrapped.

Among all spinal roots, those of the cauda equina have the longest course in the subarachnoid space and are, therefore, commonly affected. In the MSKCC series,[77] one third of 90 patients with leptomeningeal metastases had signs of cauda equina dysfunction at the initial examination; it was the presenting complaint in approximately 20 percent of patients. The symptoms and signs of cauda equina dysfunction are usually a combination of sphincter disturbance, lower extremity weakness of a lower motor neuron type (that is, areflexic, hypotonic weakness), sensory loss in the lower extremities and sacral dermatomes over the buttocks, and pain in the back and lower extremities. The reflex abnormalities, weakness, and sensory loss are often asymmetric early in the course of the disease. It should be recalled that in a patient with cauda equina involvement, one would expect to find lower extremity weakness with depressed reflexes rather than hyperreflexia, which is typical of weakness due to upper motor neuron dysfunction. Alternatively, lower extremity weakness associated with asymmetric hyporeflexia may also be due to lumbosacral plexus disease or peripheral nerve disease. Furthermore, hyporeflexia in the cancer patient may be secondary to chemotherapy, such as vinca alkaloids. The peripheral neuropathy caused by these drugs, however, is usually symmetric, rather than markedly asymmetric as commonly found in patients with focal radiculopathies or peripheral nerve dysfunction. Paresthesias, which are also frequent radicular complaints, may be vague and unfamiliar to the patient and thus be dismissed by the patient or the physician. Finally, rectal tone is frequently diminished when the cauda equina is invaded by leptomeningeal metastases.

Cerebral Symptoms and Signs

Cerebral symptoms and signs were found in 45 of 90 patients (50 percent) in the MSKCC study of leptomeningeal metastases from solid tumors (Table 7–2).[77] Although they are not as common as spinal and root disturbances, their recognition should suggest the possibility of leptomeningeal metastases rather than epidural spinal cord compression alone.

Headache, which may be secondary to raised intracranial pressure or irritation of innervated structures, is the most common cerebral complaint. Mental status change and gait difficulties also were very common. The latter is of interest since a spinal disorder must also be considered when patients offer this complaint. The most common cerebral abnormality found on neurological examination was mental status change (lethargy, memory loss, and confusion). In addition to these bicerebral disturbances, focal cerebral dysfunction was found in the form of dysphasia, seizures, hemiparesis, hemisensory disturbances, visual loss, and diabetes insipidus. Other reports of such cases have

Table 7−2 LEPTOMENINGEAL
METASTASES FROM SOLID
TUMORS IN 90 PATIENTS:
CEREBRAL SYMPTOMS AND SIGNS*

Symptoms	Number of Patients (%)	
Headache	30	(33)
Mental change	15	(17)
Difficulty walking	12	(13)
Nausea/vomiting	10	(11)
Unconsciousness	2	(2)
Dysphasia	2	(2)
Dizziness	2	(2)

Signs	Number of Patients (%)	
Mental change	28	(31)
Seizures	5	(6)
Generalized	3	(3)
Focal	2	(2)
Papilledema	5	(6)
Diabetes insipidus	2	(2)
Hemiparesis	1	(1)

*From Wasserstrom, WR, Glass, JP, and Posner, JB, [77] p 760, with permission.

Table 7−3 LEPTOMENINGEAL
METASTASES FROM SOLID
TUMORS IN 90 PATIENTS:
CRANIAL NERVE SYMPTOMS
AND SIGNS*

Symptoms	Number of Patients (%)	
Diplopia	18	(20)
Hearing loss	7	(8)
Visual loss	5	(6)
Facial numbness	5	(6)
Decreased taste	3	(3)
Tinnitus	2	(2)
Hoarseness	2	(2)
Dysphagia	1	(1)
Vertigo	1	(1)

Signs	Number of Patients (%)	
Ocular muscle paresis (III, IV, VI)	18	(20)
Facial weakness (VII)	15	(17)
Diminished hearing (VIII)	9	(10)
Optic neuropathy (II)	5	(6)
Trigeminal neuropathy (V)	5	(6)
Hypoglossal neuropathy (XII)	5	(6)
Blindness	3	(3)
Diminished gag (IX, X)	3	(3)

*From Wasserstrom, WR, Glass, JP, and Posner, JB, [77] p 761, with permission.

found similar examples of cerebral disturbances.[42, 63, 82, 83] Finally, convulsive and nonconvulsive seizures may also be manifestations of cerebral involvement.[11]

Cranial Nerve Symptoms and Signs

Cranial nerve symptoms and signs were present in 50 of 90 patients (56 percent) with leptomeningeal metastases in the MSKCC series (Table 7−3).[77] While 38 percent of patients had cranial nerve symptoms as the presenting complaint, 56 percent had cranial nerve abnormalities at the time of diagnosis. Diplopia was overwhelmingly the most common of these symptoms; similarly, diplopia and dysconjugate gaze were the most common cranial nerve abnormalities among a group of patients with leptomeningeal lymphoma reported from Stanford.[42] Hearing loss and facial weakness are other common cranial neuropathies encounted.

Comparison of data presented in Tables 7−1 through 7−3 demonstrates that spinal/radicular symptoms and signs (present in 80 percent) were the most frequent

initial complaints and findings on neurological examination of patients with leptomeningeal metastases.[77] Lower extremity weakness, the most common of these, is among the most vexing to evaluate because it may be due to cerebral dysfunction, spinal cord disease, cauda equina or lumbosacral plexus dysfunction, peripheral neuropathy or non-neurological systemic causes. In evaluating gait difficulties in the oncology patient, one must especially consider the following etiologies: intraparenchymal brain metastases, epidural spinal cord compression, leptomeningeal metastases, peripheral neuropathy secondary to chemotherapy, cachexia, large tumor burden, and a variety of toxic-metabolic disturbances. More than one of these conditions may coexist in patients with leptomeningeal metastases. Many cancer patients will have had multiple forms of chemotherapy and be suffering from advanced cancer. In this clinical setting, the history and physical examination may be helpful but laboratory and diagnostic imaging studies usually are needed to confirm the clinical impression and exclude unexpected causes. To evaluate the spinal axis and exclude epidural spinal cord compression, which represents a medical emergency, myelography,[58, 62] CT scanning,[50, 61] and, most recently, MRI[19, 68, 74, 87] have been used. (See Chapter 5.)

LABORATORY AND DIAGNOSTIC IMAGING STUDIES

Cerebrospinal Fluid

Examination of the cerebrospinal fluid (CSF) is the single most useful laboratory test for the diagnosis of leptomeningeal metastases.[76, 77, 84] A lumbar puncture is routinely performed if there is no contraindication such as impending herniation from an intracranial mass or bleeding diathesis. In the setting of leptomeningeal metastases, the initial lumbar puncture CSF analysis usually reveals some abnormalities when tested for opening pressure, cell count, protein, glucose, and cytology. Although a CSF cytology that is positive for malignant cells is specific for leptomeningeal metastases, the other abnormalities often found, including an abnormally high opening pressure, elevated protein and/or white cell count, and a decrease in the CSF glucose, are nonspecific. The CSF findings in two series of patients with leptomeningeal invasion from solid tumors and from lymphoma are shown in Tables 7–4 and 7–5.

In the study of leptomeningeal metastases from solid tumors[77] (Table 7–4), among 90 patients with leptomeningeal cancer, all but 3 percent showed at least one abnormality on the initial routine CSF analysis. On repeated lumbar punctures, only one patient (1 percent) had persistently completely normal CSF analyses for all routine parameters. As in the case of lymphoma, however, false-negative CSF cytologies in such patients are commonly encountered. The initial CSF yielded a positive cytology in only 54 percent of cases. When multiple CSF analyses were performed, a positive cytology for malig-

nant cells was found in nearly 90 percent of cases; still, the diagnosis of leptomeningeal metastases from solid tumors could not be confirmed by CSF cytology in approximately 10 percent of patients. There were four cases in which the CSF cytology from the lumbar space was consistently negative but the ventricular fluid (two cases) or the cisternal fluid (two cases) yielded malignant cells. Others have reported variations in the yield of CSF cytology and other routine parameters as CSF is sampled at different levels of the neuraxis.[47]

In leptomeningeal lymphoma[84] (Table 7–5), the initial lumbar puncture was completely normal with regard to all routine parameters in only 3 percent of 33 patients. Although 97 percent of the patients showed some abnormality, the CSF cytology was diagnostic of lymphoma in only 54 percent of cases on the initial

Table 7–4 LEPTOMENINGEAL METASTASES FROM SOLID TUMORS IN 90 PATIENTS: CSF FINDINGS*

Parameter	Initial No. (%)	Total on All Punctures No. (%)
Pressure > 160 mm CSF	45 (50)	64 (71)
Cells > 5/mm³	51 (57)	65 (70)
Protein > 50 mg/dl	73 (81)	80 (89)
Glucose < 40 mg/dl	28 (31)	37 (41)
Positive cytology	49 (54)	82 (91)
Normal	3 (3)	1 (1)

*From Wasserstrom WR, Glass JP, and Posner JB,[77] p 762, with permission.

Table 7–5 CSF FINDINGS IN 33 PATIENTS WITH LEPTOMENINGEAL LYMPHOMA*

Positive Findings	On First Lumbar Puncture No. (%)	Total on All Punctures No. (%)
Pressure > 150 mm H_2O	17 (52)	22 (66)
White blood cells > 4/mm³	22 (67)	24 (73)
Positive cytology	18 (54)	22 (67)
Protein > 50 mg/100 ml	23 (70)	29 (88)
Glucose < 50 mg/100 ml	11 (33)	19 (58)
No abnormalities	1 (3)	0 (0)

*From Young, RC et al,[84] p 437, with permission).

lumbar puncture. Following repeated lumbar punctures, only 67 percent had a CSF cytology diagnostic of lymphoma; one third of patients had persistently negative CSF cytology. Others also have found a high incidence of a persistently false-negative CSF cytology despite involvement of the CNS from systemic lymphoma.[42]

The difficulties with regard to CSF cytological diagnosis of leptomeningeal leukemia are similar to those of lymphoma and other lymphoproliferative diseases; it is often difficult for the pathologist to distinguish reactive cells from leukemic cells.[25, 45, 59] Thus the brain, spinal cord, and nerve roots may be invaded by leukemic cells despite a negative CSF cytology in such cases.

The problem of "false-negative" CSF cytologies in patients with leptomeningeal metastases has been recognized since 1904.[22] Also, although most patients with malignant primary or metastatic intraparenchymal brain tumors have negative cytologies, occasionally the CSF of such patients reveals a positive cytology. Thus the clinical and pathological significance of a positive or negative CSF cytology under various circumstances needs to be defined.

Glass and colleagues[28] studied the correlation between CSF cytological examination during life and neuropathological findings at autopsy in an effort to determine the pathological significance and, therefore, the clinical implications of a positive CSF cytology. Among 66 patients in whom only parenchymal or dural neoplasms, without pathological evidence of leptomeningeal involvement, were found at autopsy, these authors found a positive CSF cytology in only one case. In this patient, the cytology reverted to negative while under treatment, suggesting that leptomeningeal disease may have been successfully eliminated prior to death. These findings suggest that a parenchymal primary or metastatic brain tumor will not yield a positive CSF cytology unless the leptomeninges have been seeded. Another study,[15] however, reported that parenchymal tumors could cause a positive CSF cytology without leptomeningeal seeding.

Glass and coworkers[28] also studied the rate of false-negative CSF cytologies in

cases of leptomeningeal metastases. Of 51 patients with pathologically proven leptomeningeal involvement, the CSF cytology was positive in 59 percent during life.[28] Furthermore, the frequency of positive CSF cytology correlated with the extent of leptomeningeal invasion. For example, among patients found to have only focal leptomeningeal invasion, CSF cytologies were positive in only 38 percent of cases, but they were positive in 66 percent of those with diffuse leptomeningeal metastases. Of the 30 patients who had a positive CSF cytology, 25 (83 percent) had diffuse leptomeningeal metastases at autopsy. These results suggest, therefore, that when a CSF cytological examination is found to have malignant cells, it can be inferred that the patient has a high probability of diffuse and multifocal leptomeningeal metastases.

Glass and colleagues[28] found a false-negative cytology in 21 (41 percent) of 51 patients with documented leptomeningeal disease at autopsy; among them were 13 cases with disseminated leptomeningeal spread. They concluded that *a negative CSF cytology does not exclude the presence of diffuse leptomeningeal spread,* a finding which has been corroborated by several other clinical studies.[25, 42, 51, 76, 77, 84]

On the issue of false-positive cytology, the same researchers[28] found two cases. Both patients had lymphoma and infection at the time of lumbar puncture; case one had sepsis and case two had herpes zoster. The reason for the false-positive cytologies was unknown but it has been reported by other authors in the setting of lymphoma and CNS infections.[20, 48, 60]

The question is often asked, "How many lumbar punctures should be performed when evaluating the patient suspected of having leptomeningeal metastases if the initial CSF cytology is negative?" As noted above, in the setting of solid tumors, of 90 patients with proven leptomeningeal cancer, the initial lumbar puncture yielded a positive cytology in 49 (54 percent); an additional 27 (30 percent) positive cytologies were found on the second lumbar puncture, and subsequent lumbar punctures yielded a positive cytology in two additional cases. The rate of persistently false-negative CSF cytologies was near 10 percent.[77] In the case of lymphoma, the rate of false-negative cytology may be somewhat higher.[42, 84] Therefore, when the diagnosis of leptomeningeal metastases is suspected, is the initial lumbar puncture is negative for malignant cells, it is generally recommended (if not contraindicated) that patients undergo a minimum of three lumbar punctures, if necessary, and that these samples for cytologic analysis be at least 5 to 10 cc each.[8, 42]

As noted above, the frequent finding of a false-negative CSF cytology for malignant cells in the setting of leptomeningeal lymphoma or leukemia is often a significant clinical problem. Monoclonal antibodies may be helpful in differentiating normal from malignant cells in the cerebrospinal fluid.[16, 17] Recently, monoclonal antibodies have identified inflammatory mononuclear cells in the cerebrospinal fluid as predominantly T cells.[45] Thus B-cell lymphoproliferative neoplasms involving the leptomeninges may be differentiated from reactive pleocytosis.[25] This technique may improve the ability to confirm leptomeningeal invasion in cases of lymphoproliferative disease.

BIOCHEMICAL MARKERS

There are several biochemical substances produced by neoplasms that could potentially be useful in early detection of malignancy. In the serum, perhaps the most commonly assayed is carcinoembryonic antigen (CEA), which has emerged as a useful marker to screen patients for recurrence of a variety of different neoplasms.[43] In the CSF, there have been several studies to determine if the measurement of CEA and other biochemical markers has any role in the evaluation and management of patients with suspected leptomeningeal invasion.[26, 54, 55, 64, 75, 80]

CEA is a glycoprotein produced by both normal and malignant cells.[43] Originally thought to be a specific marker for gastrointestinal malignancies,[29] it has more recently been recognized to be elevated in a variety of malignant and nonmalignant conditions.[43] It is usually detectable in the

serum of normal individuals at low concentrations. In the CSF of normal individuals it is either not detectable or found at only trace concentrations.[38, 64, 69] Despite earlier reports to the contrary,[70, 81] CEA has been found in the CSF of patients with serum CEA concentrations greater than 100 ng/ml; therefore, simultaneous measurement of plasma and cerebrospinal fluid CEA is recommended because at plasma levels greater than 100 ng/ml, CEA has been found to enter the CNS through an intact blood-brain barrier in the absence of CNS disease.[64]

Beta-glucuronidase is an intracellular enzyme that is normally present in both gray and white matter of the brain and is found in relatively high concentrations within the pia-arachnoid and choroid plexus.[64] It is not unexpected, therefore, for it to be found under normal conditions in the CSF.[1] In the presence of malignancy in the CNS, however, the level of beta-glucuronidase has been found to rise.[1] Further studies have shown that the level of CSF beta-glucuronidase is often elevated in the setting of leptomeningeal metastases but this elevation is not specific for this disease because elevated levels have also been found in cases of acute and chronic CNS infections.[64, 75]

Both CEA and beta-glucuronidase frequently have been studied in the CSF of patients suspected of having CNS metastases from adenocarcinoma, leukemia, lymphoma, and other malignancies.[64, 75, 80] Recent studies have shown that measurement of cerebrospinal fluid CEA may be useful in the evaluation of patients with leptomeningeal tumor.[64] Serial measurements of CEA may be useful in identifying patients with leptomeningeal relapse of breast cancer before other evidence of relapse.[80] Unlike beta-glucuronidase, CEA appears not to be consistently elevated in cases of chronic infectious meningitis.[64] It has been suggested that CSF, CEA, and beta-glucuronidase are both useful tumor markers for the detection of leptomeningeal metastases but not for intraparenchymal brain metastases or epidural tumor.[64] CSF levels of CEA were more accurate in detecting leptomeningeal metastases from lung carcinomas than those from breast cancer and melanoma. Neither

CSF CEA nor beta-glucuronidase has been found to be very sensitive in the diagnosis of leptomeningeal lymphoma, however.[64]

Other biochemical markers in the CSF have been studied. An abnormal lactic dehydrogenase (LDH) isoenzyme pattern was found in some individuals with leptomeningeal metastases.[77] The CSF LDH-5/LDH-1 ratio was abnormal in 15 of 20 patients with leptomeningeal cancer in whom it was assayed. An elevated CSF lactic acid also was found in many patients with leptomeningeal cancer, as compared with controls.

CSF and serum immunoglobulins and beta$_2$-microglobulin have been assayed in patients with neoplastic diseases involving the CNS. In patients with lymphoproliferative diseases and occasional patients with nonlymphoid neoplasms, researchers found several abnormalities involving CSF and serum oligoclonal bands and an elevated IgM index.[26] The results, however, were not sufficiently sensitive or specific to establish a diagnosis of CNS neoplastic involvement with certainty. They also found increased levels of beta$_2$-microglobulin in many cases of neoplastic involvement of the CNS.[26] However, this assay was associated with both false-positive and false-negative results. Furthermore, these authors found that the CSF beta$_2$-microglobulin level increased during intrathecal treatment and/or CNS irradiation. Finally, CSF levels of beta$_2$-microglobulin, the IgG index, and the IgM index rose in infectious complications in the CNS.

The cerebrospinal levels of vasopressin (ADH) and adrenocorticotrophic hormone (ACTH) have been assayed in patients suspected of harboring CNS metastatic disease from small-cell lung cancer.[54, 55] As with the other biochemical markers described, the utility of these assays has been questioned due to their lack of specificity and sensitivity in accurately diagnosing leptomeningeal metastases. Attempting to explain this lack, Pedersen and colleagues[55] have cited evidence suggesting that with regard to production of biochemical markers, many tumors may be polyclonal; different metastatic clones might produce varying quantities of biochemical markers, creating an inherent difficulty in reliable marker measurement. Thus, given the lack of specificity and sensitivity of the biochemical tumor markers in the evaluation of patients with suspected leptomeningeal metastases, they must be interpreted in the context of the other clinical and laboratory findings.

Diagnostic Imaging Studies

The most frequently used modalities for imaging the central nervous system are myelography, CT, and MRI. Myelography has been a frequently utilized imaging technique for visualizing leptomeningeal metastases.[42, 51, 77] Characteristic findings on myelography include thickening of nerve roots and nodules along the cauda equina due to metastases (Fig. 7–3.) Myelography was diagnostic in 13 of 49 patients in the MSKCC series.[77]

Although changes may be seen on contrast-enhanced head CT scanning, this modality has not been found to be sensitive in the diagnosis of leptomeningeal tumor.[24] The changes most frequently encountered are meningeal enhancement, obliteration of sulci and cisterns, ventriculomegaly, and enhancing cortical nodules.[36] Normal head CT scans, however, are often encountered in the presence of leptomeningeal metastases. One study[39] recently reported that contrast-enhanced cranial CT was normal in 44 percent of patients with leptomeningeal cancer. Spinal CT scanning following the introduction of intrathecal water-soluble contrast material may be more sensitive than myelography, however, in demonstrating the presence of nodules and thickening along nerve roots and the cauda equina.

The role of MRI in the diagnosis and management of leptomeningeal metastases is rapidly evolving. In a recent study,[21] noncontrast MRI of the brain was compared to contrast-enhanced cranial CT. Many abnormalities seen on CT, such as sulcal and cisternal enhancement and ependymal or subependymal metastases, were not as readily recognized on the noncontrast MRI, or could not be differentiated from radiation effects or ventriculomegaly alone. In the study cited above,[39] which compared cranial CT with nonen-

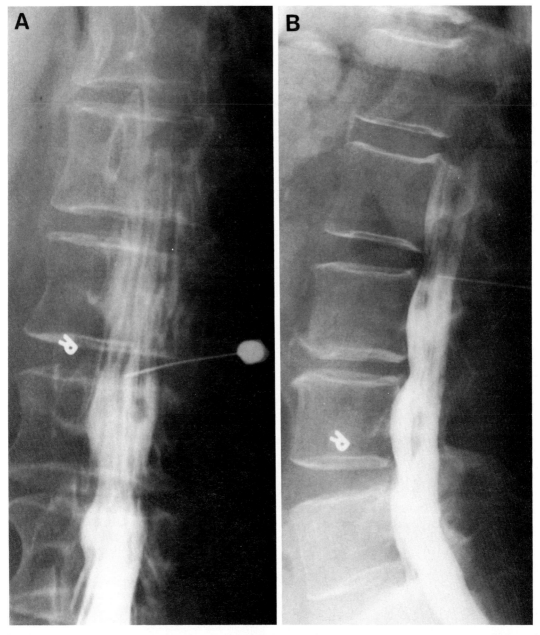

Fig. 7–3. Myelogram demonstrating leptomeningeal metastases from breast cancer. The patient had cauda equina symptoms and signs and the myelogram reveals metastatic nodules involving the cauda equina. (A) Anteroposterior view. The largest filling defect is seen just above the spinal needle. (B) Lateral view.

hanced cranial MRI in the evaluation of leptomeningeal cancer, nonenhanced MRI of the brain was normal in 65 percent of cases.

Similarly in the spine, noncontrast MRI has been found relatively insensitive in detecting leptomeningeal metastases.[39, 73] In a study of 16 patients undergoing myelography in the evaluation of leptomeningeal cancer, there were no false-negative myelograms; but with nonenhanced spinal MRI, definite abnormality of the subarachnoid space was found in only 27 percent of patients who had positive myelograms.[39] These authors state that high-grade obstruction or subarachnoid block due to leptomeningeal neoplasm may be present with no apparent alteration in the nonenhanced MR signal in the spinal canal.[39]

Alternatively, with the use of contrast-enhanced MRI with gadolinium-DTPA, leptomeningeal metastases are much more readily visualized (Fig. 7–4).[7, 72, 73] The sensitivity of gadolinium-enhanced MRI scans for leptomeningeal metastases appears to match that of myelography and postmyelography CT.[72] However, as in the case of myelography, the gadolinium-enhanced MRI may be normal in the setting of leptomeningeal metastases; thus CSF cytology continues to be helpful in the evaluation of these patients.[72] Further experience is needed with contrast-enhanced MRI to determine the full potential of this imaging modality in the evaluation of these patients.

Cerebral angiography occasionally may be helpful. It was abnormal in 4 of 11 patients in whom it was performed.[77] The most frequent abnormality was irregular narrowing of the blood vessels at the base of the brain. This finding, however, is not

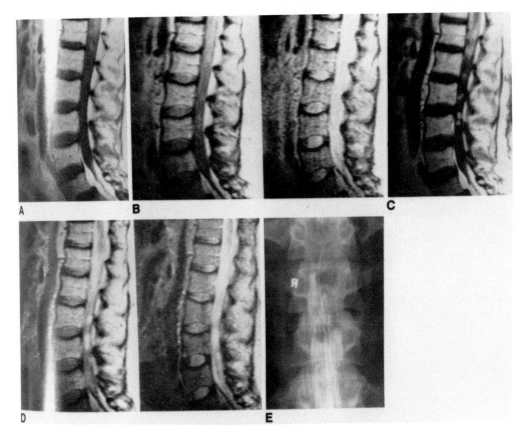

Figure 7–4. A 28-year-old man with known cerebral glioblastoma presenting with back pain and bilateral lower extremity weakness. The clinical history, examination, myelogram, and positive CSF cytology were all consistent with leptomeningeal metastases. Sagittal lumbar MR images are shown in A through D. (A) T1- weighted noncontrast image was considered negative except for poor definition of the conus and proximal nerve roots. In retrospect, vague nodules may be present in the subarachnoid space. (B) Proton-density (left panel) and T2-weighted (right panel) images were also considered equivocal; there was a suggestion of high intensity near the conus. (C) T1-weighted image after contrast administration shows enhancing subarachnoid tumor encasing the nonenhancing distal spinal cord. Multiple metastases are seen. (D) Proton-density (left panel) and T2-weighted (right panel) scans after contrast administration show that the lesions enhance (white nodular areas in the spinal canal). (E) Myelogram confirms the presence of multiple nodules and block at the level of the conus. (From Sze, G, et al,[73] with permission.)

specific for leptomeningeal metastases and may be difficult to differentiate from vasculitis. With the advent of contrast-enhanced MRI, the more invasive angiography is expected to be supplanted.

Although not specific, electrophysiological studies may occasionally help in evaluating patients with leptomeningeal metastases. The electroencephalogram may be diffuse or focally slow and seizure activity may be seen.[51] Electrophysiological studies of the peripheral nervous system (i.e., spinal roots) may identify subclinical abnormalities in these patients.

The following case illustrates the protean manifestations of leptomeningeal cancer and the difficulties sometimes encountered in confirming the diagnosis with laboratory methods.

Case Illustration

A 24-year-old man with a history of diffuse histiocytic lymphoma was referred for low back pain and gait difficulty. The patient reported that he had had intermittent but progressive low back pain for 3 to 4 weeks and during the past week developed left leg pain and most recently neck and right arm pain. His gait difficulty began 1 to 2 weeks previously. Initially he noted left leg numbness and weakness but more recently his right leg seemed to be getting weaker. In addition, there was some difficulty with the strength of his right hand. During the past two weeks he had also noted increasing difficulty sustaining an erection of his penis. He denied headache, diplopia, dysarthria, change in cognitive function, bowel or bladder difficulties, fever, chills, or other symptoms of infection.

His past medical history was significant only for lymphoma, which was originally diagnosed 18 months previously. He had received several cycles of chemotherapy, some of which had included vinca alkaloids. A recent extent of disease evaluation showed bone marrow involvement by lymphoma and enlarging retroperitoneal adenopathy.

Physical examination revealed a chronically ill young man with normal vital signs. He had palpable cervical and axillary adenopathy and an enlarged spleen. The remainder of the general physical examination was unremarkable. The neurological examination revealed a nor-

mal mental status, normal funduscopic examination, and normal cranial nerve function. The neck was supple and deep tendon reflexes were asymmetric, with the biceps and triceps reflexes absent on the right side but present on the left. Both brachioradialis reflexes were absent. The left patellar reflex was absent while being intact on the right. Both ankle jerks were depressed. No Babinski signs were elicited and the superficial abdominal reflexes were present and symmetric. The right upper extremity strength was 4/5 proximally and 4−/5 distally. The left leg strength was 4−/5 throughout and the right leg strength was 4/5. No fasciculations were seen and there was no atrophy. Sensory examination showed a stocking-glove sensory loss to pin, vibration, and temperature. There was also decreased pin sensation in the right proximal upper extremity and markedly decreased sensation over the sacral dermatomes of the buttocks. The anal sphincter was lax.

The clinical impression was that the patient had leptomeningeal metastases from lymphoma. Routine laboratory studies were unremarkable. Total spine films did not demonstrate a compression fracture or paravertebral mass. Because epidural spinal cord compression could not be excluded on the basis of the examination alone, the patient was treated with corticosteroids and a total spinal myelogram with metrizamide, was followed by CT scanning. There was no evidence of epidural tumor or leptomeningeal seeding on the radiological studies. The CSF studies revealed a protein of 84 mg per dl, glucose 51 mg per dl, 25 nucleated cells (1 percent polymorphonuclear cells, 90 percent lymphocytes, 9 percent monocytes). Cytology was negative for malignant cells and infectious disease studies (routine, AFB, fungal studies, and cryptococcal antigen) were all negative.

In the absence of laboratory confirmation of leptomeningeal metastases, the patient underwent two more lumbar punctures during the following week. In each case, there was persistent CSF pleocytosis, elevated protein, and negative cytology for malignant cells. The infectious disease workup was repeated (including serum Lyme titer and FTA-ABS) and again found to be negative. Repeat CSF examination showed glucose to be 50 and 38 mg per dl with simultaneous blood sugars of 90 and 110 mg per dl. During this period of time, the patient developed progressive bilateral upper extremity weakness and lower extremity weakness. The deep tendon reflexes that had been present initially were lost. He developed memory difficulties. He began to complain of diplopia and was found to have a partial left third nerve palsy with inability to adduct and elevate the eye. A questionable left facial paresis was also seen. A contrast-enhanced head CT scan was performed and was normal.

After one week of hospitalization, despite the lack of definitive laboratory confirmation, leptomeningeal lymphoma was considered the most likely diagnosis and treatment was initiated for this. Despite whole neuraxis radiation therapy and intrathecal chemotherapy (his CSF cytologies remained negative for malignant cells), his neurological condition deteriorated and he died two weeks later of respiratory failure.

At postmortem examination, this patient's leptomeninges were studded with lymphoma, with the heaviest concentration in the spinal axis. The cranial nerves were involved and lymphoma was found to cuff leptomeningeal blood vessels. Areas of cerebral infarction were seen on histopathological examination.

Comment. This case illustrates the difficulties often encountered in the evaluation of patients with leptomeningeal metastases. Initially only radicular abnormalities were found but with further observation, cranial nerve and cerebral symptoms and signs developed, which helped to confirm the clinical impression. The laboratory workup showed no definite signs of leptomeningeal lymphoma but the CSF was persistently abnormal in terms of cell count, protein, and glucose determinations. Thus, when the other causes of chronic meningitis were confidently excluded and the clinical examination confirmed the presence of multiple levels of neuraxis involvement, it was elected to treat this patient for leptomeningeal metastases. It should be noted that the clinical diagnosis also was supported by the histological type of lymphoma that showed bone marrow involvement, a risk factor for leptomeningeal invasion.

APPROACH TO THE PATIENT SUSPECTED OF HAVING LEPTOMENINGEAL METASTASES

As has been emphasized throughout this chapter, the clinical manifestations of leptomeningeal metastases are, by the very nature of the disease, multifocal and, therefore, protean. Occasional cancer patients with no neurological complaints undergo lumbar punctures for unrelated reasons and malignant cells are found. Patients may have solitary symptoms or signs as the initial manifestation of leptomeningeal involvement. In other cancer patients with multifocal involvement of the nervous system, there may be a high index of suspicion that the patient has leptomeningeal metastases, but the CSF may fail to reveal malignant cells that would confirm the clinical impression. Thus no single approach can be recommended. In the absence of definitive laboratory confirmation, only guidelines can be offered and the decision making and management modified on the basis of the patient's individual circumstances.

The diagnosis of leptomeningeal cancer is usually suspected in the cancer patient with the appropriate clinical history and examination. In addition to the clinical data, the clinician should consider the primary tumor type, the extent of disease elsewhere, and the risk factors for the development of leptomeningeal metastases; all of these factors may provide clinical evidence for or against the diagnosis. Laboratory data such as CSF cytology will usually confirm the clinical impression, but as seen above, CSF cytology may continue to be negative.

In the patient presenting with spinal symptoms and signs, leptomeningeal metastases may be considered if the patient has symptoms or signs of intracranial disease or other signs of multifocal involvement that cannot be explained on the basis of epidural spinal cord compression alone. In the setting of coexisting cerebral or cranial nerve disturbances, a head CT scan will identify a mass lesion or hydrocephalus. It also may demonstrate enhancing meningeal or superficial cortical nodules or basilar enhancement that may further suggest the diagnosis of leptomeningeal metastases.

If the clinical presentation suggests the possibility of epidural spinal cord compression, then plain films and MRI or myelography will identify an epidural mass. If myelography is performed, CSF may be obtained at the time of myelography. If MRI shows no epidural spinal cord or cauda equina compression to explain the patient's clinical findings, then (if there is no contraindication) a lumbar puncture with CSF studies sent for cell count, protein, glucose, cytology and infectious disease studies (including bacterial, AFB, fungal studies, cryptococcal antigen, and VDRL) may confirm the clinical impression of leptomeningeal metastases. If the initial cytology is negative, two or three repeat CSF analyses for routine studies, cytology, and infectious disease evaluation may be performed. If the CSF cytologies are persistently negative for malignant cells, and infectious etiologies (including Lyme disease and syphilis) and noninfectious causes of chronic meningitis[78] have been excluded, then, if not already performed, a contrast-enhanced MRI or myelogram may demonstrate multiple tumor nodules on nerve roots, providing evidence for the presence of leptomeningeal cancer.

If the diagnosis cannot be confirmed by laboratory studies, repeat CSF analyses and repeat head CT scans may be helpful. If the patient has leptomeningeal metastases, some laboratory evidence supporting this diagnosis is usually seen, such as a markedly depressed CSF glucose or persistent CSF pleocytosis, in the absence of infectious or other non-neoplastic etiology.

If the clinical evidence for leptomeningeal cancer is not strong, then relatively specific laboratory findings such as positive CSF cytology, enhancing metastases on CT scanning, or metastatic neoplasms on nerve roots should be demonstrated before a diagnosis is made.[77] Given the difficult diagnostic and management issues in cases where a definitive clinical and laboratory diagnosis is not forthcoming, it is recommended that consultation with an experienced neurological clinician and other specialists, as the circumstances indicate, be obtained.

THERAPY

Treatment of leptomeningeal metastases must be directed to both the intracranial compartment and spinal axis because malignant cells circulate throughout the entire subarachnoid space. Radiotherapy, intrathecal chemotherapy, and systemic chemotherapy have each been used alone and in combination.[8] For example, systemic high-dose methotrexate with leukovorin rescue[6] and high-dose cytosine arabinoside[27] have been used for leptomeningeal leukemia. Although radiotherapy is generally effective in treating leptomeningeal cancer, it usually cannot be delivered to the entire neuraxis without significant bone marrow suppression. Thus radiotherapy directed to symptomatic sites, in combination with intrathecal chemotherapy consisting of methotrexate, (ARA-C), cytosine arabinoside or thiotepa, is often used.

Intraventricular administration of chemotherapy provides better distribution of drug throughout the neuraxis than does intralumbar administration.[66] Two independent studies have shown the clinical advantage of intraventricular chemotherapy in overt leptomeningeal leukemia.[9, 65] In both studies, patients served as their own controls: In the first, the median duration of remission was increased from 9.5 months in the intralumbar-treated period to 16 months in the intraventricular-treated period (p < 0.05);[9] in the other study, the monthly incidence of CNS relapses in the intraventricular-treated period was one fourth that of the intralumbar-treated period (p < 0.05).[65]

In a randomized trial of intrathecal chemotherapy (methotrexate versus methotrexate plus cytosine arabinoside) for the treatment of leptomeningeal metastases from solid tumors in 42 patients,[35] 25 patients received chemotherapy via the lumbar route and 17 were treated via the intraventricular route. Twenty-two received CNS radiotherapy; 20 did not. Response was seen in 61 percent of those receiving methotrexate alone and 45 percent of those receiving methotrexate plus cytosine arabinoside (p > 0.1). Responses were found in 61 percent of those receiving intraventricular chemotherapy as compared with 45 percent of those receiving intralumbar chemotherapy (p > 0.1) Concurrent administration of CNS radiation therapy yielded a significantly better response than chemotherapy alone (73 percent vs. 35 percent; p < 0.05).

Toxicities from treatment include neurotoxicity, mucositis, and bone marrow suppression from radiotherapy and intrathecal chemotherapy. Acute and subacute neurotoxicity may be reduced by administering intraventricular chemotherapy according to a "concentration × time" regimen. For example, 1 mg of intraventricular methotrexate every 12 hours for 3 days rather than a single dose of 12 mg per m^2 intraventricular methotrexate results in a similar remission duration for some leptomeningeal neoplasms and less neurotoxicity.[10] Systemic toxicities from intrathecal methotrexate may also be reduced by administering oral or parenteral leukovorin.

The treatment of leptomeningeal metastases and toxicities associated with various forms of therapy (e.g., leukoencephalopathy) have been recently reviewed.[8] The median survival of patients with leptomeningeal metastases from solid tumors has been reported to be 4 to 6 months.[8, 77]

REFERENCES

1. Allen, N and Reagan, E: Beta-glucuronidase activities in cerebrospinal fluid. Arch Neurol 11:144–154, 1964.
2. Argov, Z and Siegal, T: Leptomeningeal metastases: Peripheral nerve and root involvement—clinical and electrophysiological study. Ann Neurol 17:593–596, 1985.
3. Aroney, RS, Dalley, DN, Chan, WK, Bell, DR, and Levi, JA: Meningeal carcinomatosis in small cell carcinoma of the lung. Am J Med 71:26–32, 1981.
4. Azzarelli, B, Mirkin, LD, Goheen, M, Muller, J, and Crockett, C: The leptomeningeal vein: A site of re-entry of leukemic cells into the systemic circulation. Cancer 54:1333–1343, 1984.
5. Balducci, L, Little, DD, Khansur, T, and Steinberg, MH: Carcinomatous meningitis in small cell lung cancer. Am J Med Sci 287:31–33, 1984.
6. Balis, FM, Savitch, J, Reaman, G, and others: Remission induction of meningeal leukemia with high-dose intravenous methotrexate. J Clin Oncol 3:485–489, 1985.
7. Barloon, TJ, Yuh, WTC, Yang, CJC, and Schultz, DH: Spinal subarachnoid tumor seeding from intracranial metastasis: MR findings. J Comput Assist Tomogr 11:242–244, 1987.
8. Bleyer, WA and Byrne, TN: Leptomeningeal cancer in leukemia and solid tumors. Current Problems in Cancer 12:185–238, 1988.
9. Bleyer, WA and Poplack, DG: Intraventricular versus intralumbar methotrexate for central nervous system leukemia. Med Pediatr Oncol 6:207–213, 1979.
10. Bleyer, WA, Poplack, DG, and Simon, RM: "Concentration × Time" methotrexate via a subcutaneous reservoir: A less toxic regimen for intraventricular chemotherapy of central nervous system neoplasms. Blood 51:835–842, 1978.
11. Broderick, JP and Cascino, TL: Nonconvulsive status epilepticus in a patient with leptomeningeal cancer. Mayo Clin Proc 62:835–837, 1987.
12. Bunn, PA, Schein, PS, Banks, PM, and DeVita, VT: Central nervous system complications in patients with diffuse histiocytic and undifferentiated lymphoma: Leukemia revisited. Blood 47:3–10, 1976.
13. Cairncross, JG and Posner, JB: Neurological complications of malignant lymphoma. In Vinken, PJ and Bruyn, GW (eds): Handbook of Clinical Neurology, Vol 39. North-Holland Publishing, Amsterdam, 1980, pp 27–62.
14. Carpenter, MB: Meninges and cerebrospinal fluid. In Carpenter, MB (ed): Human Neuroanatomy. Williams & Wilkins, Baltimore, 1976, pp 1–19.
15. Choi, HH and Anderson, PJ: Diagnostic cytology of cerebrospinal fluid by the cytocentrifuge method. Am J Clin Pathol 72:931–943, 1979.
16. Coakham, HB, Brownell, B, Harper, EI, Garson, JA, Allen, PM, Lane, EB, and Kemshead, JT: Use of monoclonal antibody panel to identify malignant cells in cerebrospinal fluid. Lancet 1:1095–1097, 1984.
17. Coakham, HB, Harper, EI, Garson, JA, Brownell, B, and Lane, EB: Carcinomatous meningitis diagnosed with monoclonal antibodies. Br Med J 288:1272, 1984.
18. Costigan, DA and Winkelman, MD: Intramedullary spinal cord metastasis: A clinicopathological study of 13 cases. J Neurosurg 62:227–233, 1985.
19. Daffner, RH, Lupetin, AR, Dash, N, Deeb, ZL, Sefczek, RJ, and Schapiro, RL: MRI in detection of malignant infiltration of bone marrow. AJR 146:353–358, 1986.
20. Davies, SF, Gormus, BJ, Yarchoan, R, et al: Cryptococcal meningitis with false-positive cytology in the CSF: Use of T-cell rosetting to exclude meningeal lymphoma. JAMA 239:2369–2370, 1978.
21. Davis, PC, Friedman, NC, Fry, SM, Malko, JA, Hoffman, JC, and Braun, IF: Leptomeningeal metastasis: MR imaging. Radiology 163:449–454, 1987.
22. Dufour, MH: Meningite sarcomateuse diffuse avec encahissement de la moelle et des racines: Cytologie positive et special du liquide cephaloradichien. Rev Neurol (Paris) 12:104–106, 1904.

23. Edwards, MS, Levin, VA, Seager, ML, and Wilson, CB: Intrathecal chemotherapy for leptomeningeal dissemination of medulloblastoma. Childs Brain 8:444–451, 1981.

24. Enzmann, DR, Krikorian, J, Yorke, C, and Hayward, R: Computed tomography in leptomeningeal spread of tumor. J Comput Assist Tomgr 2:448–455, 1978.

25. Ernerudh, J, Olsson, T, Berlin, G, Gustafsson, B, and Karlsson, H: Cell surface markers for diagnosis of central nervous system involvement in lymphoproliferative diseases. Ann Neurol 20:610–615, 1986.

26. Ernerudh, J, Olsson, T, Berlin, G. and von Schenck, H: Cerebrospinal fluid immunoglobulins and beta$_2$-microglobulin in lymphoproliferative and other neoplastic diseases of the central nervous system. Arch Neurol 44:915–920, 1987.

27. Frick, J, Ritch, PS, Hansen, RM, et al: Successful treatment of meningeal leukemia using systemic high-dose cytosine arabinoside. J Clin Oncol 2:365–368, 1984.

28. Glass, JP, Melamed, M, Chernik, NL, and Posner, JF: Malignant cells in cerebrospinal fluid (CSF): The meaning of a positive CSF cytology. Ann Neurol 29:1369–1375, 1979.

29. Gold, P and Freeman, SO; Demonstration of tumor-specific antigens in human colonic carcinomata by immunologic tolerance and absorption techniques. J Exp Med 121:439–466, 1965.

30. Gonzalez-Vitale, JC and Garcia-Bunuel, R: Meningeal carcinomatosis. Cancer 37:2906–2911, 1976.

31. Grain, GO and Karr, JP: Diffuse leptomeningeal carcinomatosis. Clinical and pathologic characteristics. Neurology 5:706–722, 1955.

32. Grem, JL, Burgess, J, and Trump, DL: Clinical features and natural history of intramedullary spinal cord metastasis. Cancer 56:2305–2314, 1985.

33. Griffin, JW, Thompson, RW, and Mitchinson, MJ: Lymphomatous leptomeningitis. Am J Med 51:200–208, 1971.

34. Herman, TS, Hammond, N, Jones, SE, et al: Involvement of the central nervous system by non-Hodgkin's lymphoma: The Southwest Oncology Group experience. Cancer 43:390–397, 1979.

35. Hitchins, RN, Bell, DR, Woods, RL, et al: A prospective randomized trial of single-agent versus combination chemotherapy in meningeal carcinomatosis. J Clin Oncol 5:1655–1662, 1987.

36. Jaeckle, KA, Krol, G, and Posner, JB: Evolution of computed tomographic abnormalities in leptomeningeal metastases. Ann Neurol 17:85–89, 1985.

37. Johnson, DL and Schwarz, S: Intracranial metastases from malignant spinal-cord astrocytoma: Case report. J Neurosurg 66:621–625, 1987.

38. Kido, D, Dyce, B, Haverback, BJ, and Rumbaugh, C: Carcinoembryonic antigen in patients with untreated central nervous system tumors. Bulletin of the Los Angeles Neurological Society 41:47–54, 1976.

39. Krol, G, Sze, G, Malkin, M, and Walker, R: MR of cranial and spinal meningeal carcinomatosis: Comparison with CT and myelography. AJR 151:583–588, 1988.

40. Levitt, LJ, Dawson, DM, Rosenthal, DS, et al: CNS involvement in non-Hodgkin's lymphomas. Cancer 45:545–552, 1980.

41. Litam, JP, Cabanillas, F, Smith, TL, et al: Central nervous system relapse in malignant lymphomas: Risk factors and implications for prophylaxis. Blood 54:1249–1257, 1979.

42. Mackintosh, FR, Colby, TV, Podolsky, WJ, et al: Central nervous system involvement in non-Hodgkin's lymphoma: An analysis of 105 cases. Cancer 49:586–595, 1982.

43. McIntire, KR: Tumor markers. In DeVita Jr, VT, Helman, S, and Rosenberg, SA (eds): Cancer: Principles and Practice of Oncology. JB Lippincott, Philadelphia, 1985, pp 375–388.

44. Mead, GM, Kennedy, P, Smith, JL, Thompson, J, Macbeth, FRM, Ryall, RDH, Williams, CJ, and Whitehouse, JMA: Involvement of the central nervous system by non-Hodgkin's lymphoma in adults: A review of 36 cases. Q J Med 60:699–714, 1986.

45. Moench, TR and Griffin, DE: Immunocytochemical identification and quantitation of the mononuclear cells in cerebrospinal fluid, meninges, and brain during acute viral meningoencephalitis. J Exp Med 159:77–88, 1984.

46. Moore, EW, Freireich, EJ, Shaw, RK, and Thomas, LB: The central nervous system in acute leukemia. Arch Intern Med 105: 451–467, 1960.

47. Murray, JJ, Greco, FA, Wolff, SN, and Hainsworth, JD: Neoplastic meningitis: Marked variations of cerebrospinal fluid composition in the absence of extradural block. Am J Med 75:289–294, 1983.

48. Naylor, B: The cytologic diagnosis of cerebrospinal fluid. Acta Cytol 8:141–149, 1964.

49. Nugent, JL, Bunn, PA, Matthews, MJ, et al: CNS metastases in small cell bronchogenic carcinoma—increasing frequency and changing patterns with lengthening survival. Cancer 44:1885–1893, 1979.

50. O'Rourke, T, George, CB, Redmond, J, et al: Spinal computed tomography and computed tomographic metrizamide myelography in the early diagnosis of metastatic disease. J Clin Oncol 4:576–583, 1986.

51. Olson, ME, Chernik, NL, and Posner, JB: Infiltration of the leptomeninges by systemic cancer: A clinical and pathologic study. Arch Neurol 30:122–137, 1974.

52. Parsons, M: The spinal form of carcinomatous meningitis. Q J Med 41:509–518, 1972.

53. Patchell, RA and Posner, JB: Neurologic complications of systemic cancer. Neurol Clin 3:729–750, 1985.

54. Pedersen, AG, Hammer, M, Hansen, M, and Sorensen, PS: Cerebrospinal fluid vasopressin as a marker of central nervous system

metastases from small-cell bronchogenic cancer. J Clin Oncol 3:48–53, 1985.

55. Pedersen, AG, Hansen, M, Hummer, L, and Rogowski, P: Cerebrospinal fluid ACTH as a marker of central nervous system metastases from small cell carcinoma of the lung. Cancer 56:2476–2480, 1985.

56. Perez-Soler, R, Smith, TL, and Cabanillas, F; Central nervous system prophylaxis with combined intravenous and intrathecal methotrexate in diffuse lymphoma of aggressive histologic type. Cancer 57:971–977, 1986.

57. Posner, JB: Neurologic complications of systemic cancer. DM 25:1–60, 1978.

58. Posner, JB: Back pain and epidural spinal cord compression. Med Clin North Am 71:185–204, 1987.

59. Price, RA and Johnson, WW: The central nervous system in childhood leukemia: I. The arachnoid. Cancer 31:520–533, 1973.

60. Rawlinson, DG, Billingham, ME, Berry, PF, et al: Cytology of the cerebrospinal fluid in patients with Hodgkin's disease or malignant lymphoma. Acta Neuropathol (Berlin) (Suppl)VI:187–191, 1975.

61. Redmond, J, Freidl, KE, Cornett, P, Stone, M, O'Rourke, T, and George, CB: Clinical usefulness of an algorithm for the early diagnosis of spinal metastatic disease. J Clin Oncol 6:154–157, 1988.

62. Rodichok, LD, Ruckdeschel, JC, Harper, GR, et al: Early detection and treatment of spinal epidural metastases: The role of myelography. Ann Neurol 20:696–702, 1986.

63. Rosen, ST, Aisner, J, Makuch, RW, et al; Carcinomatous leptomeningitis in small cell lung cancer: A clinicopathologic review of the National Cancer Institute experience. Medicine 61:45–53, 1982.

64. Schold, SC, Wasserstrom, WR, Fleisher, M, Schwartz, MK, and Posner, JB: Cerebrospinal fluid biochemical markers of central nervous system metastases. Ann Neurol 8:597–604, 1980.

65. Shapiro, WR, Posner, JB, Ushio, Y, et al: Treatment of meningeal neoplasms. Cancer Treat Rep 61:733–743, 1977.

66. Shapiro, WR, Young, DF, and Mehta, BM: Methotrexate: Distribution in cerebrospinal fluid after intravenous, ventricular and lumbar injections. N Engl J Med 293:161–166, 1975.

67. Siegal, T, Mildworf, B, Stein, D, and Melamed, E: Leptomenigeal metastases: Reduction in regional cerebral blood flow and cognitive impairment. Ann Neurol 17:100–102, 1985.

68. Smoker, WRK, Godersky, JC, Knutzon, RK, Keyes, WD, Norman, D, and Bergman, W: The role of MR imaging in evaluating metastatic spinal disease. AJR 149:1241–1248, 1987.

69. Snitzer, LS and McKinney, E: Carcinoembryonic antigen in cerebrospinal fluid (abstr). Proceedings of the American Society for Clinical Oncology 17:249, 1976.

70. Snitzer, LS, McKinney, EG, Tejada, F, Seigel, M, Rosomoff, H, and Zubrod, G; Cerebral metastases and carcinoembryonic antigen in CSF (letter). N Engl J Med 293:1101, 1975.

71. Sorensen, SC, Eagen, RT, and Scott, M: Meningeal carcinomatosis in patients with primary breast or lung cancer. Mayo Clin Proc 59:91–94, 1984.

72. Sze, G: Gadolinium-DTPA in spinal disease. Radiol Clin North Am 26:1009–1024, 1988.

73. Sze, G, Abramson, A, Krol, G, et al: Gadolinium-DTPA in the evaluation of intradural extramedullary spinal disease. AJNR 9:153–163, 1988.

74. Sze, G, Krol, G, Zimmerman, RD, and Deck, MDF: Gadolinium-DTPA: Malignant extradural spinal tumors. Radiology 167:217–223, 1988.

75. Tallman, RD, Kimbrough, SM, O'Brien, JF, Goellner, JR, and Yanagihara, T: Assay for beta-glucuronidase in cerebrospinal fluid: Usefulness for the detection of neoplastic meningitis. Mayo Clin Proc 60:293–298, 1985.

76. Theodore, WH and Gendelman, S: Meningeal carcinomatosis. Arch Neurol 38:696–699, 1981.

77. Wasserstrom, WR, Glass, JP, and Posner, JB: Diagnosis and treatment of leptomeningeal metastases from solid tumors: Experience with 90 patients. Cancer 49:759–772, 1982.

78. Wilhelm, C and Ellner, JJ: Chronic meningitis. Neurol Clin 4:115–141, 1986.

79. Winkelman, MD, Adelstein, DJ, and Karlins, NL: Intramedullary spinal cord metastasis: Diagnostic and therapeutic considerations. Arch Neurol 44:526–531, 1987.

80. Yap, B-S, Yap, H-Y, Fritsche, HA, Blumenschein, G, and Bodey, GP; CSF carcinoembryonic antigen in meningeal carcinomatosis from breast cancer. JAMA 244:1601–1603, 1980.

81. Yap, B-S, Yap, H-Y, Benjamin, RS, Bodey, GP, and Freireich, EJ: Cerebrospinal fluid carcinoembryonic antigen in breast cancer patients with meningeal carcinomatosis (abstr). Proceedings of the American Society for Clinical Oncology 19:98, 1978.

82. Yap, H, Tashima, CK, Blumerschein, GR, and Eckles, N: Diabetes inspidus in breast cancer. Arch Intern Med 139:1009–1011, 1979.

83. Yap, H-Y, Seng, B-S, Tashima, CK, DiStefano, A, and Blumenschein, GR: Meningeal carcinomatosis in breast cancer. Cancer 42:283–286, 1978.

84. Young, RC, Howser, DM, Anderson, T, and others: Central nervous system complications of non-Hodgkin's lymphoma. Am J Med 66:435–443, 1979.

85. Yuill, GM: Leukemia: Neurologic involvement. In Vinken, PJ and Bruyn, GW (eds): Handbook of Clinical Neurology, Vol 39. North-Holland Publishing, Amsterdam, 1980, pp 1–25.

86. Yung, W-K, Horten, BC, and Shapiro, WR: Meningeal gliomatosis: A review of 12 cases. Ann Neurol 8:605–608, 1980.

87. Zimmer, WD, Bergquist, TH, McLeod, RA, et al: Bone tumors: Magnetic resonance imaging versus computed tomography. Radiology 155:709–718, 1985.

Chapter 8

NONCOMPRESSIVE
MYELOPATHIES
SIMULATING SPINAL
CORD
COMPRESSION

There are many forms of myelopathy due to causes other than compressive lesions. Table 8–1 lists some of those forms of myelopathy that must be considered in the differential diagnosis of spinal cord compression. This chapter reviews the clinical features of the more common causes of noncompressive myelopathy.

TRANSVERSE AND ASCENDING MYELITIS

We first consider postinfectious or parainfectious myelitis, postvaccination myelitis, multiple sclerosis, and acute and subacute necrotizing myelitis.[6, 65, 103] Collectively, these diseases of unknown etiology are the most common causes of acute transverse myelitis and ascending myelitis.[28, 196] Although each may have a different antecedent, these diseases share a similar pathology and are thought to have an inflammatory pathogenesis. Unlike the viral myelitides, which show a predilection for the gray matter, this group of diseases usually involves white matter tracts, or both white and gray matter (transverse myelopathy).[6, 28]

Postinfectious and Postvaccination Myelitis

Although the antecedent conditions are separable, postinfectious (sometimes termed parainfectious) myelitis shares a very similar clinical course and pathology with that of postvaccination myelitis.[89, 126, 153, 161, 239] Some of the exanthematous infections and vaccinations that are antecedents to myelitis are shown in Table 8–2. Although the most common antecedent infections are viral illnesses, bacterial mycoplasma[147] and other infections may also trigger myelitis.[45, 110, 158, 161, 183, 225, 270] In many cases, a myelopathy clinically and pathologically indistinguishable from postinfectious myelitis occurs without an apparent infection or vaccination.[28]

PATHOGENESIS

It is now recognized that postinfectious and postvaccination myelitis are not due to viral invasion of the central nervous system but that, on the contrary, immunological mechanisms play an important role in pathogenesis of the myelitis.[162, 204] Although the precise mechanisms of CNS injury are unknown, the histopathological similarity between postinfectious and postvaccination myelitis and experimental allergic encephalomyelitis has suggested to many investigators that an autoimmune response to a CNS antigen such as myelin basic protein may be responsible.[198, 202, 203, 270] Alternatively, it has been suggested that circulating immune complexes may play a role in the pathogenesis of these disorders by inducing a vascular injury.[202, 203] The time interval between exposure to the infection or vaccination and the development of the neurological

Table 8–1 NON-COMPRESSIVE CAUSES OF MYELITIS AND MYELOPATHY*

Postinfectious or Parainfectious Myelitis
Postvaccinal
"Influenzal" and subsequent to viral infection
Spontaneous acute myelitis (acute disseminated encephalomyelitis of unknown cause)
Demyelinating Myelitis of Unknown Etiology
Multiple sclerosis
Neuromyelitis optica
Acute necrotizing myelitis
Primary Infectious Myelitis
Viral Myelitides
Poliomyelitis
Postpoliomyelitis syndrome
Myelitis with acute viral encephalomyelitis
Herpes zoster
Rabies
Subacute myoclonic spinal neuronitis
HTLV-1
AIDS myelopathy
Bacterial and Spirochetal Myelitides
Acute suppurative myelitis with spinal abscess
Tuberculoma of spinal cord
Syphilitic myelitis
Lyme disease
Rickettsial, fungous, and parasitic myelitides
Typhus and spotted fever
Actinomycosis, coccidioidomycosis, aspergillosis, torulosis
Trichinosis, falciparum malaria, schistosomiasis
Myelopathy Secondary to Acute Intraspinal Infection
Acute bacterial meningitis
Tuberculous meningitis
Toxic Myelopathy
Ortho-cresyl phosphate
Following aortography
Arsenic
Lathyrism
Organic iodide contrast media
Penicillin
Spinal anesthetics and arachnoiditis
Myelopathy Owing to Physical Agents
Irradiation
Electrical injury to the central nervous system
Metabolic and Nutritional Myelopathy
Diabetes mellitus
Cyanocobalamin deficiency
Pellagra
Complex deficiencies without single identified nutrient
Myelopathy of chronic liver disease
Myelopathy Owing to Diseases of the Blood Vessels
Arteriosclerosis
Dissecting aortic aneurysm
Coarctation of the aorta
Periarteritis nodosa
Systemic lupus erythematosus
Sjogren's syndrome
Vascular malformations of the spinal cord
Paraneoplastic myelopathy

*Adapted from Plum, F and Olson, ME. [196]

Table 8–2 SOME ANTECEDENTS TO PARAINFECTIOUS MYELITIS

Viral Disease
Rubeola (measles)
Rubella (German measles)
Mumps
Influenza
Mycoplasma pneumonia
Infectious mononucleosis
Varicella
Vaccinations
Tetanus
Poliomyelitis
Rabies
Smallpox

disorder varies but is commonly 7 to 10 days.[196]

PATHOLOGY

The clinical manifestations of postinfectious and postvaccination myelitis usually include symptoms, signs, and/or laboratory evidence of brain involvement. However, in occasional cases the spinal cord is the predominant (or only) site of involvement. In such cases, although the clinical examination may only reveal signs of myelopathy, both the brain and spinal cord usually are involved on pathological examination.

As noted above, the pathological findings of postinfectious and postvaccination myelitis are the same.[47, 198] On gross examination the spinal cord may be normal or swollen. On histopathological inspection of gray and white matter, the most prominent findings are found in the blood vessels and the perivascular regions.[103] Hyperemia, perivascular cellular exudate and edema, and hemorrhage usually are found around arterioles, venules, and capillaries.[161, 198] The perivenous areas infiltrated by inflammatory cells typically show regions of demyelination that may coalesce with other areas so that the perivascular localization is not apparent. In regions of severe inflammation, necrosis may be seen.[103, 105, 204]

CLINICAL FEATURES

The clinical features of postinfectious and postvaccination myelitis are highly variable. Systemic symptoms including fever, malaise, nausea, vomiting, and muscular aching, suggesting an infectious etiology, may appear first. When the spinal cord is the major clinical site of neurological involvement, paresthesias may be reported in the lower extremities. Although back pain and/or radicular pain may herald the illness, the myelopathy may develop without pain.

Any level of the spinal cord may be involved, but the thoracic region is the most frequent. The myelopathy may be accompanied, or occasionally preceded by, a polyradiculopathy. Symptoms and signs of cord involvement usually evolve acutely, with the majority of patients developing maximal neurological deficit within several days. The specific signs (weakness, sensory loss, and sphincter dysfunction) are dependent upon the tracts involved and whether the involvement is transverse, ascending, or multifocal.

Routine laboratory studies are usually normal or nonspecific. The CSF may be normal, but typically shows a moderate lymphocytic pleocytosis. Other signs of CNS inflammation may include a slightly elevated protein (usually less than 120 mg/deciliter) and elevated IgG and the presence of oligoclonal bands.[196, 204] If polyradiculitis is part of the clinical presentation, or if there is a subarachnoid block secondary to cord swelling, then the protein may be further elevated. The CSF glucose concentration is normal.[196] CT scan may be normal or may reveal multiple contrast-enhancing lesions in the cortex and/or periventricular areas when the brain is involved.[144] MRI of the brain may reveal areas of demyelination.[68] The role of spinal MRI, especially with contrast agents, appears to be promising.

THERAPY

Although there is no specific therapy shown to be effective in the vast majority of cases of postinfectious/postvaccination myelitis, the use of corticosteroids, or ACTH has been helpful for many.[6] Many physicians prescribe oral corticosteroids (e.g., 1 mg/kg/day prednisone) for a two-week period, followed by tapering off over one week.[256] Alternatively, parenteral corticosteroids may be used. If corticosteroids are used, attention should be directed to untoward effects including mental status changes, hypertension, glucose intolerance, immunosuppression, impaired wound healing, and possible gastrointestinal bleeding.

Urinary retention may require intermittent catheterization or an indwelling catheter, and careful attention is needed to prevent development of a urinary tract infection. If bladder dysfunction persists, urodynamic studies usually are undertaken to determine the specific mechanism of impairment. Constipation is a common problem and may be due to ileus. When the ileus has resolved and oral feedings have resumed, a stool softener or enemas may be needed. Attention also must be given to preventing skin breakdown, as in other patients with spinal cord injury.

Multiple Sclerosis

The clinical manifestations of multiple sclerosis are protean. Although the history, findings on neurological examination, or laboratory studies (MRI or evoked responses) often demonstrate a multifocal distribution of lesions, the spinal cord is a common site of initial clinical involvement. In one series,[67] for example, sensory cord symptoms (43 percent) were the most common presenting complaint (Table 8–3). Other spinal symptoms such as Lhermitte's sign, gait difficulties, extremity weakness, and sphincter disturbances also were very common, so that the spinal cord was considered the site of initial involve-

Table 8–3 INITIAL SYMPTOMS OF MULTIPLE SCLEROSIS IN 1,000 PATIENTS SEEN IN THE MS CLINIC, LONDON, ONTARIO*

Sensory cord	43%	Motor acute	7%
Retrobulbar neuritis	17	Sensory face	5
Gait	13	Pain	5
Motor slow	12	Limb ataxia	5
Diplopia	11	Bladder	3
Lhermitte's sign	9	Vertigo	3
Balance	9	Transverse myelitis	2

*From Ebers, GC,[67] p 1268, with permission.

ment in over one half of patients presenting with multiple sclerosis.[67]

PATHOLOGY

In a classic study on the neuropathology of multiple sclerosis, Lumsden[145] drew attention to the presence of demyelinated plaques (on postmortem examination) in the spinal cords of most multiple sclerosis patients. Lumsden also commented on the relative symmetry of demyelination in multiple sclerosis, with similar lesions on both sides of the midline in many cases (Fig. 8–1).

Fog[76] has noted that fan-shaped plaques in the lateral columns are especially common, and suggested that demyelination is most likely to occur in the vicinity of veins within the spinal cord. More recently, Oppenheimer[178] observed that plaques in the cervical cord are about twice as common as those at lower levels. On the basis of the distribution of lesions in the transverse plane, he suggested that mechanical stresses, transmitted to the cord via the denticulate ligaments, might play a role in determining the site of lesions in the spinal cord in multiple sclerosis. This suggestion remains controversial.

CLINICAL FEATURES

Clinical features of the spinal form of multiple sclerosis (cases characterized by solely spinal symptomatology) have been described. A study[199] found 109 cases of spinal multiple sclerosis out of a pool of 1,271 multiple sclerosis patients (9 percent). This figure is somewhat lower than the 25 percent reported by others,[130] whose patients were characterized by current symptoms only, not excluding patients with a history of extraspinal symptoms. There was a slight preponderance of females among the 109 cases.[199] Both studies note in the spinal form of multiple sclerosis a higher age at onset compared with other forms, and a higher percentage of cases with progressive course.[130, 199] Signs and symptoms of pyramidal tract and posterior column dysfunction are especially prominent, although sensory ataxia, impairment of sensibility for light touch and temperature, and sphincter/sexual impairment also occur. Many patients with spinal forms of multiple sclerosis harbor subclinical demyelinated plaques in other regions of the CNS. Why these lesions remain asymptomatic remains conjectural.[264]

An important question concerns the fre-

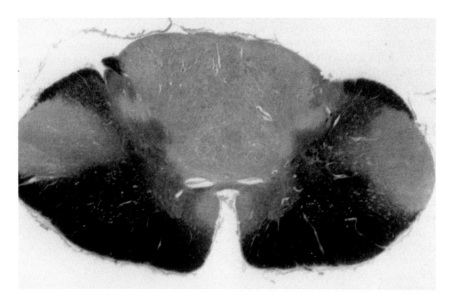

Figure 8–1. Multiple sclerosis involving the spinal cord. Note the nearly total demyelination of posterior and lateral columns. (Courtesy of Dr. Lysia Forno.)

quency with which multiple sclerosis will develop in patients who present with isolated spinal cord syndromes. Some authors have suggested that, in a series of patients without evidence of cord compression, clinically definite multiple sclerosis will develop in a higher proportion of patients with chronic progressive myelopathies than in patients with acute myelopathies. In an autopsy series,[150] multiple sclerosis was found in 34 percent of patients with undiagnosed, chronic progressive myelopathies. Other researchers[188] have observed oligoclonal bands and/or abnormal visual evoked potentials in 44 percent of patients with chronic progressive myelopathy.

Hume and Waxman[104] examined visual, somatosensory, and brainstem auditory evoked potentials in 222 patients referred to Yale-New Haven Hospital because of suspected multiple sclerosis. Thirty-two had a history and signs of isolated spinal cord disease. Of these four developed clinically definite multiple sclerosis (McAlpine criteria) on $2\frac{1}{2}$-year follow-up; all four of these patients had had positive visual or brainstem-evoked potentials, demonstrating slowed conduction outside the spinal cord at the time of presentation. Three of the 32 recovered and showed no further symptoms; none of these patients had positive evoked potentials. Notably, 3 of these 32 patients referred for suspected multiple sclerosis harbored structural lesions causing cord compression (cervical disc disease, cervical cord tumor, foramen magnum meningioma); in each of these cases the visual and brainstem-evoked potentials were normal. These patients illustrate the danger in making a premature diagnosis of spinal multiple sclerosis, especially when the visual and brainstem-evoked potentials are normal.[104]

A study of acute myelopathies[26] found abnormal visual evoked responses in only 10 percent. A follow-up study[212] on patients presenting with acute myelitis and subacute transverse myelopathy found multiple sclerosis in only about 10 percent of cases; a subsequent study[211] observed normal visual, brainstem auditory, and median somatosensory evoked potentials in 12 patients with complete, acute transverse myelitis; suggesting that acute transverse myelitis usually is a monophasic illness, distinct from multiple sclerosis.

In a series of 121 patients with isolated noncompressive spinal cord syndromes,[160] brain and spinal MRI showed lesions in the appropriate spinal cord region in 64 percent of patients with a cervical syndrome, and 28 percent of patients with thoracic or lumbar syndrome. In patients with *chronic* progressive spinal cord syndromes, MRI revealed cerebral lesions in 72 percent; most lesions were similar to those characteristic of multiple sclerosis. MRI revealed lesions in the white matter of the cerebral hemispheres in 79 percent of patients with chronic relapsing spinal cord syndromes. In patients with *acute* spinal cord syndromes (defined as a single clinical episode, fully developed within 14 days of onset), MRI of the brain was abnormal in 56 percent, often showing lesions indistinguishable from those seen in multiple sclerosis. The authors point out that the finding of multiple lesions at presentation cannot be used to make a diagnosis of clinically definite multiple sclerosis because the criteria of time and number are not met; serial MRI scanning, showing dissemination of lesions, or a second clinical bout, is required.[187, 197] Other investigators also have found cranial MRI helpful in the evaluation of patients with myelopathy of undetermined etiology when demyelinating disease is the cause.[164]

Unexpected spinal cord compression occasionally can be demonstrated in patients with remitting and/or mild symptoms of spinal cord dysfunction. As noted above, 3 patients with spinal cord compression were among 32 patients referred to a teaching hospital because of suspected spinal multiple sclerosis. In a series[160] of 130 patients referred to a neurological hospital for evaluation of a spinal cord syndrome in which a compressive cause was considered unlikely, 9 (2 of whom had negative myelograms, 1 and 3 months earlier) had compressive lesions demonstrated by MRI. Several of these patients had a remitting spastic paraparesis that had been previously diagnosed as multiple sclerosis. None of these patients had symptoms or signs referable to levels of the neuraxis above the foramen magnum. This demonstration of unexpected compressive lesions in patients with remitting myelopathies emphasizes the importance of carefully considering cord compression in patients with undiagnosed spinal cord syndromes, and of rethinking the diagnosis if there is progression of signs.

Although the clinical presentation of spinal multiple sclerosis may resemble postinfectious myelitis, the evolution of myelopathy in multiple sclerosis more frequently occurs over a few weeks rather than hours or days. Furthermore, unlike some cases of postinfectious myelitis, pain usually is not a prominent complaint in multiple sclerosis. The CSF sometimes shows signs of inflammation with pleocytosis and elevations of protein (usually to levels less than 100 mg per deciliter). IgG is usually elevated in CSF and oligoclonal bands are often present. MRI imaging of the spine may demonstrate evidence of demyelination (Fig. 8–2).

THERAPY

No specific therapy has been proven to alter the natural history of multiple sclerosis. Both ACTH and corticosteroids may shorten the course of an acute relapse but long-term use has been discouraged.[155] Several reports suggest that high-dose intravenous corticosteroids may be effective in treating multiple sclerosis and this approach is being studied in clinical trials.[163] Some of the side effects associated with the use of corticosteroids are discussed in the section on therapy of postinfectious myelitis.

Cytotoxic therapies for multiple sclerosis also are under study. High-dose cyclophosphamide and ACTH appear to have some effect in halting progressive multiple sclerosis, although the favorable response is usually temporary, lasting 6 to 24 months.[37, 265] The efficacy of cyclophosphamide in multiple sclerosis has been questioned by some clinicians.[138] In view of its immunosuppressive effects and other side effects, it is recommended only in patients with particularly aggressive multiple sclerosis, and should be used only after the risk-benefit ratio is carefully weighed. It should be administered by clinicians well versed in its use, preferably in the setting of clinical trials. Recent results suggest that total lymphoid irradi-

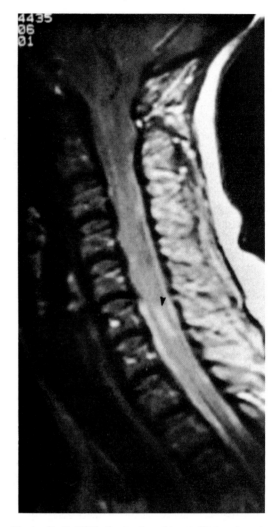

Figure 8–2. MRI of spinal cord in multiple sclerosis. Note the demyelinating plaque (white) in the spinal cord in the lower cervical spine. (From Sze, G, [247] with permission.)

ation may be of some value,[44, 60] but this modality remains experimental. Several additional investigational treatment protocols are undergoing trial and it is expected that effective new modalities of therapy may become available for multiple sclerosis.

Devic's Disease (Neuromyelitis Optica)

Devic's disease (neuromyelitis optica) has been considered by various authors as a variant of multiple sclerosis, a form of acute disseminated encephalomyelitis, or a distinct disorder. It is characterized by involvement of the spinal cord (usually although not invariably in the thoracic region) and the optic nerve(s) or chiasm.[154, 263] Devic's disease is characterized pathologically by a greater degree of axonal degeneration than is usual in multiple sclerosis. The spinal cord can present a frankly necrotic picture, in some cases leading to cavitation.

Spinal cord and optic nerve/chiasm involvement occur almost simultaneously. While optic neuritis and spinal cord involvement can occur together in multiple sclerosis, Devic's disease presents a distinct constellation, characterized by a more common presentation at the extremes of age (before 10 and after 50 years of age). The necrotizing pathology of this disorder is unusual for multiple sclerosis. The CSF is characterized by a pleocytosis, often associated with an increase of protein of up to 200 mg per deciliter.

The clinical presentation reflects the sites of pathology. Thus, unilateral or bilateral visual impairment is followed within days or weeks by a transverse or ascending myelitis. Visual impairment often progresses rapidly, over the course of several hours. Paraparesis or paraplegia, together with a sensory level, develop with a similar rapid time course. In some cases, temporary remissions are followed by worsening. As would be expected from the necrotizing character of the lesions, remission is less likely than in typical multiple sclerosis. Nevertheless, in several cases there have been claims of nearly total recovery.

Acute Necrotizing Myelitis

This rare disorder clinically presents as an acute or subacute transverse myelopathy.[212, 254] Thus motor, sensory, and sphincter paralysis evolve over a matter of hours or days; occasionally the optic nerves may be involved.[6] Sensory disturbances tend to be more prominent early symptoms than are motor complaints.[103] Motor weakness rapidly evolves into an areflexic, flaccid paralysis. Some patients report a prior infectious illness, usually an upper respiratory infection.[103]

Acute necrotizing myelitis is distinguished from the other forms of myelitis above by its distinctive pathological findings.[103] The CSF demonstrates evidence of inflammation. Pathological characteristics include perivenous demyelination and diffuse necrosis of all spinal cord elements.[103] The appearance of the acute lesion, necrotizing hemorrhagic myelitis, resembles necrotizing hemorrhagic leukoencephalitis.[6] The rostro-caudal extent of the lesions may involve several segments. Acutely, the spinal cord may be swollen but eventually atrophy supervenes. Potentially, these gross pathological findings may be seen on imaging studies such as MRI.

VIRAL MYELITIS

Most viruses that invade the spinal cord demonstrate a predilection for gray matter with relative sparing of white matter. Viral myelitis may be classified according to the location of spinal cord damage. For example, anterior horn cell damage is due to the poliomyelitis virus,[27] and posterior horn cell disease occurs as a result of infection by herpes zoster.

With the notable exceptions of HTLV-I myelopathy and AIDS myelopathy, the white matter tracts are characteristically spared in comparison with the major clinical and pathological involvement found in the gray matter. This observation is important in distinguishing viral myelitis from other causes of myelopathy. For example, in cases of neoplastic or non-neoplastic spinal cord compression, white matter dysfunction is often a predominant finding. Furthermore, in cases of inflammation of the spinal cord where white matter tracts bear the brunt of involvement, one should initially consider causes other than viral myelitides (such as parainfectious and postvaccination myelitides, multiple sclerosis, and paraneoplastic myelopathy). In addition, involvement of multiple roots, as may occur with sacral radiculitis due to herpes simplex type 2, may be difficult to differentiate from myelopathy or conus medullaris involvement. The major clinical features of viral myelitis that are important in the differential diagnosis of spinal cord compression are discussed below.

Acute Anterior Poliomyelitis

The clinical syndrome of acute anterior poliomyelitis is a febrile illness associated with flaccid motor weakness or paralysis and signs of meningeal inflammation.[109] Prior to the advent of the polio vaccine, epidemic paralytic poliomyelitis due to one of three antigenic types of poliovirus occurred. (In areas where widespread vaccination has not been performed or where it has lapsed, epidemic polio is, of course, still a major threat.) Even in regions in which the vaccination program has been successful, sporadic cases still occur.[174, 175, 189, 207] For example, in the United States between 1969 and 1982, 208 cases of paralytic poliomyelitis were reported.[5, 109, 175] Although rare, the poliomyelitis virus has not been eradicated and one can expect occasionally to encounter the clinical syndrome of acute anterior poliomyelitis. Similar clinical syndromes, usually milder, may be caused by other enteroviruses, echoviruses, and Coxsackie viruses groups A and B.[49, 107, 133, 148, 245, 260] Only the most common spinal manifestations of paralytic poliomyelitis will be reviewed here. For a more complete account, the reader is referred elsewhere.[5, 174, 175, 189, 196, 207]

CLINICAL AND LABORATORY FEATURES

Most individuals with poliovirus infection have no symptoms or mild gastrointestinal or flu-like symptoms during the viremic phase of the disease. If an effective immune response is not mounted, aseptic meningitis and/or paralytic poliomyelitis may occur. The early spinal manifestations of the disease are characterized by fever, tenderness and spasm of the muscles, as well as headache, neck and back pain, and other signs of meningeal irritation. Diffuse fasciculations of muscles may be present. Motor paralysis may occur abruptly, evolving over hours to tetraplegia, or show a more indolent course over several days. The pattern of weakness is usually asymmetric and may, of course, involve bulbar muscles as well as those innervated by spinal motor neurons. Although hyperreflexia initially may be present, areflexia usually develops as flaccid paralysis ensues. Sensory loss is rarely found although sensory complaints in the form of dysesthesias and paresthesias may be present. Transient urinary retention is seen in 50 percent of adults.[109] Transient papilledema lasting 2 to 10 weeks is seen in 5 percent of seriously paralyzed cases.[196]

Although initially the CSF may be normal in 10 percent of cases, it typically shows signs of inflammation: pleocytosis, elevated protein, normal sugar levels, and normal pressure. The CSF white cell counts may exceed 2,500; initially, the spinal fluid contains predominantly polymorphonuclear cells but later evolves to contain primarily lymphocytes. The spinal fluid protein does not usually rise above 150 mg per deciliter. However, in cases associated with papilledema, the protein may be much higher and persists for several months.[196]

DIFFERENTIAL DIAGNOSIS

The syndrome of acute poliomyelitis from poliovirus must be distinguished from a variety of other paralytic diseases. Acute polyneuritis (Guillain-Barré syndrome) usually presents with symmetric areflexic weakness and no meningeal signs, fever, or signs of systemic illness; sensory changes are often present. Furthermore, the CSF in Guillain-Barré syndrome exhibits increased protein but rarely shows significant pleocytosis.

Epidemic neuromyasthenia (Iceland disease, benign myalgic encephalomyelitis) is an obscure illness with a clinical syndrome similar to that of poliomyelitis.[146] It usually occurs in outbreaks in residential communities or in hospitals during the summer months.[109] It is characterized by fever, headache, and aching muscles. Muscle paresis develops in 10 to 80 percent of cases but, unlike the weakness seen in poliomyelitis, there is no muscle atrophy, and preserved reflexes or hyperreflexia rather than hyporeflexia is the rule.[109] Sensory complaints are often reported. Brainstem signs, emotional instability, and urinary retention also may be found.[109, 196] The CSF is usually entirely normal. The causative agent is unknown.[109]

Although usually less severe, the clinical syndrome of anterior poliomyelitis caused by the enteroviruses, echoviruses, and Coxsackie viruses is clinically indistinguishable from that caused by the poliomyelitis virus.[196] In areas where polio vaccination programs have all but eradicated this disease, these enteroviruses are responsible for the majority of cases of paralytic poliomyelitis syndrome.[109] Because the clinical and spinal fluid findings are similar, differentiation must be made on the basis of virus isolation or serological studies. With rare exception (e.g., Coxsackie A7 and some other enteroviruses), most cases of nonpolio enteroviral poliomyelitis do not occur as epidemics.[109, 260] A polio-like syndrome also has been reported secondary to mumps virus,[132] infectious mononucleosis,[169] and rabies virus.[105, 126]

Postpoliomyelitis Syndrome

Many years following an attack of acute paralytic poliomyelitis, a slowly progressive syndrome of muscle weakness that has been termed the postpoliomyelitis syndrome may develop.[50–52, 170] Because it has been estimated that 25 percent of patients with antecedent paralytic poliomyelitis will develop this late sequela,[40] nearly 60,000 individuals in the United States are at risk to develop this syndrome. The weakness, of a lower motor neuron type, is often most prominent in the areas of original paralysis. It is associated with fatigue and pain. The lack of upper motor neuron signs distinguishes this disease from amyotrophic lateral sclerosis.[109]

Recent pathological studies of spinal cords from patients with prior poliomyelitis (mean 20 years prior to autopsy) have been performed.[194] The histopathological findings in those suffering from the postpoliomyelitis syndrome did not differ from those without the syndrome. In both settings, there was evidence of atrophy of motor neurons, severe gliosis, and only mild to moderate perivascular and parenchymal inflammation. The pathogenesis of the disorder is uncertain,[109, 194] though it is suggested that late denervation of muscles previously reinnervated during the recovery phase from paralytic poliomyelitis is involved in its causation.[39]

Herpes Zoster

Herpes zoster, an acute viral infection involving a dorsal root ganglion, may extend into the spinal cord to cause a posterior horn myelitis at one or several cord segmental levels.[196] In addition, segmental (radicular) weakness at the level(s) of sensory involvement as a result of anterior poliomyelitis is a relatively frequent finding.[108, 119, 196, 249] More rarely, a zoster-associated myelitis involving ascending and descending white matter tracts may occur.[16, 87, 95, 108, 196] Among 1,210 cases of herpes zoster seen at the Mayo Clinic over a nine-year period, only one case of zoster-associated myelitis was reported.[251]

The pathogenesis of zoster-associated myelitis is uncertain.[16] The mechanisms suggested include direct viral invasion of the cord,[101, 157] an associated vasculitis and thrombosis[103, 213] and an immunologic parainfectious cause.[13] The development of zoster-associated myelitis may immediately follow the cutaneous vesicular eruption or may be delayed by several weeks to months.[16] The neurological abnormalities found on examination depend upon the specific tracts involved. There may be progressive, relentless cord destruction with an ascending myelopathy.[101, 213] The CSF generally shows a pleocytosis, elevated protein, and normal glucose level.

It is important to note that secondary or symptomatic zoster[103] may develop at a segmental level of underlying spinal disease. For example, occasionally neoplastic epidural spinal cord compression may present with herpes zoster at the level of metastasis.[84] Thus in diagnosing zoster-associated myelopathy, one should consider the possibility that another underlying disease process is responsible for the neurological deficit.

The optimal treatment of zoster-associated myelitis has not been defined. Because virus has been isolated from the CSF and spinal cords of some patients, the administration of antiviral agents has been advocated.[16]

HTLV-I Associated Myelopathy

The retrovirus human T-lymphotropic virus type I (HTLV-I) recently has been implicated as the causative agent of a slowly progressive myelopathy characterized by symmetric upper motor neuron paraparesis, sphincter disturbances, and mild sensory signs.[152] In Japan, this myelopathy has been found to be associated with leukemia-like cells in the blood and CSF and has been identified as HTLV-I-associated myelopathy (HAM).[83, 111, 257] A progressive myelopathy with similar clinical features has been recognized for many years in the tropics and has been termed tropical spastic paraparesis (TSP).[179, 257] Since HTLV-I antibodies have been found in most patients with TSP, in many instances TSP and HAM may be the same disease.[31, 173, 209] However, a positive serology without neurological disease may be seen in up to 26 percent of some populations studied, and it has been suggested that the presence of an HTLV-I antibody does not necessarily indicate a causal relationship.[31] Furthermore, in some cases, a distinction between TSP and HAM should be made. For example, when in epidemic form, TSP has been attributed to toxic and nutritional factors such as lathyrism, cassava consumption, malnutrition, and cyanide intoxication.[210, 257] It has been claimed that HAM may be associated with a more favorable response to steroids than are some cases of TSP.[31]

CLINICAL FEATURES

The clinical presentation is usually progressive lower extremity weakness, often associated with lumbar or thoracic pain with or without lower extremity discomfort. Paresthesias are common but prominent sensory disturbances are unusual. Bladder dysfunction is common. The signs and symptoms are usually bilateral and symmetric but may be asymmetric. Although weakness usually involves the legs more prominently than the arms, spasticity is typically found in all extremities. The

course evolves over several months in most patients but may occasionally be less than one month.[257] Most patients in recent series are women.[152, 179, 257]

Patients with myelopathy found to be seropositive for HTLV-I usually have antibodies in the serum and CSF.[23, 152, 257]The retrovirus HTLV-I also has been found to be associated with acute T-cell leukemia.[111, 173, 271] In one recent report, patients with chronic progressive myelopathy who were positive for HTLV-I also showed evidence for adult T-cell leukemia-like cells.[179]

Although it is uncertain whether the myelopathy is secondary to direct viral invasion or another mechanism,[111, 179] HTLV-I nucleic acid sequences have been found in blood and CSF and viral antigens were found in the CSF of patients with chronic progressive myelopathy.[23] This observation and others have strengthened the argument that HTLV-I may be the cause of nervous system disease in such patients.[30] With the increase in frequency of individuals seropositive for HTLV-I, the HTLV-I associated myelopathy may be encountered more frequently in the United States.[208]

THERAPY

The therapy of HAM is unsatisfactory. Corticosteroid therapy may be temporarily effective in some patients. Because the HTLV-I antibody titers and IgG fall, both in the serum and CSF, in patients treated with corticosteroids, it has been suggested that HTLV-I antibody may be important in the pathogenesis of the disorder. Alternatively, plasmapheresis, which may also be a temporarily effective treatment, does not lower the HTLV-I antibody titer in the CSF. These findings and the observation that serum and CSF HTLV-I antibody titers do not correlate with disease severity have cast doubt on the role of HTLV-I antibody in the pathogenesis of HAM.[152]

AIDS-Related Myelopathies

Patients with acquired immunodeficiency syndrome (AIDS) may develop myelopathies secondary to compression from

infection or neoplasm or may develop myelopathies induced by infection with the
human immunodeficiency virus or other
infectious diseases.[86, 88, 156] Whereas in
adults with AIDS, vacuolar myelopathy
may lead to a progressive myelopathy, in
pediatric patients bilateral corticospinal
tract degeneration may occur with a distinct histopathology;[61] such children may
develop progressive quadriparesis.

Vacuolar myelopathy[193, 237] may occur
in patients with AIDS, and is often seen in
patients with AIDS-related dementia[156]
(Figs. 8–3 and 8–4). The lateral and
posterior columns of the thoracic spinal
cord appear to be predominantly affected.[193] The histopathological features are
similar to those of subacute combined
degeneration of the spinal cord secondary
to vitamin B_{12} deficiency. While earlier
studies suggested that direct viral invasion
is involved in the pathogenesis of this
disorder,[134, 135, 156] more recent investigations using immunohistochemistry and *in
situ* hybridization found that vacuolar
myelopathy occurred independent of productive HIV-1 infection in the spinal
cord.[88, 215]

The most common clinical manifestations of vacuolar myelopathy are progressive spastic paraparesis, incontinence,
and ataxia.[193] When peripheral neuropathy is also present, the deep tendon reflexes may be absent and there may be
distal sensory loss and/or paresthesias. Of
the 20 patients in one study,[193] dementia
was present in 14 (70 percent). Because
compressive myelopathies may clinically
resemble vacuolar myelopathies, MRI and/
or myelography is usually performed in
such patients before a diagnosis is
made.[135]

In addition to vacuolar myelopathy, patients with AIDS are at risk for the development of a variety of infections that
damage the spinal cord.[156, 214] Herpes
simplex types I and II and varicella-zoster
virus has been found to cause myeloradic-
ulopathies in patients with AIDS.[32, 125, 156]
Cytomegalovirus also has been reported to
cause an ascending myelitis and ra-
diculomyelitis.[88, 168, 253] Mycobacterial
meningomyelitis and spinal toxoplasmo-
ses are other identifiable CNS infectious
complications of AIDS.[99a, 272] In addition

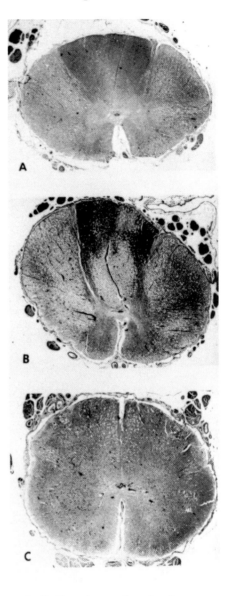

Figure 8–3. Vacuolar myelopathy shown in a patient with AIDS. The lower thoracic spinal cord (B) is
most severely affected with marked, confluent vacuo-
lation of the posterior and lateral columns. The upper
thoracic (A) and lumbar (C) spinal cord areas are less
severely involved. (Hematoxylin-eosin stain, X 7.92.)
(From Petito, CK et al,[193] p 876, with permission.)

to direct viral invasion of the spinal cord by
opportunistic infections, patients with
AIDS suffer from poor nutrition, and toxic
and metabolic derangements, that may be
responsible for some cases of myelopathy.[88, 156] Finally, patients with AIDS
have an increased risk of primary CNS

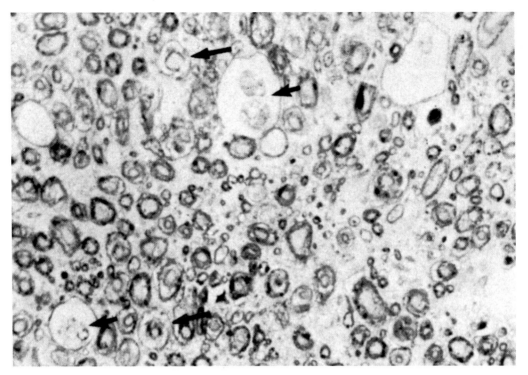

Figure 8–4. A 1 micron plastic embedded section of the lateral column of a patient with moderately severe AIDS-related vacuolar myelopathy. Vacuoles surrounded by thin myelin sheath are shown. Two vacuoles contain lipid-laden macrophages (short arrows). A few myelin sheaths show intramyelin swelling (long arrows). (Toluidine blue stain, X 1085.) (From Petito, CK, et al, [193] p 877, with permission.)

lymphoma and other systemic neoplasms that may cause spinal cord compression.[22, 100, 237]

SPIROCHETAL DISEASE OF THE SPINAL CORD

Syphilis

Involvement of the nervous system by syphilis has been a major public health problem and again appears to be increasing with the development of AIDS.[114] In a recent study of HIV-infected and HIV-noninfected patients, *Treponema pallidum*, the cause of syphilis, was located from the CSF in 30 percent of patients with primary or secondary syphilis.[143] The importance of syphilis in the evaluation of spinal cord disease was best expressed by Merritt, Adams, and Solomon[159] (page 144), who state, "In summary it should be said that with the combination of chronic

meningitis, arterial disease, and granuloma formation, it is not surprising that almost every conceivable cord disease may be simulated clinically by spinal syphilis."

The spirochete *Treponema pallidum* usually invades the CNS, resulting in an acute syphilitic meningitis, during the secondary stage of the disease.[103, 159] Following a latent period of variable duration, the tertiary stage, which is subdivided into meningovascular syphilis and parenchymal syphilis, may occur. The meningovascular form is characterized pathologically by an arteritis, the location of which determines the clinical neurological manifestations.[159] The clinical syndromes of spinal cord involvement from the meningovascular disease may be classified as syphilitic meningomyelitis, syphilitic pachymeningitis, syphilitic spastic paraplegia (Erb's spastic paraplegia), and syphilitic amyotrophy.[103] Among these meningovascular forms, syphilitic meningomyelitis is the most common.[103] It is characterized pathologically by a granulomatous involvement of blood vessels, Heubner's arteritis. As mentioned, the clinical syndromes are secondary to the areas of the spinal cord that are infarcted. Thus patients may present with a Brown-Séquard syndrome or an anterior spinal artery syndrome. Alternatively, scattered smaller infarctions may cause a variety of spinal presentations. In cases of syphilitic pachymeningitis, the pachymeninges and leptomeninges are the site of granulomatous inflammation. Some patients have only progressive spastic paraparesis, with preservation of sensory function, which was formerly called Erb's spastic paraplegia; this must be differentiated from motor neuron disease and familial spastic paraplegia. Syphilitic meningovascular involvement also may give rise to a syndrome of amyotrophy as a result of nerve root involvement. This may or may not be associated with spastic paraplegia. Some authors question the relationship between syphilitic pachymeningitis and syphilitic amyotrophy.[4]

The parenchymal form of neurosyphilis involving the spinal cord is tabes dorsalis. More common than meningovascular forms of spinal syphilis,[4] tabes dorsalis is a parenchymal disease of the nervous system secondary to invasion by *Treponema pallidum*. Pathologically, changes in the posterior roots, thickening of the leptomeninges, and gliosis of the posterior columns are typically seen[103] (Fig. 8–5). The dominant symptoms and signs are lightning pains, ataxia, urinary incontinence, absent lower extremity deep tendon reflexes, and impaired vibratory and position sensibilities in the lower extremities. The ataxia is secondary to a sensory disturbance. Argyll-Robertson pupils, constricting in accommodation but not to light, also are typically present. Some patients experience severe abdominal pain and diarrhea.

Although the CSF is usually abnormal in neurosyphilis, some authorities report that it may be entirely normal by conventional testing in a significant number of patients.[171] Specific laboratory findings and the clinical constellation of neurosyphilis are discussed elsewhere in detail.[55, 114, 143, 180, 234]

The following is a case illustration of a syphilitic meningitis.

Case Illustration

A 34-year-old woman presented with a 4-week history of back and leg pain followed by headache and gait difficulty. There was also a history of maculopapular rash during this period, and night sweats. On physical examination she had no adenopathy or splenomegaly but did have

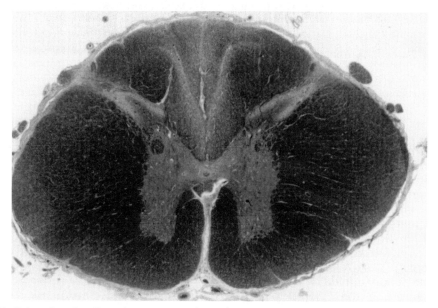

Figure 8–5. Tabes dorsalis. Note the symmetric loss of myelin in posterior columns. (Courtesy of Dr. Lysia Forno.)

maculopapular rash. Neurological examination revealed papilledema on funduscopic examination and hypotonic lower extremity weakness (4/5) with depressed-to-absent lower extremity reflexes. She had a waddling gait due to proximal lower extremity weakness and could not stand on toes or heels. There was slight sensory disturbance to touch and pin over the right distal lower extremity.

An MR scan of the entire spine with gadolinium demonstrated enhancement of the cauda equina and clumping or nodularity of the nerve roots. A lumbar puncture demonstrated an opening pressure of 340 mm, with a CSF pleocytosis, protein 85 mg per deciliter, glucose 50 mg per deciliter, and positive VDRL. The serum VDRL was positive, as was the serum FTA-ABS. CSF IgG was 38 mg per deciliter (normal < 5 mg per deciliter) and oligoclonal bands were present. The skin lesions were biopsied and showed perivascular plasma cells highly suggestive of spirochetal infection. A diagnosis of secondary syphilis with syphilitic meningitis was made, and the patient showed neurological recovery following high-dose intravenous penicillin.

Comment. This case illustrates a rare neurological manifestation of syphilitic meningitis. This patient had evidence of increased intracranial pressure and a cauda equina syndrome caused by syphilis. The MRI was done without and with gadolinium to look for leptomeningeal enhancement because the papilledema and cauda equina syndrome were considered suspicious for meningeal involvement. Although this clinical constellation of multifocal involvement of the CNS is often found in leptomeningeal cancer,[25] it is clear that other forms of chronic meningitis may cause a similar clinical picture.

THERAPY

Although there is general agreement that penicillin is the drug of choice for neurosyphilis, there is considerable controversy over the form and dosage.[143, 171] The CDC has included the use of IM benzathine penicillin G and IM aqueous procaine penicillin G, as well as IV aqueous crystalline penicillin G, as potentially effective regimens.[41] Despite these recommendations, subtreponemicidal levels of penicillin are found in the CSF of patients treated with benzathine penicillin[234] and the adequacy of benzathine and procaine penicillin regimens has been questioned.[114] Careful neurological follow-up is important to determine the efficacy of therapy. Repeated CSF examinations following treatment are recommended to verify improvement of the CSF parameters.[4, 234]

Lyme Disease

Lyme disease is caused by the spirochete *Borrelia burgdorferi*, which has been found to be transmitted by ticks and other arthropod vectors.[242–244] Lyme disease recently has been recognized to manifest a wide variety of neurological complications.[181, 205, 244] Although the disease's clinical manifestations have been classified into three stages, many patients do not demonstrate symptoms or signs of all three.[180]

The first stage of the disease often begins soon after infection and consists of a flu-like illness associated with erythema chronicum migrans, the characteristic skin lesion. The second stage usually begins within a few weeks to months of infection and may include neurological and/or cardiac involvement. When neurological involvement occurs, there is often evidence of meningitis, cranial neuritis, radiculitis, and/or peripheral neuropathy.[180] The third stage, which may commence within several months to years after the initial infection, is often manifested as arthritis. However, neurological involvement may dominate this stage.

Although a demyelinating disease resembling multiple sclerosis and a variety of neuropsychiatric syndromes have been reported during the third stage,[75, 180, 205] recent studies have challenged the etiologic role of *Borrelia burgdorferi* in the development of multiple sclerosis.[46, 94] Rarely, transverse myelitis also has been reported to dominate the neurological picture in late Lyme disease.[180] Acute transverse myelitis occasionally may occur as a presenting neurological manifestation of Lyme disease, within several days of the appearance of erythema chronicum migrans.[219]

Because in many geographical areas Lyme disease is very common and serum immunoreactivity against *Borrelia burgdorferi* is widespread, it may be difficult to determine confidently whether a specific neurological disorder is due to Lyme disease. In an attempt to identify CNS disorders due to Lyme disease, researchers have reported that intrathecal production of specific antibodies appears to be a marker for active CNS involvement.[94]

As in the case of syphilis, involvement of the nervous system by Lyme disease may respond to antibiotic therapy.[75, 180, 219] Ceftriaxone and penicillin have been used for CNS involvement.[94, 226]

TOXIC AND DEFICIENCY MYELOPATHIES

Myelopathies may occur secondary to toxic exposures and metabolic and nutritional deficiency states. In many cases, the symptoms and signs of myelopathy are overshadowed by those of other organs affected. For example, although lead may cause a myelopathy, its toxic effect on the brain in children, and on peripheral nerves in adults, may be far more prominent findings. This section lists some of the more commonly encountered causes of toxic and deficiency-state myelopathies. As further experience is gained with other substances, this list is expected to lengthen.

Toxic Myelopathies

ORTHO-CRESYL PHOSPHATE

Ortho-cresyl phosphates, used as industrial solvents, are highly toxic to the central and peripheral nervous system when ingested.[42] During the era of Prohibition, jake paralysis, an acute peripheral neuropathy secondary to the ingestion of ginger jake adulterated with triortho-cresyl phosphate, was seen.[196] More recently, outbreaks have occurred when lubricating oil containing triortho-cresyl phosphate contaminated olive oil was found.[235] The clinical picture is usually that of an acute peripheral neuropathy developing over a period of weeks, accompanied or followed by myelopathy. On pathological inspection, Wallerian degeneration is seen of both peripheral and central nervous system fibers.[15, 103]

MYELOPATHY FOLLOWING AORTOGRAPHY

On rare occasions, aortography has been followed by myelopathy.[122, 123] The mechanism is uncertain and in some cases might be secondary to embolic infarction or vasospasm of the spinal cord; in other instances, the contrast material has been considered toxic to the spinal cord.[103, 196]

The myelopathy may present as immediate spasms in the lower extremities during the injection of contrast material.[1] The patient may have a sensory level and loss of bowel and bladder function, as well as a flaccid paraplegia.[196] When due to anterior spinal artery infarction, posterior column function (position and vibration) may be spared.

LATHYRISM

Lathyrism, a disease most often encountered in India and North Africa, is a relatively acute neurological syndrome of pain, sensory complaints, and weakness of the lower extremities that evolves into an ataxic, spastic paraplegia. (Lathyrism has been considered a cause of tropical spastic paraparesis.[210]) On pathological inspection, the anterior and lateral columns reveal degeneration.[7, 53] Its specific etiology and pathogenesis have not been elucidated, but it is considered secondary to consumption of vetches such as *Lathyrus sativas*.[103]

MYELOPATHY DUE TO INTRATHECAL AGENTS

Myelopathy may follow the injection of a variety of agents into the subarachnoid space. Penicillin, which was frequently administered intrathecally in the past, may cause radiculitis, arachnoiditis, and transverse myelitis.[196, 231, 246, 261] In the past, methylene blue was injected into the subarachnoid space to detect sites of CSF leak.[196] This compound was found to cause a myelitis and radiculitis, apparently without arachnoiditis.[70, 228]

Spinal Anesthetics. Although the frequency of this complication varies widely, both acute and delayed myelopathies have been reported to occur following the administration of spinal anesthetics.[54, 63, 182, 252] The pathogenesis is unknown and has been considered secondary to the anesthetic[190] or contaminants such as phenol or detergents within the anesthetics.[182, 268] In an acute myelopathy, paralysis may occur immediately following spinal anesthesia. On pathological examination, the spinal cord has been reported to show softening, petechial hemorrhages, and inflammatory cells.[117, 120, 182]

Intrathecal Chemotherapy

Both acute and delayed myelopathy have been reported following the intrathecal administration of methotrexate, cytosine arabinoside, and thiotepa.[93, 142, 222, 266, 269] The myelopathy may occur between 30 minutes and 48 hours (or, occasionally, up to 1 to 2 weeks) following administration.[118] The clinical presentation often is associated with leg pain, paraplegia, sensory level, and neurogenic bladder.[66, 118, 142] Improvement of the myelopathy, which can be partial or complete, may occur within days to months following its onset, or the myelopathy may be permanent.[118]

Myelopathy may occur either with intrathecal chemotherapy for the treatment of malignant leptomeningeal disease or in the setting of prophylactic therapy. It appears to be unrelated to the administration of other systemic drugs or CNS irradiation.[80] Its pathogenesis is unknown but may be secondary to demyelination or another toxic phenomenon.[222]

SPINAL ARACHNOIDITIS

Spinal arachnoiditis is an uncommon disorder in which a nonspecific inflammatory reaction of the leptomeninges and fibrosis cause both root and spinal cord symptoms and signs. Although the etiology of the inflammatory reaction often is never uncovered, spinal arachnoiditis may occur secondary to intrathecal administration of contrast material, antibiotics, and other agents.[20, 96, 115, 141, 196, 267]

On pathological examination of the spinal cord and meninges, the findings of inflammation and fibrosis may be widespread along the neuraxis or may be more circumscribed.[103] The spinal subarachnoid space may be obliterated from the process.[136] There may be a predilection for the thoracic spine.[6] In addition, there may be loculated cystic areas that cause spinal cord and root compression. Although the pathogenesis of neurological dysfunction may be secondary to compression in some cases, vascular disturbances secondary to arachnoiditis also may occur.[103]

The clinical presentation of spinal arachnoiditis is most commonly that of multifocal spinal disease manifested by a combination of radicular and/or spinal cord symptoms and signs. Neuropathic pain, which may be burning in the distribution of one or several spinal roots, is a common presenting symptom. Weakness of a lower motor neuron type may be seen, especially in cases of cauda equina involvement.[6] In lumbosacral arachnoiditis, the straight-leg-raising sign is frequently positive and neck flexion may cause pain in the lower extremities. If the spinal cord becomes involved, a progressive myelopathy with features of spasticity and ataxia may ensue.

The CSF is nearly always abnormal, with elevation of protein and pleocytosis common. Myelography with or without follow-up CT scanning usually reveals a characteristic appearance.[92, 97] Patients with arachnoiditis may be sensitive to the administration of intrathecal contrast material, which may cause further irritation.[92, 196] Tethered and clumped nerve roots and distortion of the thecal sac may be seen on noncontrast MRI studies.[216, 217] Using gadolinium-DTPA, enhancement has recently been seen in some cases.[247] It is hoped that MRI will replace myelography in the evaluation of patients with arachnoiditis, and thereby avoid the administration of potentially irritating intrathecal contrast material.

The management of spinal arachnoiditis is difficult. While corticosteroids and surgery have been used, they remain controversial.[6, 64, 229]

RADIATION MYELOPATHY

Radiation myelopathy may occur following radiation therapy in which the spinal cord is included within the radiation port. Despite advances in knowledge concerning the effects of radiation on the spinal cord, severe forms of radiation myelopathy are still occasionally encountered. For example, it has been found that some patients will develop chronic progressive radiation myelopathy despite the fact that they have received a dose of spinal irradiation considered safe for most individuals.[33, 116] Furthermore, some agents, such as hyperbaric oxygenation, may increase the risk of radiation myelopathy.[255] Based upon its clinical manifestations, radiation myelopathy has been classified into four distinct syndromes (Table 8-4).[201]

Transient Radiation Myelopathy

Transient radiation myelopathy is characterized by the subjective complaints of paresthesias and electric-like shock sensations on neck flexion (Lhermitte's sign).[137, 273] This form of myelopathy is a frequent sequela of standard doses of radiation to the spinal cord when neoplasms of the neck and upper thoracic region are irradiated. Typically, the symptoms begin 2 to 37 weeks (average, 16 weeks) following radiation therapy and spontaneously resolve after a period usually lasting 2 to 36 weeks (average 16 weeks).[113, 218] Although Lhermitte's sign does not typically portend the later development of progressive spinal cord dysfunction, it may be an early manifestation of chronic progressive radiation myelopathy.[113]

Clinical features consist of painful electric-like shock sensations, elicited by neck flexion or extension, which involve the body below the neck. Although the regions of the body involved are quite variable, typically affected individually or in combination are the trunk, anterior or posterior

lower extremities, and upper extremities (Fig. 8-6). The sensations usually are bilateral.

On neurological examination no abnormalities are found. The differential diagnosis for the cause of Lhermitte's sign includes spinal metastasis and unrelated disorders such as cervical spondylosis and disc herniation,[56] subacute combined degeneration,[19, 82, 223] post-traumatic syndrome,[43] multiple sclerosis,[121, 264] and cisplatin chemotherapy.[262] The pathogenesis of the disorder is thought to be reversible damage to myelin in the ascending sensory tracts of the spinal cord, which allows axons to be abnormally sensitive to mechanical deformation.[113, 236]

Lower Motor Neuron Dysfunction. The second form of radiation myelopathy, which appears to be very rare, presents as signs of lower motor neuron dysfunction.[201] In the patients described, painless amyotrophy and weakness, usually of the lower extremities, develops subacutely 3 to 8 months following high-dose radiation therapy to the spinal cord.[90, 128, 221] Sensory abnormalities are not found and sphincters remain intact. Electrodiagnostic studies demonstrate normal motor conduction velocities and denervation on electromyogram. The CSF protein may be elevated.[218] The course is usually subacutely progressive but ultimately self-limited. The pathogenesis is unknown but the clinical constellation resembles the subacute motor neuronopathy that occurs secondary to ionizing radiation and/or activation of a latent virus.[227]

Acute Transverse Myelopathy. The third form of radiation myelopathy is that of an acutely developing paraplegia or quadriplegia presumably secondary to infarction of the spinal cord. It may be secondary to radiation-induced vascular pathology.[201] This form of radiation myelopathy is exceedingly rare and is not included in all reviews of the subject.[218]

Chronic Progressive Radiation Myelopathy

The fourth type of radiation myelopathy is a chronic progressive disorder that has been widely recognized clinically and studied pathologically.[77, 151, 184, 185, 224] Its pathogenesis is controversial but recent

Table 8-4 CLASSIFICATION OF RADIATION MYELOPATHY

Transient myelopathy (Lhermitte's sign)
Lower motor neuron dysfunction
Acute transverse myelopathy
Chronic progressive radiation myelopathy

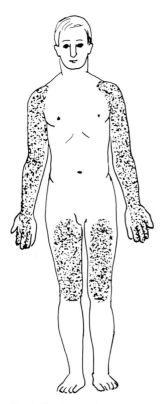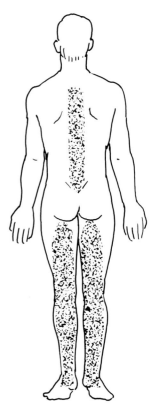

Figure 8—6. Anatomical areas commonly involved in electrical paresthesias (Lhermitte's sign) in cases of transient radiation myelopathy.

evidence suggests that progressive damage to vascular endothelium may be the primary event leading to spinal cord ischemia.[58]

Although the interval of time between radiation therapy to the spinal cord and the onset of symptoms is variable, most typically the neurological symptoms begin 5 months to many years (average, 14 months) following therapy.[201] Sensory symptoms beginning in the lower extremities, described as burning paresthesias and alterations in pain and temperature sensation, are often reported.[201] As noted above, Lhermitte's sign may herald the development of chronic progressive myelopathy, but in this case it generally arises after a higher dose of radiation therapy and after a more prolonged latent period (usually more than one year) than that seen in the transient form of radiation myelopathy.[113]

The neurological examination usually reveals spastic lower extremity weakness. Sphincter disturbance also develops. A Brown-Séquard syndrome is sometimes seen, or other forms of transverse myelopathy (incomplete) may predominate. An ascending sensory level may evolve over several weeks or months. Symptoms and signs are usually slowly progressive over several months but may ultimately stabilize.

The main pathological findings consist of asymmetric demyelination of the lateral columns and, to a lesser extent, demyelination of the anterior and posterior columns of white matter. The gray matter generally shows evidence of coagulative necrosis at the level of irradiation. Secondary ascending and descending tract degeneration (Wallerian degeneration) is seen. Vascular changes described include hyalinization of arterial walls, subendothelial intimal swelling, and luminal narrowing and thrombosis.[35, 218] The primary insult that causes the myelopathy has been debated; some authors favor a radiation-induced vascular etiology[85] while others suggest a direct radiation-induced neural injury.[35]

The diagnosis of chronic radiation myelopathy requires the exclusion of compressive lesions by neuroradiological studies. Plain films are normal or noncontributory, although incidental spondylosis may be seen. Myelography is usually normal but may demonstrate spinal cord atrophy. The latter may be the most specific sign on myelography. Occasionally a swollen cord may be found, which may raise a question of intramedullary metastasis.[218] MRI may have a role in the evaluation of radiation myelopathy and its differentiation from intramedullary metastasis. The CSF may be normal but the protein is often elevated.[201]

In an experimental model of radiation myelopathy, high-dose corticosteroids produced some benefit in the neurological function of animals.[58] Occasional clinical reports suggest that corticosteroids may have a role in the management of this disorder.[85]

ELECTRICAL INJURIES

Spinal cord damage secondary to electrical injuries may be either acute or delayed. The cervical spinal cord is frequently the site of injury because the electrical current often passes from hand to hand.[186] Acute injuries may be secondary to heating of tissue or to ischemia. Both gray matter and white matter tracts may be damaged, so that sensory, motor, and sphincter disturbances may occur. The motor weakness may be secondary to anterior horn cell damage resulting in amyotrophy. Such findings may be self-limited or may regress.[196]

Occasionally, a delayed progressive spinal cord syndrome develops following electrical injury; this syndrome may be difficult to differentiate clinically from spinal muscular atrophy or amyotrophic lateral sclerosis.[72, 106, 186] The pathogenesis of this delayed progressive myelopathy is not well understood; it may be secondary to

vascular occlusive changes as seen in some cases of delayed myelopathy following radiation therapy.[6]

Metabolic and Nutritional Myelopathy

SUBACUTE COMBINED DEGENERATION OF THE CORD

This treatable disease was first described in detail at the turn of this century.[220] Unlike some other deficiency myelopathies in which either the posterior or lateral columns may be involved alone, the designation combined degeneration refers to the fact that both the lateral and posterior columns are usually involved pathologically and clinically.[129] The disease results from vitamin B_{12} deficiency and is often, but not invariably, associated with megaloblastic anemia.[139]

Degenerative and demyelinative changes occur in the white matter of the posterior and lateral columns of the spinal cord (Fig. 8–7). The white matter of the brain may show similar changes. The peripheral nerves also may show signs of demyelination and axonal degeneration.[258]

The initial neurological manifestations are generally sensory complaints, including paresthesias involving the distal extremities.[71] Many patients first note pins-and-needles tingling or numbness in the feet, followed by the hands. These symptoms, which may be due to sensory peripheral neuropathy and/or damage to ascending white matter tracts, are usually progressive and ascend the extremities. Vibration and position sensation are disturbed and the Romberg usually becomes positive. The motor symptoms generally are weakness and stiffness in the lower extremities. The degree of spasticity and ataxia depends upon the relative degree of involvement of the descending and ascending tracts respectively. Thus the patient may have primarily a spastic gait, an ataxic gait, or a combined spastic, ataxic gait. The deep tendon reflexes depend upon the relative degree of central and peripheral nervous system involvement. Babinski signs eventually develop if the disease is not recognized and treated.

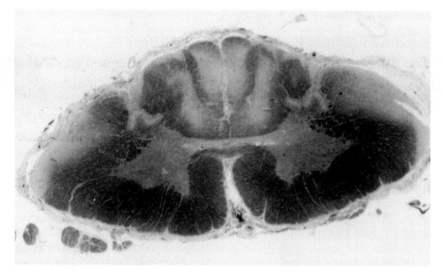

Figure 8—7. Subacute combined degeneration affecting the spinal cord. Note lateral and posterior column involvement. (Courtesy of Dr. Lysia Forno.)

Sphincter disturbances are atypical.[71] When the brain is involved, a variety of neuropsychiatric findings may occur, along with visual and other cerebral manifestations.[139] Diagnosis depends upon the recognition of the clinical syndrome, measurement of serum vitamin B_{12} level, and a two-stage Schilling test. Treatment consists of parenteral administration of vitamin B_{12}.

NUTRITIONAL MYELOPATHY

Unlike subacute combined systems disease, the myelopathy of nutritional deprivation may be due to a variety of (and possibly multiple) deficiencies.[48, 59, 91, 210, 238] Erbsloh and Abel[69] have classified the nutritional myelopathies as: (1) posterolateral myelopathy manifesting itself as mainly an ataxic syndrome; (2) anterolateral myelopathy presenting with a spastic syndrome; and (3) combined ataxic and spastic syndromes. Nutritional and vitamin deficiencies also are responsible for some of the reported cases of tropical spastic paraparesis and tropical ataxic neuropathy.[210]

Although clinical manifestations vary, Hughes[103] has summarized the most com-

monly encountered syndromes. Some patients present with a progressive spastic paraparesis that may evolve to quadriparesis. Bowel and bladder function are involved in advanced cases, as are mental changes. Sensory findings are less frequent. Pathological studies[91] have revealed bilateral corticospinal tract degeneration, and posterior column degeneration may also be seen.

Clinical and pathological findings similar to those of nutritional myelopathy have been attributed to nicotinic acid deficiency (pellagra) but probably are due to several vitamin deficiencies as well as caloric malnutrition.[69, 71] There have been rare reports of myelopathy developing in the setting of chronic alcoholism. Whether this is a direct effect of alcohol *per se* or secondary to associated nutritional deficiencies, liver disease, or other factors is unknown.[62]

MYELOPATHY ASSOCIATED WITH LIVER DISEASE

While encephalopathy is a common manifestation of liver failure, in rare individuals, myelopathy secondary to liver disease is encountered. The myelopathy usually occurs in the setting of a surgical portacaval anastomosis or a spontaneously developing shunt.[17, 81, 131] Hepatic encephalopathy is usually an associated feature but chronic progressive myelopathy secondary to hepatic failure may be the sole neurological abnormality.[195, 275]

The disorder appears to occur predominantly in men.[81] In one review,[81] myelopathy occurred 1 to 120 months following surgical shunting procedures. The clinical features are those of a chronically progressive symmetric spastic paresis. Difficulty in walking is often, therefore, an early complaint. Sphincter dysfunction is also frequently seen, whereas sensory disturbances are not prominent.[103] On pathological inspection, the spinal cord shows bilateral corticospinal tract degeneration; posterior column degeneration also may be seen.[103, 195] The spastic paresis is usually progressive over a course of many years. The pathogenesis of the disorder is unknown.

SPINAL CORD INFARCTION

Although spinal cord infarction had been considered an extremely rare disease, its frequency appears to be increasing. An autopsy study of 3,737 cases at the National Hospital, Queen Square, between 1909 and 1958 found 9 cases (5 arterial occlusion and 4 venous thrombosis) of nonhemorrhagic spinal cord infarction and only 2 cases of hemorrhage.[24] In this older series based on patients in a neurological hospital, the common causes of vascular disease (that is, hypertension and atherosclerosis) were not found to be the etiology in any of the cases; rather, dislocation of the odontoid (1 case), herniated cervical intervertebral disc (3), dissecting aortic aneurysm (1), and subacute necrotic myelitis secondary to thrombosis of spinal veins (4) were the causes found.

A more recent study at a general hospital found 52 cases of hypoxic myelopathy among 1,200 consecutive autopsies over a 5-year period.[259] The discrepancy in the frequency found in these two studies may be because the latter study was done in a general hospital where more systemic diseases that predispose to spinal cord infarction are found, and where more invasive procedures that may be complicated by

spinal cord infarction take place. Causes of spinal cord infarction include aortic dissection, hypotension, atherosclerosis, collagen vascular disease and other inflammatory/infectious diseases, diabetes, trauma, caisson disease, spondylosis, and various surgical or other invasive procedures[57, 98, 103, 196, 206] (Table 8–5). An interesting but rare cause of spinal cord embolization and infarction is fibrocartilaginous embolization.[29, 172]

ARTERIAL INFARCTION

First described early in this century[200, 240] anterior spinal artery infarction is far more common than infarction in the territory of the posterior spinal artery. The anatomical distribution of anterior spinal artery infarction is shown in Chapters 1 and 2.

Patients with anterior spinal artery infarction typically develop, below the level of the lesion, acute paralysis and dissociated sensory loss and loss of sphincter function. The symptoms develop abruptly. Radicular pain in a girdle distribution or lower extremity pain of a throbbing, burning character is often reported to last for two or three days. Usually the motor paralysis below the level of infarction is initially flaccid and areflexic owing to spinal shock. Tendon reflexes usually return and spasticity may supervene. Babinski signs are usually absent initially but later develop. A sensory level is typically found to pain and temperature with preservation of posterior column function. Sacral sensation may be spared. Urinary retention usually occurs immediately following infarction.[233]

Anterior spinal artery infarction is most common in the thoracic area because this is the watershed area for blood flow in the rostro-caudal axis.[98] Thus aortic artery dissection or clamping of the aorta for surgical procedures may cause infarction leading to a sensory level for pain and temperature near the T4 level. A Brown-Séquard syndrome may occur if only half of the spinal cord has been infarcted.

Posterior spinal artery infarction is rare.[192] The damage extends into the posterior horns of the spinal cord, resulting in global anesthesia at the affected level(s).[34]

Table 8–5 CAUSES OF SPINAL CORD INFARCTION*

	Ischemic	Emboli
Heart	Hypotension	Subacute bacterial endocarditis
	Cardiac arrest	Atrial myxoma
Aorta	Atherosclerosis	Aortic angiography
	Aortic surgery (with clamping)	Cholesterol emboli
	Dissecting aneurysm	Saddle emboli
	Coarctation of aorta	Aortic trauma
		Intra-aortic balloon counterpulsation
Vertebra	Vertebral occlusion	Vertebral angiography
	Vertebral dissection	
	Sickle cell anemia	
	Fracture and spinal dislocations	
Intercostal arteries	Thoracoplasty	
	Coarctation operation	
Radicular arteries	Arteriosclerosis	Aortic emboli
	Ligation during surgery	Spinal angiography
	Cervical spondylosis	
	Cervical sprain	
	Caisson disease	
	Plasmacytoma	
	Reticulum cell sarcoma	
	Lumbar sympathectomy	
	Aneurysm artery of Adamkiewicz	
Anterior median spinal artery	Atherosclerosis	Aorta embolization
	Diabetes	
	Syphilis	
	Cervical disc	
Sulcal arteries	Hypertensive lacunae disease	Aorta embolization
	Diabetes	Renal embolization
	Polyarteritis nodosa	
	Infection, TB, syphilis	
Pial microcirculation	In association with AVM	Emboli from AVM
	Adhesive arachnoiditis	
	Neoplastic spread	
	Subarachnoid hemorrhage	
	Infective and granulomatous meningitis	

*From Buchan, AM and Barnett, HJM, [34] p 712, with permission.

Below the level of infarction, there is loss of vibratory and position sensation.

In addition to anterior and posterior spinal artery infarctions, lacunar infarctions also have been found in the spinal cords of patients with hypertension and atherosclerosis.[74] These lesions are considered the spinal counterpart to lacunae in the basal ganglia.[34] Transient ischemic attacks of the spinal cord also have been reported. These seem to be most commonly due to arteriovenous malformations that steal blood into the low-pressure AVM away from the normal tissue.[250] The symptoms of transient ischemia are due either to shunting blood away from normal spinal cord tissue or to compression of the spinal cord when the AVM distends.[34]

VENOUS INFARCTION

Venous infarction of the spinal cord may be either hemorrhagic or nonhemorrhagic. Although venous infarction may occur in the setting of severe systemic disease such as sepsis or carcinomatosis, many patients have an associated vascular malformations.[34, 102, 149]

The typical clinical presentation of a hemorrhagic venous infarction is sudden onset of back, leg, or abdominal pain, evolving over 1 to 2 days to progressive flaccid weakness and loss of sensation below the level of the hemorrhagic infarction, and loss of sphincter function.[102] Because the venous hemorrhagic infarction does not respect the distribution of the anterior spinal artery alone, the sensory loss is usually not that of a dissociated sensory disturbance. Nonhemorrhagic venous infarction of the spinal cord may have a subacute evolution consisting of painless progressive lower extremity weakness, sphincter disturbance, and sensory loss below the level of the lesion.[124] Unlike hemorrhagic venous infarction, all the reported cases of nonhemorrhagic venous infarction have been at T3 or below.[34]

LABORATORY EVALUATION

As emphasized above, vascular diseases of the spinal cord are sufficiently unusual that other diseases such as compressive lesions and inflammatory disorders must be considered first. Meylography excludes extramedullary compressive lesions and MRI can provide anatomical information concerning both the spinal cord and extramedullary tissues. An AVM may be found. Developments in MRI are expected to permit the antemortem diagnosis of these disorders.

Evaluation of CSF is useful to exclude inflammatory conditions (both infectious and noninfectious) and demyelinating disease. The CSF in vascular disease of the spinal cord may demonstrate a nonspecific elevation of protein and pleocytosis. A careful systemic workup for associated conditions such as underlying neoplastic disease, infection, or collagen vascular disease should be performed when clinically indicated.

AUTOIMMUNE DISEASES

The spinal cord may be the target of a variety of systemic autoimmune diseases that by their very nature demonstrate a predilection for multiorgan injury. Among others, Sjogren's syndrome, sytemic lupus erythematosus, rheumatoid arthritis, polyarteritis nodosa, Wegener's granulomatosis, lymphomatoid granulomatosis, Takayasu's arteritis, isolated angiitis of the CNS, spinal cord arteritis, giant cell (temporal) arteritis, Behçet's disease, and progressive systemic sclerosis have been reported to involve the CNS.[11, 36, 38, 165, 166,]

[232] In many cases, there is already evidence of a systemic vasculitis. Alternatively, injury of the central and/or the peripheral nervous system may herald the onset of the disease; in such cases, involvement of the brain, the peripheral nervous system, or both may dominate the neurological manifestations. Rarely, the spinal cord may be the sole manifestation of systemic arteritis. Isolated spinal cord arteritis may rarely be seen in association with heroin addiction.[232] The reader is referred to review articles and textbooks of rheumatology and internal medicine for a more detailed discussion of autoimmune disorders.[166, 167]

Sjogren's Syndrome

Sjogren's syndrome is an autoimmune disease that is considered to affect approximately 2 percent of the population.[10] It characteristically involves the lacrimal and salivary glands, resulting in xerophthalmia and xerostomia. Multiple visceral organs also may be involved, including the central and peripheral nervous system.[11, 73]

A recent study[10] reported that approximately 20 percent of patients with primary Sjogren's syndrome developed CNS involvement. In such cases, episodic multifocal involvement of the brain and spinal cord may evolve over time. Thus the presentation of such patients may mimic the clinical course of multiple sclerosis. In addition to cerebral, brainstem, and cerebellar disturbances, patients may demonstrate an acute or subacute transverse myelopathy, chronic progressive myelopathy, neurogenic bladder, and other spinal cord syndromes.[127] In the study above,[10] the spinal cord was involved in 85 percent of cases with CNS involvement.

The CSF findings in patients with CNS involvement by Sjogren's syndrome mimic those found in multiple sclerosis.[10] For example, there may be CSF pleocytosis, oligoclonal bands, and elevated IgG indices. Evoked responses may also be abnormal at multiple sites, as typically seen with demyelinating diseases.[10] MRI of the spinal cord and brain also may demonstrate abnormalities similar to those seen in multiple sclerosis.[9, 10.] Although the pathogenesis of CNS involvement is uncertain, an immune vasculopathy has been considered.[11]

The diagnosis of CNS involvement by Sjogren's syndrome may be difficult if the underlying disease has not been recognized. Involvement of multiple organs such as salivary and lacrimal glands, lungs, kidneys, thyroid, muscle, and peripheral nerves may suggest the diagnosis and help distinguish this disease from multiple sclerosis.[10, 11] Furthermore, the presence of antibodies to Ro(SS-A) or La(SS-B) and other serologic abnormalities are often found in these patients.[10, 144]

Case Illustration

A 54-year-old woman with a past medical history significant for discoid lupus and Raynaud's phenomenon developed neck pain and pain radiating into the left arm when her neck was hyperextended during a shampoo. An orthopedic consultation found a left C6 radiculopathy and she was placed in a cervical collar. Two weeks later she developed numbness of the left lower face and ascending numbness beginning in the left lower extremity, which then extended into the right leg and later ascended up through the trunk to the ulnar aspect of both hands, forearms, and axillae. She was admitted to the hospital for evaluation.

General physical examination was unremarkable. Neurological examination demonstrated slight hyperpathia over the second and third divisions of the left fifth cranial nerve. There were also hyperpathia and causalgia bilaterally from the first thoracic segment caudally with preservation of temperature and position sensation. On extension of the neck, dysesthesias appeared in the lower back. Motor, cerebellar, and gait examinations were normal. There was a depressed left brachioradialis reflex and plantar responses were flexor.

Laboratory studies revealed a sedimentation rate of 40, and a positive ANA with a titer of 1:128 consisting of a diffuse and nucleolar pattern. CSF revealed normal cell count, protein, and glucose, and the IgG index was normal. There were two faint oligoclonal bands in the CSF, which were also present in the serum. Cervical spine film showed narrowing of the disc space at the C5−6 level. MRI (0.15 Tesla unit) of the brain and cervical spine showed an equivocal small linear periventricular hyperintensity in the left parietal area of unknown significance, and compression of the spinal cord at the C5−6 level due to disc protrusion and spondylosis. Triple evoked responses including somatosensory latencies from the upper and lower extremities were normal. Rheumatological consultation revealed no evidence for systemic lupus erythematosus or autoimmune illness involving the CNS. A neurosurgical opinion was obtained and although the presentation was considered atypical, a tentative diagnosis of spinal cord compression and cervical radiculopathy was made and the patient was discharged with a soft cervical collar.

Five days later she was readmitted with progressive right leg weakness and a right Babinski sign but no evidence of left leg weakness. She had pain in both hands and forearms, and dysesthesias and reduced pin sensation below the C7 level bilaterally. A myelogram demonstrated congenital spinal stenosis with superimposed spinal cord compression at the C5−6 level due to disc protrusion and spondylosis with bilateral foraminal encroachment at the same level. Repeat MRI of the brain showed no evidence of the previously seen area of hyperintensity in the left parietal area. The clinical presentation was considered atypical for cervical spondylosis, but in the absence of a definitive alternative diagnosis and with concern that the spinal cord compression could be responsible, the patient underwent an anterior cervical discectomy and fusion of C5−6.

Postoperatively the patient's myelopathy was significantly improved but she continued to complain of progressive sensory disturbances of the upper extremities and described a progressive tight girdle-like sensation of the chest. A repeat MRI of the brain and cervical spine 4 months postoperatively demonstrated several areas of hyperintensity in both cerebral hemispheres and no evidence of spinal cord compression. Electrodiagnostic studies of the upper extremities demonstrated no evidence of peripheral neuropathy or denervation. Somatosensory evoked responses of the upper extremities revealed conduction disturbances within the cervical spinal cord.

Over the next several weeks, the patient developed progressive position sense disturbances of the hands, with secondary pseudoathetoid movements. A repeat rheumatological evaluation included serological studies for Sjogren's syndrome, the results of which were positive. A biopsy of minor salivary glands was interpreted as consistent with this diagnosis. The patient was placed on a course of steroids and cyclophosphamide for several months with clinical stabilization of her neurological syndrome. However, MRI continued to show evidence of evolving subclinical cerebral lesions.

Comment. This case illustrates the frequent difficulty of differentiating intramedullary spinal cord disease from spinal cord compression. Although this patient did have spinal cord compression secondary to cervical spondylosis, which may have aggravated the intramedullary spinal cord disease, the latter was primarily responsible for her neurological condition, as ultimately shown by her clinical course. Only with continued close observation and the recognition at the time of surgery that the spondylosis alone might not have been completely responsible for her neurological condition was the diagnosis of neurological involvement by Sjogren's syndrome made. The case also illustrates that a systemic disease such as Sjogren's syndrome may present clinically with spinal cord dysfunction alone.

Systemic Lupus Erythematosus

Systemic lupus erythematosus (SLE) is typically a systemic disease with multiorgan involvement. In occasional patients, however, the CNS is the principal site of clinical involvement, with minimal evidence of skin or articular disease.[79] Furthermore, although less common than cerebral and brainstem involvement, myelopathy has been well documented as a complication of SLE.[206]

Among patients with SLE, the most common cause of myelopathy has been found to be vascular disease.[112] In 26 cases of transverse myelopathy in the setting of SLE,[8] the myelopathy, which could occur at any time during the course of SLE, evolved rapidly in the majority of cases. A sensory level, sphincter disturbance, and paresis or paralysis below the lesion was commonplace. On pathological examination, extensive destruction of the thoracic and lumbar segments was usually seen, with angiitis and thrombosis of blood vessels secondary to SLE. Prognosis

for recovery with this form of myelopathy is considered to be poor.[206]

Other cases of myelopathy in patients with SLE may resemble acute transverse myelopathy.[12, 191, 206] As in other cases of acute transverse myelopathy, the pathogenesis of those cases associated with SLE is unknown.[206]

Occasionally, myelopathy in the setting of SLE may clinically resemble multiple sclerosis.[79, 206, 230] In such cases the patient may show improvement in neurological function, as in some bouts of multiple sclerosis. Patients with SLE also have been reported to develop a necrotic and demyelinative myelopathy and demyelinative optic neuritis.[14, 206]

PARANEOPLASTIC MYELOPATHY

Paraneoplastic myelopathy refers to spinal cord disease in patients with malignancy where the myelopathy is not due to compression from tumor, effects of treatment, metabolic or electrolyte imbalance, or identifiable disease unrelated to the malignancy (e.g, spondylosis, vitamin B_{12} deficiency)[176] (Table 8–6). Paraneoplastic myelopathies must be considered in the cancer patient with a progressive myelopathy for which no alternative cause is discovered.

First described by Mancall and Rosales,[149] the etiology and pathogenesis of paraneoplastic myelopathies is unknown.[177] On pathological examination of the spinal cord, necrotizing myelopathy is characterized by nearly symmetric necrosis involving both gray and white matter.[99] Both myelin sheaths and axons are in-

Table 8–6 CLASSIFICATION OF SPINAL CORD LESIONS IN CANCER PATIENTS

Metastatic Cancer
  Epidural
  Leptomeningeal
  Intramedullary
Toxicity from Therapy
  Radiation Myelopathy
  Myelopathy due to Chemotherapy
  Infectious Disease
  Vascular Disease
  Paraneoplastic Syndromes
  Diseases Unrelated to Cancer or Its Therapy

volved and there is a predilection for the thoracic spinal cord.[177] Vascular necrotic changes also may be seen but the pathological changes within the spinal cord are not characteristic of those of ischemic myelopathy.[196]

The clinical picture of paraneoplastic necrotizing myelopathy is that of a rapidly ascending sensorimotor myelopathy. The course is typically short, with death ensuing within a few months.[177] Paraneoplastic myelopathy has most frequently occurred in the setting of a variety of carcinomas and lymphoma.[177] As discussed in Chapter 6, the diagnosis may be difficult to distinguish from intramedullary metastasis, radiation myelopathy, and other diseases because there is no specific laboratory test for paraneoplastic myelopathy. Its rarity compared with the frequent incidence of metastatic disease to the spine or complications of therapy should be recognized by the clinician when this diagnosis is considered.[177]

NEURONAL DEGENERATIONS

There are several neuronal degenerations that may involve the spinal cord and are thus considered in the differential diagnosis of spinal cord compression. Some of these disorders are genetic in origin (Table 8–7) and others are of unknown etiology and pathogenesis (for example, motor neuron disease).

The clinical presentation of most of these disorders share several features. Most begin insidiously and are slowly progressive. In those cases of genetic origin, patients may report a history of clumsiness or inability to compete in athletics or perform in the military at an early age. Other signs, such as pes cavus and scoliosis, may precede the clinical presentation.

**Table 8–7 SOME NEURONAL
DEGENERATIONS OF GENETIC ORIGIN**

Spinocerebellar ataxia (Friedereich's ataxia)
Hereditary motor neuron disease
Werdnig-Hoffmann disease
Hereditary spastic paraplegia
Charcot-Marie-Tooth disease
Adrenomyeloneuropathy

A family history of neurological disease may be obtained. Unlike the case of spinal cord compression, pain is not usually a prominent early feature. Symptoms and signs of involvement of the brain and/or peripheral nerves are frequently encountered, if carefully sought. There may be other signs of systemic involvement such as heart disease in Friedereich's ataxia or endocrine disturbance in adrenomyeloneuropathy. The reader is referred to textbooks of neurology and other sources for a complete discussion.

ACUTE AND SUBACUTE TRANSVERSE MYELOPATHY OF UNKNOWN ETIOLOGY

Despite exhaustive attempts to diagnose the etiology and pathogenesis of acute or subacute noncompressive transverse myelopathy, there are many cases in which no specific diagnosis can be made at the time of clinical presentation. This has led to the concept of noncompressive transverse myelopathy (TM), which is defined as a clinical syndrome of bilateral intramedullary dysfunction, which may be ascending or static and often involves several spinal segmental levels; the syndrome occurs without prior history of neurological disease.[140, 212] *Because there is usually no specific laboratory test for transverse myelopathy, the diagnosis of noncompressive TM is often a clinical one after the exclusion of known (and often treatable) causes such as cord compression secondary to neoplasm, abscess, or degenerative joint disease.*

Although the etiology is often unknown, some neuropathological processes that may give rise to TM include: postinfectious and postvaccination myelitis, multiple sclerosis, and acute necrotizing myelitis;[2, 3, 21, 183] viral invasion of the spinal cord;[18, 101] spinal cord infarction;[34, 98, 241] radiation myelopathy;[33, 77, 116, 224] vascular malformations;[78, 274] and paraneoplastic syndrome.[149, 176, 227] Even after a clinical diagnosis of TM is made, the specific etiology and pathogenesis may remain obscure despite a detailed evaluation; thus the clinician may not be able to distin guish between the various causes of TM and must consider TM as a clinical syndrome of diverse etiology.

The clinical challenge in diagnosing TM is seen in a study from the Massachusetts General Hospital.[212] Of 164 patients presenting with acute myelopathy or myelitis, 82 were ultimately found to have an anatomical mass lesion (usually metastatic cancer) responsible for the myelopathy. Because many of the patients reviewed had been initially diagnosed as having TM but were later found to have tumors impinging on the spinal cord, the researchers would only include in their study those patients who had undergone a myelogram to exclude a compressive lesion. This study underscores *the necessity to exclude compressive lesions of the cord that are treatable before a diagnosis of TM is made.*

The clinical features of 52 patients with TM have been reported in detail.[212] The age at diagnosis ranged from 4 to 83 years and there was no sex preponderance. A recent acute infectious illness was reported to antedate the onset of TM in one third of patients. The initial symptoms are shown in Table 8–8. In some patients, these symptoms occurred in combination. Paresthesias often began distally and ascended. When pain was the presenting complaint, it usually occurred at the segmental level of neurological dysfunction. The temporal profile of the myelopathy varied in these 52 patients; 21 percent of the patients developed a myelopathy within 12 hours, 69 percent progressed smoothly over a period of 1 to 14 days, and 10 percent had a stuttering progressive course over a period of 10 days to 4 weeks. Spinal shock was seen in some of the patients with catastrophic onset.

The difficulty in clinically distinguishing intramedullary disease from extramedullary compressive disease has already been reviewed. In a manner similar to patients with TM, patients with epidural abscess or spinal tumor usually present with back pain and a relatively rapid neurological deterioration. Although neoplasms generally run a more chronic course than the inflammatory myelitides, spinal tumors may have a brief course. Although the history of recent infection may be helpful in a diagnosis of postinfectious myelitis, patients with epidural abscess often have a history of recent infection as well. These observations underscore the importance of a high index of suspicion for cord compression and emphasize the role of laboratory and imaging studies in differentiating compressive lesions such as epidural abscess or neoplasm from transverse myelopathy. In arriving at a diagnosis of noncompressive myelitis or myelopathy, the clinician must ask at each juncture, "Can this patient be harboring a compressive lesion?"

The optimal treatment of acute and subacute transverse myelopathy of unknown etiology remains uncertain. In the Massachusetts General Hospital series,[212] half of the patients with adequate follow-up received no specific treatment other than bed rest and analgesia as required. An equal number of patients received adrenocorticotrophic hormone or corticosteroids. Some of the general principles involving the management of patients with myelopathy are discussed in the section on postinfectious myelitis.

The prognosis for neurological recovery following TM varies from good to poor. Factors that have been found to affect outcome include the tempo of neurological deterioration and the presence of back

Table 8–8 SUMMARY OF CLINICAL DATA FROM 52 PATIENTS WITH ACUTE AND SUBACUTE NONCOMPRESSIVE TRANSVERSE MYELOPATHY*

	Number (%) of Patients
Preceding febrile illness	18 (35%)
Initial symptoms	
Paresthesias	24 (46%)
Back pain	18 (35%)
Leg weakness	7 (13%)
Sphincter disturbance	3 (6%)
Time to maximal deficit	
< 1 day	13 (25%)
1 to 10 days	30 (57%)
> 10 days	9 (17%)
Multiple sclerosis	7 (13%)
Outcome	
Good	16 (31%)
Fair	20 (38%)
Poor	12 (23%)
Total	52

*From Ropper, AH and Poskanzer, DC,[212] p 58, with permission.

pain. Patients with a gradual or stuttering progressive myelopathy had a good (41 percent) or fair (46 percent) outcome in the series cited above.[212] However, a poor outcome was found in 64 percent of those with a rapid catastrophic onset and in 53 percent of those with back pain heralding the onset. Of the 52 patients, 7 (13 percent) were diagnosed as having multiple sclerosis on follow-up examinations.[212]

REFERENCES

1. Abeshouse, BA and Tiongson, AT: Paraplegia, a rare complication of translumbar aortography. J Urol 75:348–355, 1956.
2. Abramsky, O and Teitelbaum, D: The autoimmune features of acute transverse myelopathy. Ann Neurol 2:36–40, 1977.
3. Adams, RD and Kubick, CS: The morbid anatomy of the demyelinating diseases. Am J Med 12:510–546, 1952.
4. Adams, RD and Victor, M: Nonviral infections of the nervous system. In Adams, RD and Victor, M (eds): Principles of Neurology, ed 3. McGraw-Hill, New York, 1985, pp 510–544.
5. Adams, RD and Victor, M: Viral infections of the nervous system. In Adams, RD and Victor, M (eds): Principles of Neurology, ed 3. McGraw-Hill, New York, 1985, pp 545–568.
6. Adams, RD and Victor, M: Diseases of the spinal cord. In Adams, RD and Victor, M (eds): Principles of Neurology, ed 3. McGraw-Hill, New York, 1985, pp 665–698.
7. Adams, RD and Victor, M: Disorders of the nervous system due to drugs and other chemical agents. In Adams, RD and Victor, M (eds): Principles of Neurology, ed 3. McGraw-Hill, New York, 1985, pp 826–858.
8. Adrianakos, AA, Duffy, J, Suzuki, M, and Sharp, JT: Transverse myelopathy in systemic lupus erythematosus: Report of three cases and review of the literatutre. Ann Intern Med 83:616–624, 1975.
9. Alexander, EL, Beall, SS, Gordon, B, et al: Magnetic resonance imaging of cerebral lesions in patients with the Sjogren syndrome. Ann Intern Med 108:815–823, 1988.
10. Alexander, EL, Malinow, K, Lejewski, JE, et al: Primary Sjogren's syndrome with central nervous system disease mimicking multiple sclerosis. Ann Intern Med 104:323–330, 1986.
11. Alexander, EL, Provost, TT, Stevens, MB, and Alexander, GE: Neurologic complications of primary Sjogren's syndrome. Medicine 61:247–257, 1982.
12. Andrews, JM, Cancilla, PA, and Kimm, J: Regressive spinal cord signs in a patient with disseminated lupus erythematosus. Bulletin of the Los Angeles Neurological Society 35:78–85, 1970.
13. Applebaum, E, Kreps, SI, and Sunshine, A: Herpes zoster encephalitis. Am J Med 32:25–31, 1972.
14. April, RS and Vansonnenberg, E: A case of neuromyelitis optica (Devic's syndrome) in systemic lupus erythematosus: Clinicopathologic report and review of the literature. Neurology 26:1066–1070, 1976.
15. Aring, CS: The systemic nervous affinity of triorthocresyl phosphate (Jamaica ginger palsy). Brain 65:34–47, 1942.
16. Barnes, DW and Whitley, RJ: CNS diseases associated with varicella zoster virus and herpes simplex virus infection. Neurol Clin 4:265–283, 1986.
17. Bechar, M, Freud, M, Kott, E, et al: Hepatic cirrhosis with post-shunt myelopathy. J Neurol Sci 11:101–107, 1970.
18. Bell, EJ and Russel, SJM: Acute transverse myelopathy and ECHO-2 virus infection. Lancet 2:1226–1227, 1963.
19. Benninger, TR and Patterson, VH: Lhermitte's sign as a presenting symptom of B_{12} deficiency. Ulster Med J 53:162–163, 1984.
20. Bergeron, RT, Rumbaugh, CL, Frang, H, et al: Experimental pantopaque arachnoiditis in the monkey. Radiology 99:95–101, 1971.
21. Berman, M, Feldman, S, Alter, M, et al: Acute transverse myelitis: Incidence and etiologic considerations. Neurology 31:966–971, 1981.
22. Bermudez, MA, Grant, KM, Rodvien, R, and Mendes, F: Non-Hodgkin's lymphoma in a population with or at risk for acquired immunodeficiency syndrome: Indications for intensive chemotherapy. Am J Med 86:71–76, 1989.
23. Bhagavati, S, Ehrlich, G, Kula, RW, et al: Detection of human T-cell lymphoma/leukemia virus type I DNA and antigen in spinal fluid and blood of patients with chronic progressive myelopathy. N Engl J Med 318:1141–1147, 1988.
24. Blackwood, W: Discussion on the vascular disease of the spinal cord. Proc R Soc Med 51:543, 1958.
25. Bleyer, WA and Byrne, TN: Leptomeningeal cancer in leukemia and solid tumors. Current Problems in Cancer 12:185–238, 1988.
26. Blumhardt, LD, Barrett, G, and Halliday, AM: The pattern visual evoked potential in the clinical assessment of undiagnosed spinal cord disease. In Corjon, JE, Maugiere, F and Revol, M (eds): Clinical Applications of Evoked Potentials in Neurology. Raven Press, New York, 1982, pp 463–471.
27. Bodian, D: Histopathologic basis of clinical findings in poliomyelitis. Am J Med 6:563–578, 1949.
28. Booss, J and Esiri, MM: Viral Encephalitis: Pathology, Diagnosis and Management.

Blackwell Scientific Publishers, Oxford, 1986.

29. Bots, TAM, Wattendorf, AR, and Buruma, OJS: Acute myelopathy caused by fibrocartilaginous emboli. Neurology 31:1250–1256, 1981.

30. Brew, BJ and Price, RW: Another retroviral disease of the nervous system: Chronic progressive myelopathy due to HTLV-I. N Engl J Med 318:1195–1197, 1988.

31. Brew, BJ, Sidtis, JJ, Petito, CK, and Price, RW: The neurological complications of AIDS and human immunodeficiency virus infection. In Plum, F (ed): Advances in Contemporary Neurology. FA Davis, Philadelphia, 1988, pp 1–50.

32. Britton, DB, Mesa-Tejada, R, Fenoglio, CM, et al: A new complication of AIDS: Thoracic myelitis caused by herpes simplex virus. Neurology 35:1071–1074, 1985.

33. Brown, WJ and Kagan, AR: Comparison of myelopathy associated with megavoltage irradiation and remote cancer. In Gilbert, HJ and Kagan, AR (eds): Radiation Damage to the Nervous System. Raven Press, New York, 1980, pp 191–206.

34. Buchan, AM and Barnett, HJM: Infarction of the spinal cord. In Barnett, HJM, Mohr, JP, Stein, BM and Yatsu, FM (eds): Stroke: Pathophysiology, Diagnosis and Management. Churchill Livingstone, New York, 1986, pp 707–719.

35. Burns, RJ, Jones, AN, and Robertson, JS: Pathology of radiation myelopathy. J Neurol Neurosurg Psychiatry 35:888–898, 1972.

36. Calabrese, LH and Mallek, JA: Primary angiitis of the central nervous system. Medicine 67:20–38, 1987.

37. Carter, JL, Hafler, DA, Dawson, DM, et al: Immunosuppression with high-dose IV cyclophosphamide and ACTH in progressive multiple sclerosis: Cumulative 6-year experience in 164 patients. Neurology (Suppl 2)38:9–14, 1988.

38. Caselli, RJ, Hunder, GG, and Whisnant, JP: Neurologic disease in biopsy-proven giant cell (temporal) arteritis. Neurology 38:352–359, 1988.

39. Cashman, NR, Maselli, R, Wollman, R, et al: Late denervation in patients with antecedent paralytic poliomyelitis. N Engl J Med 317:7–12, 1987.

40. Cashman, NR, Siegel, IM, and Antel, JP: Postpolio syndrome: A review. Clinics Prosthetics and Orthotics 11:74–78, 1987.

41. CDC: STD treatment guidelines. MMWR (Suppl)34:94S–99S, 1985.

42. Chaduri, RN: Paralytic disease caused by contamination with tricresyl phosphate. Trans R Soc Trop Med Hyg 59:98, 1965.

43. Chan, RC and Steinboh, P: Delayed onset of Lhermitte's sign following head and/or neck injuries. J Neurosurg 60:609–612, 1984.

44. Cook, SD, Devereaux, C, Troiano, R, et al: Total lymphoid irradiation in chronic progressive multiple sclerosis: Relationship between blood lymphocytes and clinical course. Ann Neurol 22:634–638, 1987.

45. Cotton, PB and Webb-Peploe, MM: Acute transverse myelitis as a complication of glandular fever. Br Med J 1:654–656, 1966.

46. Coyle, PK: Borrelia burgdorferi antibodies in multiple sclerosis patients. Neurology 39:760–761, 1989.

47. Croft, PB: Para-infectious and post-vaccinal encephalomyelitis. Postgrad Med 45:392–400, 1969.

48. Cruickshank, EK: Effects of malnutrition on the central nervous system and the nerves. In Vinken, PJ and Bruyn, GW (eds): Handbook of Clinical Neurology, Vol 28. North-Holland Publishing, Amsterdam, 1976, pp 1–41.

49. Curnen, EC, Shaw, EW, and Melnick, JL: Diseases resembling nonparalytic poliomyelitis associated with a virus pathogenic for infant mice. JAMA 141:894–901, 1949.

50. Dalakas, MC, Elder, G, Hallett, M, et al: A long-term follow-up study of patients with postpoliomyelitis neuromuscular symptoms. N Engl J Med 314:959–963, 1986.

51. Dalakas, MC and Hallett, M: The post-polio syndrome. In Plum, F (ed): Advances in Contemporary Neurology. FA Davis, Philadelphia, 1988, pp 51–94.

52. Dalakas, MC, Sever, JL, Madden, DL, et al: Late postpoliomyelitis muscular atrophy: Clinical, virologic, and immunologic studies. Rev Infect Dis (Suppl 2)6:562–567, 1984.

53. Dastur, DK: Lathyrism. Some aspects of the disease in man and animals. World Neurology 3:721–730, 1962.

54. Davis, L, Haven, H, Givens, JH, and Emmett, J: Effects of spinal anesthetics on the spinal cord and its membranes: Experimental study. JAMA 97:1781–1785, 1931.

55. Davis, LE and Schmitt, JW: Clinical significance of cerebrospinal fluid tests for neurosyphilis. Ann Neurol 25:50–55, 1989.

56. DeJong, RN: Sensation. In Vinken, PJ and Bruyn, GW (eds): Handbook of Clinical Neurology, Vol 1. North-Holland Publishing, Amsterdam, 1969, pp 80–113.

57. DeJong, RN: The neurological manifestations of diabetes mellitus. In Vinken, PJ and Bruyn, GW (eds): Handbook of Clinical Neurology, Vol 27. North-Holland Publishing, Amsterdam, 1976, pp 99–142.

58. Delattre, JY, Rosenblum, MK, Thaler, HT, et al: A model of radiation myelopathy in the rat. Pathology, regional capillary permeability changes and treatment with dexamethasone. Brain 111:1319–1336, 1988.

59. Denny-Brown, D: Neurological conditions resulting from prolonged and severe dietary restriction. Medicine 26:41–113, 1947.

60. Devereaux, C, Troiano, R, Zito, G, et al: Effect of total lymphoid irradiation on functional status in chronic multiple sclerosis: Importance of lymphopenia early after treatment—the pros. Neurology (Suppl 2)38:32–37, 1988.

61. Dickson, DW, Belman, AL, Kim, TS, et al: Spinal

cord pathology in pediatric acquired immunodeficiency syndrome. Neurology 39:227–235, 1989.

62. Dreyfus, PM: Amblyopia and other neurological disorders associated with chronic alcoholism. In Vinken, PJ and Bruyn, GW (eds): Handbook of Clinical Neurology, Vol 28. North-Holland Publishing, Amsterdam, 1976, pp 331–347.

63. Dripps, RD and Vandam, LD: Long-term followup of patients who received 10,098 spinal anesthetics: Failure to discover major neurological sequelae. JAMA 156:1486–1491, 1954.

64. Dubuisson, D: Nerve root damage and arachnoiditis. In Wall, PD and Melzack, R (eds): Textbook of Pain. Churchill Livingstone, Edinburgh, 1984, pp 435–450.

65. Dunne, K, Hopkins, IJ, and Shield, LK: Acute transverse myelopathy in childhood. Dev Med Child Neur 28:198–204, 1986.

66. Duttera, MJ, Bleyer, WA, Pomeroy, TC, et al: Irradiation, methotrexate toxicity, and treatment of meningeal leukemia. Lancet 2:703–707, 1973.

67. Ebers, GC: Multiple sclerosis and other demyelinating diseases. In Asbury, AK, McKhann, GM and McDonald, WI (eds): Diseases of the Nervous System; Clinical Neurobiology. WB Saunders, Philadelphia, 1986, pp 1268–1281.

68. Epperson, LW, Whitaker, JN, and Kapila, A: Cranial MRI in acute disseminated encephalomyelitis. Neurology 38:332–333, 1988.

69. Erbsloh, F and Abel, M: Deficiency neuropathies. In Vinken, PJ and Bruyn, GW (eds): Handbook of Clinical Neurology, Vol 7. North-Holland Publishing, Amsterdam, 1970, pp 558–663.

70. Evans, JP and Keegan, HR: Danger in the use of intrathecal methylene blue. JAMA 174:856–859, 1960.

71. Farmer, TW: Neurologic complications of vitamin and mineral disorders. In Baker, AB and Baker, LH (eds): Clinical Neurology. Harper & Row, Hagerstown, Md, 1979, pp 1–31

72. Farrell, DF and Starr, A: Delayed neurological sequelae of electrical injuries. Neurology 18:601–606, 1968.

73. Ferreiro, JE, Robalino, BD, and Saldana, MJ: Primary Sjogren's syndrome with diffuse cerebral vasculitis and lymphocytic interstitial pneumonitis. Am J Med 82:1227–1232, 1987.

74. Fieschi, C, Gottlieb, A, and De Carolis, V; Ischaemic lacunae in the spinal cord of arteriosclerotic subjects. J Neurol Neurosurg Psychiatry 33:138–146, 1970.

75. Finkel, MF: Lyme disease and its neurological complications. Arch Neurol 45:99–104, 1988.

76. Fog, T: Topographic distribution of plaques in the spinal cord in multiple sclerosis. Archives of Neurology Psychiatry 63:382–414, 1950.

77. Fogelholm, R, Haltia, M, and Andersson, LC:

Radiation myelopathy of the cervical spinal cord simulating intramedullary neoplasm. J Neurol Neurosurg Psychiatry 37:1177–1180, 1974.

78. Foix, C and Alajouanine, T: La myelite necrotique subaigue. Rev Neurol 2:1–42, 1926.

79. Fulford, KWM, Catterall, RD, Delhanty, JJ, et al: A collagen disorder of the nervous system presenting as multiple sclerosis. Brain 95:373–386, 1972.

80. Gagliano, RG and Costanzi, JJ: Paraplegia following intrathecal methotrexate. Cancer 37:1663–1668, 1976.

81. Gauthier, G and Wildi, E: L'encephalo-myelopathie porto-systemique. Rev Neurol 131:319–338, 1975.

82. Gautier-Smith, PC: Lhermitte's sign in subacute degeneration of the cord. J Neurol Neurosurg Psychiatry 36:861–863, 1973.

83. Gessain, A, Barin, F, Vernant, JC, et al: Antibodies to human T-lymphotropic virus type-I in patients with spastic tropical paraparesis. Lancet 2:407–409, 1985.

84. Gilbert, RW, Kim, JH, and Posner, JB: Epidural spinal cord compression from metastatic tumor: Diagnosis and treatment. Ann Neurol 3:40–51, 1978.

85. Godwin-Austen, RB, Howell, DA, and Worthington, B: Observations on radiation myelopathy. Brain 98:557–568, 1975.

86. Goldstick, L, Mandybur, TI, and Bode, R: Spinal cord degeneration in AIDS. Neurology 35:103–106, 1985.

87. Gordon, IRS and Tucker, JF: Lesions of the central nervous system in herpes zoster. J Neurol Neurosurg Psychiatry 8:40–46, 1945.

88. Grafe, MR and Wiley, CA: Spinal cord and peripheral nerve pathology in AIDS: The roles of cytomegalovirus and human immunodeficiency virus. Ann Neurol 25:561–566, 1989.

89. Greenfield, JG: Acute disseminated encephalomyelitis, a sequel to "influenza." J Path Bact 33:453–462, 1930.

90. Greenfield, MM and Stark, FM: Post-irradiation neuropathy. Am J Roentgenol Radium Ther Nucl Med 60:617–622, 1948.

91. Grieve, S, Jacobson, S, and Proctor, NSF: A nutritional myelopathy occurring in the Bantu on the Witwatersrand. Neurology 17:1205–1212, 1967.

92. Grossman, CB and Post, MJD: The adult spine. In Gonzalez, CF, Grossman, CB, and Masdeu, JC (eds): Head and Spine Imaging. John Wiley & Sons, New York, 1985, pp 781–858.

93. Gutin, PH, Levi, JA, Wiernik, PH, and Walker, MD: Treatment of malignant meningeal disease with intrathecal thio-TEPA: A phase II study. Cancer Treat Rep 61:885–887, 1977.

94. Halperin, JJ, Lift, BJ, Anand, AK, and others: Lyme neuroborelliosis: Central nervous system manifestations. Neurology 39:753–759, 1989.

95. Harrison, RJ: Zoster myelitis presenting with

acute retention of urine. Proc R Soc Med 57:589–590, 1964.

96. Haughton, VM and Ho, K-C: Arachnoid response to contrast media: A comparison of iophendylate and metrizamide in experimental animals. Radiology 143:699–702, 1982.

97. Haughton, VM and Williams, AL: Computed Tomography of the Spine. CV Mosby, St Louis, 1982.

98. Henson, RA and Parsons, M: Ischaemic lesions of the spinal cord: An illustrated review. J Med 36:205–222, 1967.

99. Henson, RA and Urich, H: Cancer and the Nervous System. Blackwell, Oxford, 1982.

99a. Herskowitz, S, Siegel, SE, Schneider, AT, et al: Spinal cord toxoplasmosis in AIDS. Neurology 39: 1552–1553, 1989.

100. Hochberg, FH and Miller, DG: Primary central nervous system lymphoma. (review article). J Neurosurg 68:835–853, 1988.

101. Hogan, EL and Krigman, MR: Herpes zoster myelitis. Arch Neurol 29:309–313, 1973.

102. Hughes, JT: Venous infarction of the spinal cord. Neurology 21:794–800, 1971.

103. Hughes, JT: Pathology of the Spinal Cord. WB Saunders, Philadelphia, 1978.

104. Hume, AL and Waxman, SG: Evoked potentials in suspected multiple sclerosis: Diagnostic value and prediction of clinical course. J Neurol Sci 83:191–210, 1988.

105. Hurst, EW and Pawan, JL: Outbreak of rabies in Trinidad, without history or bites, and with symptoms of acute ascending myelitis. Lancet 2:622–628, 1931.

106. Jackson, FE, Martin, R, and Davis, R: Delayed quadriplegia following electrical burn. Milit Med 130:601–605, 1965.

107. Jarcho, LW, Fred, HL, and Castle, CH: Encephalitis and poliomyelitis in the adult due to coxsackie virus group B, type 5. N Engl J Med 268:235–238, 1963.

107a. Jemsek, J, Greenberg, SB, Taber, L, et al: Herpes zoster-associated encephalitis: Clinicopathologic report of 12 cases and review of the literature. Medicine 62:81–97, 1983.

108. Johnson, RT: Herpes zoster. In Wyngaarden, JB and Smith, LH Jr (eds): Cecil: Textbook of Internal Medicine, ed 17. WB Saunders, Philadelphia, 1985, pp 2128–2130.

109. Johnson, RT: Acute anterior poliomyelitis. In Wyngaarden, JB and Smith, LH Jr (eds): Cecil: Textbook of Internal Medicine, ed 17. WB Saunders, Philadelphia, 1985, pp 2130–2132.

110. Johnson, RT, Griffin, DE, Hirsch, RL, et al: Measles encephalomyelitis—clinical and immunological studies. N Engl J Med 310:137, 1984.

111. Johnson, RT and McArthur, JC: Myelopathies and retroviral infections (editorial). Ann Neurol 21:113–116, 1987.

112. Johnson, RT and Richardson, EP Jr: The neurological manifestations of systemic lupus erythematosus: A clinical-pathological study of 24 cases and review of the literature. Medicine 47:337–369, 1968.

113. Jones, A: Transient radiation myelopathy (with reference to Lhermitte's sign of electrical paresthesia). Br J Radiol 37:727–744, 1964.

114. Jordan, KG: Modern neurosyphilis—a critical analysis. West J Med 149:47–57, 1988.

115. Junck, L and Marshall, WH: Neurotoxicity of radiological contrast agents. Ann Neurol 13:469–484, 1983.

116. Kagan, AR, Wollin, M, Gilbert, HA, et al: Comparison of the tolerance of the brain and spinal cord to injury by radiations. In Gilbert, HA and Kagan, AR (eds): Radiation Damage to the Nervous System. Raven Press, New York, 1980, pp 183–190.

117. Kamman, GR and Baker, AB: Damage to the spinal cord and meninges following spinal anesthesia: A clinico-pathological study. Minn Med 26:786–791, 1943.

118. Kaplan, RS and Wiernik, PH: Neurotoxicity of antineoplastic drugs. Semin Oncol 9:103–129, 1982.

119. Kendall, D: Motor complications of herpes zoster. Br Med J 2:616–618, 1957.

120. Kennedy, F, Effron, AS, and Perry, G: The grave spinal cord paralyses caused by spinal anesthesia. Surg Gynecol Obstet 91:385–398, 1950.

121 Khanchandani, R and Howe, JG: Lhermitte's sign in multiple sclerosis: A clinical survey and review of the literature. J Neurol Neurosurg Psychiatry 45:308–312, 1982.

122. Killen, DA and Foster, JH: Spinal cord injury as a complication of aortography. Ann Surg 152:211–230, 1960.

123. Killen, DA and Foster, JH: Spinal cord injury as a complication of contrast angiography. Surgery 59:969–981, 1966.

124. Kim, R, Smith, HR, Henbest, ML, and Choi, BH: Nonhemorrhagic venous infarction of the spinal cord. Ann Neurol 15:379–385, 1984.

125. Klastersky, J, Cappel, R, and Snoeck, JM: Ascending myelitis in association with herpes simplex virus. N Engl J Med 287:182–184, 1972.

126. Knutti, RE: Acute ascending paralysis and myelitis due to the virus of rabies. JAMA 93:754–758, 1929.

127. Konttinen, YT, Kinnunen, E, von Bonsdorff, M, et al: Acute transverse myelopathy successfully treated with plasmapheresis and prednisone in a patient with primary Sjogren's syndrome. Arithritis and Rheumatology 30:339–344, 1987.

128. Kristensen, O, Melgard, B, and Schiodt, AV: Radiation myelopathy of the lumbosacral spinal cord. Acta Neurol Scand 56:217–222, 1977.

129. Kunze, K and Leitenmaier, K: Vitamin B_{12} deficiency and subacute combined degeneration of the spinal cord (funicular spinal disease). In Vinken, PJ and Bruyn, GW (eds): Handbook of Clinical Neurology, Vol 28. North-Holland Publishing, Amsterdam, 1976, pp 141–198.

130. Leibowitz, U, Halpern, L, and Alter, M: Clinical studies of multiple sclerosis in Israel. V.

Progressive spinal syndromes and multiple sclerosis. Neurology 17:988–992, 1967.

131. Leigh, AD and Card, WI: Hepato-lenticular degeneration. A case associated with posterolateral column degeneration. J Neuropath Exp Neurol 8:338–346, 1949.

132. Lennette, EH, Caplan, GE, and Magoffin, RL: Mumps virus infection simulating paralytic poliomyelitis. Pediatrics 25:788–797, 1960.

133. Lerner, AM and Finland, M: Coxsackie viral infections. Arch Intern Med 108:329–334, 1961.

134. Levy, JA, Shimabukuro, J, Hollander, H, et al: Isolation of AIDS associated retroviruses from cerebrospinal fluid and brain of patients with neurological symptoms. Lancet 2:586–588, 1985.

135. Levy, R and Bredesen, DE: Central nervous system dysfunction in acquired immunodeficiency syndrome. In Rosenblum, ML, Levy, RM, and Bredesen, DE (eds): AIDS and the Nervous System. Raven Press, New York, 1988, pp 29–63.

136. Lewis, VL and Rosenbaum, AE: Neurologic complications of radiologic procedures. In Asbury, AK, McKhann, GM, and McDonald, WI (eds): Diseases of the Nervous System. WB Saunders, Philadelphia, 1986, pp 1592–1603.

137. Lhermitte, J and Bollak, NM: Les douleurs a type de decharge electrique consecutives a le flexion cephalique dans la sclerose en plaque. Rev Neurol (Paris) 31:36–52, 1924.

138. Likosky, WH: Experience with cyclophosphamide in multiple sclerosis: The cons. Neurology (Suppl 2) 38:14–18, 1988.

139. Lindenbaum, J, Healton, EB, Savage, DG, et al: Neuropsychiatric disorders caused by cobalamin deficiency in the absence of anemia of macrocytosis. N Engl J Med 318:1720–1728, 1988.

140. Lipton, HL and Teasdale, RD: Acute transverse myelopathy in adults. Arch Neurol 28:252–257, 1973.

141. Lombardi, G, Passerini, A, and Migliavacca, F: Spinal arachnoiditis. Br J Radiol 35:314–320, 1962.

142. Luddy, RE and Gilman, PA: Paraplegia following intrathecal methotrexate. J Pediatr 83:988–992, 1973.

143. Lukehart, SA, Hooker, EW, Baker-Zander, SA, et al: Invasion of the central nervous system by Treponema pallidum: Implications for diagnosis and therapy. Ann Intern Med 109:855–862, 1988.

144. Lukes, SA and Norman, D: Computed tomography in acute disseminated encephalomyelitis. Ann Neurol 13:567–572, 1983.

145. Lumsden, CE: Multiple sclerosis and other demyelinating diseases. In Vinken, PJ and Bruyn, GW (eds): Handbook of Clinical Neurology, Vol 9. North-Holland Publishing, Amsterdam, 1970, p 217–319.

146. Lyle, WH and Chamberlain, RN (eds): Epidemic neuromyasthenia 1934–1977. Current approaches. Postgrad Med J 54:705–770, 1978.

147. Macfarlane, PI and Miller, V: Transverse myelitis associated with Mycoplasma pneumonia infection. Arch Dis Child 59:80–82, 1984.

148. Magoffin, RL, Lennette, EH, and Schmidt, NJ: Association of coxsackie viruses with illness resembling mild paralytic poliomyelitis. Pediatrics 28:602–613, 1961.

149. Mancall, EL and Remedios, KR: Necrotizing myelopathy associated with visceral carcinoma. Brain 87:639–655, 1964.

150. Marshall, J: Spastic paraplegia in middle age. Lancet 1:643–646, 1955.

151. Marty, R and Minckler, DS: Radiation myelitis simulating tumor. Arch Neurol 29:352–354, 1973.

152. Matsuo, H, Nakamura, T, Tsujihata, M, et al: Plasmapheresis in treatment of human T-lymphotropic virus type-I associated myelopathy. Lancet II:1109–1110, 1988.

153. McAlpine, D: Acute disseminated encephalomyelitis: Its sequelae and relationship to disseminated sclerosis. Lancet 1:846–852, 1931.

154. McAlpine, D: Familial neuromyelitis optica, occurrence in identical twins. Brain 62:227, 1939.

155. McArthur, JC: Multiple sclerosis. In Johnson, RT (ed): Current Therapy in Neurologic Disease—2. BC Decker, Toronto, 1987, pp 140–144.

156. McArthur, JC and Johnson, RT: Primary infection with human immunodeficiency virus. In Rosenblum, ML, Levy, RM and Bredesen, DE (eds): AIDS and the Nervous System. Raven Press, New York, 1988, pp 183–202.

157. McCormick, WF, Rodnitzky, RL, Schochet, SS Jr, and McKee, AP: Varicella-Zoster encephalomyelitis. Arch Neurol 21:559–570, 1969.

158. McKaig, CB and Woltman, HW: Neurologic complications of epidemic parotitis: Report of a case of parotitic myelitis. Archives of Neurology and Psychiatry 31:795, 1934.

159. Merritt, HH, Adams, RD, and Solomon, HC: Neurosyphilis. Oxford University Press, New York, 1946.

160. Miller, DH, McDonald, WI, Blumhardt, LD, et al: Magnetic resonance imaging in isolated noncompressive spinal cord syndromes. Ann Neurol 22:714–723, 1987.

161. Miller, HG, Stanton, JB, and Gibbons, JL: Parainfectious encephalomyelitis and related syndromes: A critical review of the neurological complications of certain specific fevers. Q J Med 25:427–505, 1956.

162. Miller, HG, Stanton, JB, and Gibbons, JL: Acute disseminated encephalomyelitis and related syndromes. Br Med J 1:668–672, 1957.

163. Milligan, NM, Newcombe, R, and Compston, DAS: A double-blind controlled trial of high dose methylprednisolone in patients with multiple sclerosis. 1. Clinical effects. J Neurol Neurosurg Psychiatry 50:511–516, 1987.

164. Miska, RM, Pojounas, KW, and McQuillen, MP: Cranial magnetic resonance imaging in the

evaluation of myelopathy of undetermined etiology. Neurology 37:840–843, 1987.

165. Moore, PM: Diagnosis and management of isolated angiitis of the central nervous system. Neurology 39:167–173, 1989.

166. Moore, PM and Cupps, TR: Neurological complications of vasculitis. Ann Neurol 14:155–167, 1983.

167. Moore, PM and Fauci, AS: Neurologic manifestations of systemic vasculitis. A retrospective and prospective study of the clinicopathologic features and responses to therapy in 25 patients. Am J Med 71:517–524, 1981.

168. Morgello, S, Cho, E-S, Nielsen, S, et al: Cytomegalovirus encephalitis in patients with acquired immunodeficiency syndrome. Human Pathology 18:289–297, 1987.

169. Mukherjee, SK: Involvement of anterior horn of spinal cord in infectious mononucleosis. Br Med J 1:1112, 1965.

170. Mulder, DW, Rosenbaum, RA, and Layton, DP: Late progression of poliomyelitis or forme fruste amyotrophic lateral sclerosis? Mayo Clin Proc 47:756–761, 1972.

171. Musher, DM: How much penicillin cures syphilis? (editorial). Ann Intern Med 109:849–851, 1988.

172. Naiman, JL, Donahue, WL, and Pritchard, JS: Fatal nucleus pulposus embolism of spinal cord after trauma. Neurology 11: 83–87, 1961.

173. Nakamura, T, Tsujihata, M, Shirabe, S, et al: Characterization of HTLV-I in a T-cell line established from a patient with myelopathy. Arch Neurol 46:35–37, 1989.

174. Nathanson, N and Martin, JR: The epidemiology of poliomyelitis: Enigmas surrounding its appearance, pathogenicity, and disappearance. Am J Epidemiol 110:672–692, 1979.

175. Nkowane, BM, Wassilak, S, Orenstein, WA, et al; Paralytic poliomyelitis U.S.: 1973 through 1984. JAMA 257:1335–1340, 1987.

176. Norris, FH: Remote effects of cancer on the spinal cord. In Vinken, PJ and Bruyn, GW (eds): Handbook of Clinical Neurology, Vol 38. North-Holland Publishing, Amsterdam, 1979, pp 669–677.

177. Ojeda, VJ: Necrotising myelopathy associated with malignancy: A clinicopathological study of two cases and literature review. Cancer 53:1115–1123, 1984.

178. Oppenheimer, DR: The cervical cord in multiple sclerosis. Neuropathol Appl Neurobiol 4:151–162, 1978.

179. Osame, M, Matsumoto, M, Usuku, K, et al: Chronic progressive myelopathy associated with elevated antibodies to human T- lymphotropic virus type I and adult T-Cell leukemia-like cells. Ann Neurol 21:117–122, 1987.

180. Pachner, AR: Spirochetal diseases of the CNS. Neurol Clin 4:207–222, 1986.

181. Pachner, AR, Duray, P, and Steere, AC: Central nervous system manifestations of Lyme disease. Arch Neurol 46:790–795, 1989.

182. Paddison, RM and Alpers, BJ: Role of intrathecal detergents in pathogenesis of adhesive arachnoiditis. Archives of Neurology and Psychiatry 71:87, 1954.

183. Paine, RS and Byers, RK: Transverse myelopathy in childhood. Am J Dis Child 85:151–163, 1953.

184. Pallis, CA, Louis, S, and Morgan, RL: Radiation myelopathy. Brain 84:460–476, 1961.

185. Palmer, JJ: Radiation myelopathy. Brain 95:109–122, 1972.

186. Panse, F: Electrical lesions of the nervous system. In Vinken, PJ and Bruyn, GW (eds): Handbook of Clinical Neurology, Vol 7. North-Holland Publishing, Amsterdam, 1970, pp 344–387.

187. Paty, DW, Asbury, AK, Herndon, RM, et al: Use of magnetic resonance imaging in the diagnosis of multiple sclerosis: Policy statement. Neurology 36:1575, 1986.

188. Paty, DW, Blume, WT, Brown, WF, et al: Chronic progressive myelopathy: Investigation with CSF electrophoresis, evoked potentials, and CT scan. Ann Neurol 6:419–424, 1979.

189. Paul, JR: A History of Poliomyelitis. Yale University Press, New Haven, 1971.

190. Pendergrass, EP, Schaeffer, JP, and Hodes, PJ: The Head and Neck in Roentgen Diagnosis, ed 2. CC Thomas, Springfield, Ill, 1956.

191. Penn, AS and Rowan, AJ: Myelopathy in systemic lupus erythematosus. Arch Neurol 18:337–349, 1968.

192. Perier, O, Demanet, JC, Hennaux, J, et al: Existe-t-il un syndrome des arteres spinales posterieures? Rev Neurol 103:396–409, 1960.

193. Petito, CK, Navia, BA, Cho, ES, et al: Vacuolar myelopathy pathologically resembling subacute combined degeneration in patients with acquired immunodeficiency syndrome. N Engl J Med 312:874–879, 1985.

194. Pezeshkpour, GH and Dalakas, MC: Long-term changes in the spinal cords of patients with old poliomyelitis. Arch Neurol 45:505–508, 1988.

195. Plum, F and Hindfelt, B: The neurological complications of liver disease. In Vinken, PJ and Bruyn, GW (eds): Handbook of Clinical Neurology, Vol 27. North-Holland Publishing, Amsterdam, 1976, pp 349–376.

196. Plum, F and Olson, ME: Myelitis and myelopathy. In Baker, AB and Baker, LH (eds): Clinical Neurology. Harper & Row, Hagerstown, Md, 1973, pp 1–52.

197. Poser, C, Paty, D, Scheinberg, L, et al: New diagnostic criteria for multiple sclerosis. Ann Neurol 13:227–231, 1983.

198. Poser, CM: Diseases of the myelin sheath. In Baker, AB and Baker, LH (eds): Clinical Neurology. Harper and Row, Hagerstown, Md, 1978, pp 80–104.

199. Poser, S, Hermann-Gremmeis, I, Wikstrom, J, and Poser, W: Clinical features of the spinal form of multiple sclerosis. Acta Neurol Scand 57:151–158, 1978.

200. Preobrajensky, PA: Syphilitic paraplegias with

dissociated disturbances of sensibility. J Neuropat Psikhiat 4:594, 1904.

201. Reagan, TJ, Thomas, JE, and Colby, MY: Chronic progressive radiation myelopathy: Its clinical aspects and differential diagnosis. JAMA 103:106–110, 1968.

202. Reik, L: Disseminated vasculomyelinopathy: An immune complex disease. Ann Neurol 7:291–296, 1980.

203. Reik, L: Immune-mediated central nervous system disorders in childhood viral infections. Seminars in Neurology 2:106–114, 1982.

204. Reik, L: Disorders that mimic CNS infections. Neurol Clin 4:223–248, 1986.

205. Reik, L, Steere, AC, Bartenhagen, NH, Shope, RE, and Malawista, SE: Neurologic abnormalities of Lyme disease. Medicine 58:281–294, 1979.

206. Richardson, EP Jr: Systemic lupus erythematosus. In Vinken, PJ and Bruyn, GW (eds): Handbook of Clinical Neurology, Vol 39. North-Holland Publishing, Amsterdam, 1980, pp 273–292.

207. Robbins, RC, Fox, JP, Hopps, HE, Horstmann, DM, and Quinn, TC: International symposium on poliomyelitis control. Rev Infect Dis (Suppl 6)6:S301–S601, 1984.

208. Robert-Guroff, M, Weiss, SH, Giron, JA, et al: Prevalence and antibodies to HTLV-I, -II, -III in intravenous drug abusers from an AIDS epidemic region. JAMA 255:3133–3137, 1986.

209. Roman, GC, Schoenberg, BS, Madden, DL, et al: Human T-lymphotropic virus type I antibodies in the serum of patients with tropical spastic paraparesis in the Seychelles. Arch Neurol 44:605–607, 1987.

210. Roman, GC, Spencer, PS, and Schoenberg, BS: Tropical myeloneuropathies: The hidden endemias. Neurology 35:1158–1170, 1985.

211. Ropper, AH, Miett, T, and Chiappa, KH: Absence of evoked potential abnormalities in acute transverse myelopathy. Neurology 32:80–82, 1982.

212. Ropper, AH and Poskanzer, DC: The prognosis of acute and subacute transverse myelopathy based on early signs and symptoms. Ann Neurol 4:51–59, 1978.

213. Rose, FC, Brett, EM, and Burston, J: Zoster encephalomyelitis. Arch Neurol 11:155–172, 1964.

214. Rosenblum, ML, Levy, RM, and Bredesen, DE (Eds): AIDS and the Nervous System. Raven Press, New York, 1988.

215. Rosenblum, M, Scheck, AC, Cronin, K, et al: Dissociation of AIDS-related vaculoar myelopathy and productive human immunodeficiency virus type 1 (HIV-1) infection of the spinal cord. Neurology 39:892–896, 1989.

216. Ross, JS: Inflammatory disease. In Modic, MT, Masaryk, TJ, and Ross, JS (eds): Magnetic Resonance Imaging of the Spine. Year Book Medical Publishers, Chicago, 1988, pp 167–182.

217. Ross, JS, Masaryk, TJ, Modic, MT, et al: MR imaging of lumbar arachnoiditis. AJNR 8:885–892, 1987.

218. Rottenberg, DA: Acute and chronic effects of radiation therapy on the nervous system. In Posner, JB (ed): Neuro-Oncology III, Memorial Sloan-Kettering Cancer Center. MSKCC, New York, 1981, pp 88–98.

219. Rousseau, JJ, Lust, C, Zangerle, PF, and Bigaignon, G: Acute transverse myelitis as presenting neurological feature of Lyme disease. Lancet II: 1222–1223, 1986.

220. Russell, JSR, Batten, FE, and Collier, J: Subacute combined degeneration of the spinal cord. Brain 23:39–110, 1900.

221. Sadowsky, CH, Sachs, E, and Ochoa, J: Postradiation motor neuron syndrome. Arch Neurol 33:786–787, 1976.

222. Saiki, JH, Thompson, S, Smith, F, and Atkinson, R: Paraplegia following intrathecal chemotherapy. Cancer 29:370–374, 1972.

223. Sandyk, R and Brennan, MJW: Lhermitte's sign as a presenting symptom of subacute degeneration of the cord. Ann Neurol 13:215–216, 1983.

224. Sanyal, B, Pant, GC, Subrahmaniyan, K, et al: Radiation myelopathy. J Neurol Neurosurg Psychiatry 42:413–418, 1979.

225. Scheid, W: Mumps virus and the central nervous system. World Neurol 2:117, 1961.

226. Schoen, RT: Lyme Disease. In Rakel, RE (ed): Conn's Current Therapy. WB Saunders, Philadelphia, 1989, pp 866–869.

227. Schold, SC, Cho, E-S, Somasundaram, M, and Posner, JB: Subacute motor neuronopathy: A remote effect of lymphoma. Ann Neurol 5:271–287, 1979.

228. Schultz, P and Scwarz, GA: Radiculomyelopathy following intrathecal instillation of methylene blue. Arch Neurol 22:240–244, 1970.

229. Shaw, MDM, Russell, JA, and Grossart, KW: The changing pattern of spinal arachnoiditis. J Neurol Neurosurg Psychiatry 41:97–107, 1978.

230. Shepherd, EI, Downie, AW, and Best, PV: Systemic lupus erythematosus and multiple sclerosis (abstr). Arch Neurol 30:423, 1974.

231. Siegal, S: Transverse myelopathy following recovery from pneumococcic meningitis treated with penicillin intrathecally: Report of a case with note on current methods of therapy. JAMA 129:547–550, 1945.

232. Sigal, LH: The neurologic presentation of vasculitis and rheumatologic syndromes. Medicine 66:157–180, 1987.

233. Silver, JR and Buxton, PH: Spinal stroke. Brain 97:539–550, 1974.

234. Simon, RP: Neurosyphilis. Arch Neurol 42:606–613, 1985.

235. Smith, HV and Spalding, JMK: Outbreak of paralysis in Morocco due to ortho-cresyl phosphate poisoning. Lancet 2:1019–1021, 1959.

236. Smith, KJ and McDonald, WI: Spontaneous and evoked electrical discharges from a central demyelinating lesion. J Neurol Sci 55:39–47, 1982.

237. Snider, WD, Simpson, DM, Nielsen, S, et al: Neurological complications of acquired im-

mune deficiency syndrome: Analysis of 50 patients. Ann Neurol 14:403–418, 1983.

238. Spillane, JD: Nutritional Disorders of the Nervous System. Livingstone, Edinburgh, 1947.

239. Spillane, JD and Wells, EC: The neurology of jennerian vaccination. Brain 87:1, 1964.

240. Spiller, WG: Thrombosis of the cervical anterior median spinal artery; syphilitic acute anterior poliomyelitis. J Nerv Ment Dis 36:601, 1909.

241. Steegman, AT: Syndrome of the anterior spinal artery. Neurology 2:15–35, 1952.

242. Steere, AC, Broderick, TF, and Malawista, SE: Erythema chronicum migrans and Lyme arthritis: Epidemiologic evidence for a tick vector. Am J Epidemiol 108:312–321, 1978.

243. Steere, AC, Grodzicki, RL, Kornblatt, AN, et al: The spirochetal etiology of Lyme disease. N Engl J Med 308:733–740, 1983.

244. Steere, AC, Malawista, SE, Bartenhagen, NH, and others: The clinical spectrum and treatment of Lyme disease. Yale J Biol Med 57:453–461, 1984.

245. Steigman, AJ; Poliomyelitic properties of certain nonpolio viruses: Enteroviruses and Heine-Medin disease. J Mount Sinai Hosp (NY) 25:391–404, 1958.

246. Sweet, KK, Dumont-Stanley, E, Dowling, HF, and Lepper, MH: The treatment of pneumococcic meningitis with penicillin. JAMA 127:263–267, 1945.

247. Sze, G: Gadolinium-DTPA in spinal disease. Radiol Clin North Am 26:1009–1024, 1988.

248. Sze, G, Krol, G, Zimmerman, RD, and Deck, MDF: Intramedullary disease of the spine: Diagnosis using gadolinium-DTPA-enhanced MR imaging. AJNR 9:847–858, 1988.

249. Taterka, JH and O'Sullivan, ME: Motor complications of herpes zoster. JAMA 122:737–739, 1943.

250. Taylor, JR and Van Allen, MW: Vascular manlformation of the cord with transient ischemia attacks. J Neurosurg 31:576–578, 1969.

251. Thomas, JE and Howard, FM: Segmental zoster paresis: A disease profile. Neurology 22:459–466, 1972.

252. Thorsen, G: Neurological complications after spinal anesthesia and results from 2,493 follow-up cases. Acta Chir Scand 95:Suppl 121, 1947.

253. Tucker, T, Dix, RD, Katzen, C, et al: Cytomegalovirus and herpes simplex virus ascending myelitis in a patient with acquired immunodeficiency syndrome. Ann Neurol 18:74–79, 1985.

254. Tyler, HR: Acute transverse myelitis. In Wyngaarden, JB and Smith, LH Jr (eds): Cecil: Textbook of Medicine, ed 17. WB Saunders, Philadelphia, 1985, pp 2138–2139.

255. Van den Brenk, HAS, Richter, W, and Hurley, RH: Radiosensitivity of the human oxygenated cervical spinal cord based on analysis of 357 cases receiving 4 MeV X rays in

hyperbaric oxygenation. Br J Radiol 41:205–214, 1968.

256. Vasu, RI and Whitaker, JN: Postinfectious and transverse myelitis. In Johnson, RT (ed): Current Therapy in Neurologic Disease—2. BC Decker, Toronto, 1987, pp 137–140.

257. Vernant, JC, Maurs, L, Gessain, A, et al: Endemic tropical spastic paraparesis associated with human T-lymphotropic virus type I: A clinical and seroepidemiological study of 25 cases. Ann Neurol 21:123–130, 1987.

258. Victor, M and Lear, AA: Subacute combined degeneration of the spinal cord. Am J Med 20:896–911, 1956.

259. Vinters, HV and Gilbert, JJ: Hypoxic myelopathy. Can J Neurol Sci 6:380, 1979.

260. Wadia, NH, Katrak, SM, Misra, VP, and others: Polio-like motor paralysis associated with acute hemorrhagic conjunctivitis in an outbreak in 1981 in Bombay, India: Clinical and serologic studies. J Infect Dis 147:660–668, 1983.

261. Walker, AE: Toxic effects of intrathecal administration of penicillin. AMA Archives of Neurology and Psychiatry 58:39–45, 1947.

262. Walther, PJ, Rossitch, E, and Bullard, DE: The development of Lhermitte's sign during cisplatin chemotherapy: Possible drug-induced toxicity causing spinal cord demyelination. Cancer 60:2170–2172, 1987.

263. Waxman, SG: The demyelinating diseases. In Rosenberg, R (ed): Clinical Neuroscience. Churchill Livingstone, New York, 1983, pp 609–644.

264. Waxman, SG: Clinical course and electrophysiology of multiple sclerosis. In Waxman, SG (ed): Functional Recovery in Neurological Disease. Raven Press, New York, 1988, pp 151–184.

265. Weiner, HL, Hauser, SL, Halfler, DA, et al: The use of cyclophosphamide in the treatment of multiple sclerosis. Ann NY Acad Sci 436:373–381, 1985.

266. Weiss, HD, Walker, MD, and Wiernik, PH: Neurotoxicity of commonly used antineoplastic agents. N Engl J Med 291:75–81 and 127–133, 1974.

267. Williams, AG, Seiger, RS, and Kornfield, M: Experimental production of arachnoiditis with glove powder contamination during myelography. American Journal of Neuroradiology 3:121–125, 1982.

268. Winkelman, NW: Neurological symptoms following accidental intraspinal detergent injection. Neurology 2:284–291, 1952.

269. Wolff, L, Zighelbohm, J, and Gale, RP: Paraplegia following intrathecal cytosine arabinoside. Cancer 43:83–85, 1979.

270. Wolinsky, JS: Central nervous system complications of viral infections and vaccines. In Wyngaarden, JB and Smith, LH Jr (eds): Cecil: Textbook of Medicine, ed 17. WB Saunders, Philadelphia, 1985, pp 2139–2141.

271. Wong-Staal, F and Gallo, RC: Human T-lymphotropic retroviruses. Nature 317:395–403, 1985.

272. Woolsey, RM, Chambers, TJ, Chung, HD, and McGarry, JD: Mycobacterial meningomyelitis associated with human immunodeficiency virus infection. Arch Neurol 45:691–693, 1988.

273. Word, JA, Kalokhe, UP, Aron, BS, and Elson, HR: Transient radiation myelopathy (Lhermitte's sign) in patients with Hodgkin's disease treated by mantle radiation. Int J Radiat Oncol Biol Phys 6:1731–1733, 1980.

274. Wyburn-Mason, R: Vascular Abnormalities and Tumors of the Spinal Cord and Its Membranes. Kimpton, London, 1943.

275. Zieve, L, Mendelson, DF, and Goepfert, M: Shunt encephalomyelopathy. II. Occurrence of permanent myelopathy. Ann Intern Med 53:53–63, 1960.

| EPILOGUE

The approaches to the diagnosis and management of spinal cord compression presented in this book are based upon clinical anatomy and pathophysiological principles. In most cases, patients with spinal cord disease will manifest symptoms and signs that can be understood in anatomical and pathophysiological terms and the diagnosis and management will thereby be readily established. Alternatively, diseases involving the spinal cord can have protean manifestations that may lead the clinician astray from the correct diagnosis. It is important, therefore, to recognize these pitfalls when evaluating patients who may have spinal disease. As repeatedly emphasized, the correct diagnosis usually requires repeated clinical examinations with careful attention to localizing signs and symptoms, and a willingness to consider alternative etiologies.

When spinal cord compression is suspected, the appropriate imaging studies should be promptly performed. It must be recognized, however, that with such sensitive imaging studies as spinal CT or MRI, incidental abnormal findings that may be clinically insignificant frequently will be seen. These abnormalities may erroneously lead the clinician away from the correct diagnosis and may even result in unnecessary therapies such as surgery. Occasionally CT or MRI may yield false-negative results, making it imperative to correlate the imaging studies with clinical findings. Moreover, it is important to remember that one of the most sensitive diagnostic maneuvers is the repeat neurological examination.

With meticulous attention to the patient's history, physical examination, and clinical correlation of laboratory and imaging studies, the clinician usually can distinguish spinal cord compression from other medical diseases. The rewards of success may be enormous but the penalty for error is grave. If spinal cord compression is properly diagnosed and treatment is commenced early, the patient may enjoy continued ambulation and sphincter control. If diagnosis and treatment are delayed, however, an opportunity for maintenance or recovery of spinal cord function may be lost, resulting in a life of permanent sensory loss, incontinence, and paralysis.

I APPENDIX

SEGMENTAL AND PERIPHERAL INNERVATION OF THE MUSCLES AND THEIR FUNCTION*†

Nerve/Muscle	Function	Spinal Segments
Spinal accessory	Elevates shoulder/arm	C3, C4
Trapezius	Fixes scapula	
Phrenic		C3, C4, C5
Diaphragm	Inspiration	
Dorsal scapular		
Rhomboids	Draw scapula up and in	C4, **C5,** C6
Levator scapulae	Elevates scapula	C3, C4, C5
Long thoracic		
Serratus anterior	Fixes scapula on arm raise	C5, C6, C7
Anterior thoracic		
Pectoralis major (clavicular)	Pulls shoulder forward	**C5,** C6
Pectoralis major (sternal)	Adducts and medially rotates arm	C6, **C7,** C8, T1
Pectoralis minor	Depresses scapula, pulls shoulder foward	C6, C7, C8
Suprascapular		
Supraspinatus	Abducts humerus	**C5,** C6
Infraspinatus	Rotates humerus laterally	**C5,** C6
Subscapular		
Subscapularis	Rotates humerus medially	C5, C6
Teres major	Adducts, medially rotates humerus	C5, C6, C7
Thoracodorsal		
Latissimus dorsi	Adducts, medially rotates humerus	C6, **C7,** C8
Axillary		
Teres minor	Adducts, laterally rotates humerus	C5, C6
Deltoid	Abducts arm	**C5,** C6
Musculocutaneous		
Coracobrachialis	Flexes and adducts arm	C6, **C7**
Biceps brachii	Flexes and supinates arm	C5, C6
Brachialis	Flexes forearm	C5, C6
Radial		
Triceps	Extends forearm	C6, **C7,** C8
Brachioradialis	Flexes forearm	C5, **C6**
Extensor carpi radialis (longus and brevis)	Extend wrist, abduct hand	C5, **C6**
Posterior interosseus		
Supinator	Supinates forearm	C6, C7
Extensor carpi ulnaris	Extends wrist, adducts hand	**C7,** C8
Extensor digitorum	Extends fingers at proximal phalanx	**C7,** C8
Extensor digiti quinti	Extends little finger at proximal phalanx	**C7,** C8
Abductor pollicis longus	Abducts thumb in the plane of palm	**C7,** C8
Extensor pollicis (longus and brevis)	Extend thumb	**C7,** C8
Extensor indicis	Extends index finger, proximal phalanx	**C7,** C8
Median		
Pronator teres	Pronates and flexes forearm	C6, C7
Flexor carpi radialis	Flexes wrist, abducts hand	C6, C7
Palmaris longus	Flexes wrist	C7, **C8,** T1
Flexor digitorum superficialis	Flexes middle phalanges	C7, **C8,** T1
Flexor digitorum profundus (digits 2, 3)	Flexes distal phalanges	C7, **C8**
Abductor pollicis brevis	Abducts thumb at right angles to palm	C8, **T1**
Flexor pollicis brevis (superficial)	Flexes first phalange of thumb	C8, **T1**
Opponens pollicis	Flexes, opposes thumb	C8, **T1**
Lumbricals (I, II)	Flex proximal interphalangeal joint, extend other phalanges	C8, **T1**

*From Devinsky, O and Feldmann, E: Examination of the Cranial and Peripheral Nerves. Churchill Livingstone, New York, 1988, pp. 22–25, with permission.

†Muscles are listed in the order of innervation, except when presented in groups as for the quadriceps. Boldface type signifies predominant innervation.

Nerve/Muscle	Function	Spinal Segments
Anterior interosseus		
Flexor digitorum profundus (digits 2, 3)	Flexes distal phalanges	C7, **C8**
Flexor pollicis longus	Flexes distal phalanx of thumb	C7, **C8**
Pronator quadratus	Pronates forearm	C7, **C8, T1**
Ulnar		
Flexor carpi ulnaris	Flexes wrist, adducts hand	C7, **C8**, T
Flexor digitorum profundus (digits 4, 5)	Flexes distal phalanges	C7, **C8**
Hypothenar muscles	Abduct, adduct, flex, rotate digit 5	C8, **T1**
Lumbricals (III, IV)	Flex proximal interphalangeal joint, extend other phalanges	C8, **T1**
Palmar interossei	Abduct fingers, flex proximal phalanges	C8, **T1**
Dorsal interossei	Adduct fingers	C8, **T1**
Flexor pollicis brevis (deep)	Flexes and adducts thumb	C8, **T1**
Adductor pollicis	Adducts thumb	C8, **T1**
Obturator		
Obturator externus	Adducts and outwardly rotates leg	**L2, L3,** L4
Adductor longus		
Adductor magnus	Adduct thigh	**L2, L3,** L4
Adductor brevis		
Gracilis		
Femoral		
Iliacus	Flexes leg at hip	**L1, L2,** L3
Rectus femoris		
Vastus lateralis		
Vastus intermedius	Extend leg	L2, **L3, L4**
Vastus medialis		
Pectineus	Adducts leg	**L2, L3,** L4
Sartorius	Inwardly rotates leg, flexes thigh and leg	**L2, L3,** L4
Sciatic		
Adductor magnus	Adducts thigh	L4, L5, S1
Semitendinosus	Flexes and medially rotates knee, extends hip	L5, **S1,** S2
Biceps femoris	Flexes leg, extends thigh	L5, **S1,** S2
Semimembranosus	Flexes and medially rotates knee, extends hip	L5, **S1,** S2
Tibial		
Gastrocnemius	Plantar flexes foot	S1, S2
Plantaris	Spreads, brings together, and flexes proximal phalanges	L4, L5, S1
Soleus	Plantar flexes foot	S1, S2
Popliteus	Plantar flexes foot	L4, L5, S1
Tibialis posterior	Plantar flexes and inverts foot	L4, L5
Flexor digitorum longus	Flexes distal phalanges, aids plantar flexion	L5, **S1, S2**
Flexor hallucis longus	Flexes great toe, aids plantar flexion	L5, **S1, S2**
Small foot muscles	Cup sole	S1, S2
Common peroneal		
Superficial peroneal		
Peroneus longus	Plantar flexes and everts foot	L5, S1
Peroneus brevis	Plantar flexes and everts foot	L5, S1
Deep peroneal		
Tibialis anterior	Dorsiflexes and inverts foot	**L4,** L5
Extensor digitorum longus	Extends phalanges, dorsiflexes foot	**L5,** S1
Extensor hallucis longus	Extends great toe, aids dorsiflexion	**L5,** S1
Peroneus tertius	Plantar flexes foot in pronation	L4, **L5,** S1
Extensor digitorum brevis	Extends toes	L5, S1
Superior gluteal		
Gluteus medius/minimus	Abduct and medially rotate thigh	**L4, L5,** S1
Tensor fasciae latae	Flexes thigh	**L4, L5,** S1
Inferior gluteal		
Gluteus maximus	Extends, abducts, laterally rotates thigh and extends lower trunk	**L5, S1,** S2

INDEX

269